Clinically Relevant Mycoses

Elisabeth Presterl
Editor

Clinically Relevant Mycoses

A Practical Approach

Springer

Editor
Elisabeth Presterl
Department of Infection Control and Hospital Epidemiology
Medical University of Vienna
Wien
Austria

ISBN 978-3-319-92299-7 ISBN 978-3-319-92300-0 (eBook)
https://doi.org/10.1007/978-3-319-92300-0

Library of Congress Control Number: 2018960321

This Springer imprint is published by the registered company Springer Nature Switzerland AG
The registered company address is: Gewerbestrasse 11, 6330 Cham, Switzerland

Preface

Introduction

Invasive fungal infections are rare but life-threatening disease for severely ill patients. Due to perpetually improving healthcare, there are life-saving and life-improving therapies for many hemato-oncological diseases, organ transplantation, advanced supportive intensive care, and new techniques making most complicated surgical interventions possible. However, all these patients are at risk for developing invasive fungal infections. Many efforts for better diagnosis and treatment of invasive fungal infections have been undertaken in the last 3 decades. A number of new antifungal agents have emerged during this period. Many clinical studies have been conducted to develop timely and efficient diagnosis and treatments focused on the patients particularly at risk.

Dermatomycoses are the most common fungal infections of mankind, never life-threatening but awesome and ugly. However, knowledge about these dermatomycoses and their treatment is waning.

Generally, medical students learn very little about invasive fungal infections because these are limited to a small patient population at risk. These patients are most frequently encountered in hospitals that focus on neoplastic and hematological diseases. However, many immunocompromised patients, e.g. organ recipients, are cared for in outpatients' clinics or general medicine offices and not specialized centers with a mycology lab service. Thus, the authors have agreed to write a book on fungal infections particularly meant to give a satisfactory overview and a solid background for caring, diagnosing, and treating these patients. Each author wrote a chapter using his and her particular expertise in the field of fungal infection. We thought that fungal infections although rare in the general practice are also of interest for doctors in training, doctors working in other fields than hematooncology or transplantation, and who come across patients being at risk of fungal infections or having fungal infections. Moreover, this book provides good information for senior medical students, nurses, or other highly specialized medical personal.

This book, *Clinically relevant mycoses: a practical approach*, aims to give a general overview on the clinical and scientific aspects of fungal infections. It should provide information on epidemiology, diagnostics, basics of antifungal therapy, and typical clinical syndromes like invasive Candida infection, aspergillosis, and mucormycoses, but also on special patient groups like premature neonates and children with hereditary immune defects or intensive care patients. It should be a basis for further study in the field of invasive fungal infections. The purpose of this book is to supply the basics and the evidence-based approach for the management of fungal infections.

Objective of This Book

The book provides an evidence-based practical approach to the most frequent fungal infections, diagnostics and treatment in a primary and secondary care hospitals. It gives an easy overview of basic medical and scientific background of fungal infections. Epidemiology, pathogenesis, clinical presentation, diagnostics, and treatment are carefully explained and discussed. The reader will acquire a good and clear perception of invasive fungal infection as well as the challenges in diagnostics and treatment. *Clinically relevant mycoses: a practical approach* will serve as a good tool for clinical management but also will provide the basis for putting further research questions and studies on this particular field. This book will be an invaluable companion for doctors, students of medicine and pharmacology, nurses, and other healthcare professionals.

The information contained in this book applies to all countries. It is the essential requirements for understanding fungal infections. However, different countries will have their different approach according to their specific needs, environment, incidence of fungal infection, and healthcare systems.

Anyone who needs more detailed information on invasive fungal infection and its management is recommended to contact specialized institutions dealing with high-risk patients like hemato-oncology or infectious diseases units and are referred to the high-quality textbooks and recent publications in this field.

Vienna, Austria
August, 2018

Elisabeth Presterl

Acknowledgments

We wish to acknowledge the following professional study groups for paving the way by providing professional encounter and—most enjoyable—friendship among the authors to make this work possible: Sektion Antimykotische Chemotherapie der Paul-Ehrlich-Gesellschaft, Deutsche Gesellschaft für Mykologie (DMykG), and Österreichische Gesellschaft für Antimikrobielle Chemotherapie (OEGACH). We thank particularly the ESCMID Study Group of Invasive Fungal Infection (EFISG) and the ESCMID Study Group of Nosocomial Infection (ESGNI) for being a platform of discussion, research support, and scientific exchange for their members:

Elisabeth Presterl on behalf of EFISG and ESGNI
Birgit Willinger on behalf of EFISG
Christina Forstner on behalf of EFISG
Magda Diab-El Schahawi on behalf of ESGNI
Markus Ruhnke on behalf of EFISG
Rosa Bellmann-Weiler on behalf of ESGNI
Cornelia Lass-Flörl on behalf of EFISG and ESGNI
Olivier Lotholary on behalf of EFISG
Romain Guery on behalf of EFISG
Fanny Lanternier on behalf of EFISG
Volker Rickerts on behalf of EFISG
Andreas Groll on behalf of EFISG
Luigi Segagni-Lusignani on behalf of ESGNI
Aleksandra Barac on behalf of EFISG and ESGNI

Contents

Part III Special Issues

Part I

General

1 What Is the Target? Clinical Mycology and Diagnostics

Birgit Willinger

1.1 Epidemiology

More than 600 different fungi, yeasts and filamentous fungi, some of them are most commonly known as moulds and dermatophytes, have been reported to infect humans, ranging from common to very serious infections, including those of the mucosa, skin, hair and nails, and other ailments.

Particularly, invasive fungal infections (IFI) are found in patients at risk. Both yeasts and moulds are able to cause superficial, deep and invasive disseminated infections, whereas dermatophytes cause infections of the skin, nails and hair. Dermatophytoses are caused by the agents of the genera *Epidermophyton*, *Microsporum*, *Nannizia* and *Trichophyton*.

Invasive infections encompass mainly immunocompromised patients, e.g. patients with the acquired immunodeficiency syndrome or immunosuppressed patients due to therapy for cancer and organ transplantation or undergoing major surgical procedures. As the patient population at risk continues to expand so also does the spectrum of opportunistic fungal pathogens infecting these patients. Invasive fungal infections may also be serious complications of traumatic injury characterized by fungal angioinvasion and resultant vessel thrombosis and tissue necrosis [1, 2]. In contrast to other settings, posttraumatic IFI occurs through direct inoculation of tissue with spores at the site of injury [3]. Both yeasts and moulds are able to cause superficial, deep and invasive disseminated infections, whereas dermatophytes cause infections of the skin, nails and hair.

1.1.1 Yeasts

Yeasts are fungi with a more or less ball-like shape. Yeasts multiply by budding but may form hyphae or pseudohyphae. Many infections are caused by yeasts with the *Candida* being the most common representative. In the last decades, the expansion of molecular phylogenetics has shown that some genera are polyphyletic, which means that some species are of different genetic origin and therefore unrelated. The genus *Candida* is now associated with at least ten different telemorphic genera including *Clavispora*, *Debaryomyces*, *Issatchenkia*, *Kluyveromyces* and *Pichia* [4]. More than 100 *Candida* species are known, whereas the majority of infections are caused by *C. albicans*, *C. glabrata*, *C. parapsilosis*, *C. tropicalis* and *C. krusei* [5]. Other emerging species causing infections have been described. For example, *C. auris* is an emerging multidrug-resistant pathogen that is capable of causing invasive fungal infections, particularly among hospitalized patients with significant medical comorbidities [6].

B. Willinger
Division of Clinical Microbiology, Department of Laboratory Medicine, Medical University of Vienna, Vienna, Austria
e-mail: birgit.willinger@meduniwien.ac.at

E. Presterl (ed.), *Clinically Relevant Mycoses*, https://doi.org/10.1007/978-3-319-92300-0_1

Other important genera are *Cryptococcus*, *Malassezia* and *Trichosporon*. Cryptococcal infections occur with a near worldwide distribution in immunosuppressed hosts. This infection is typically caused by *Cryptococcus neoformans*, an encapsulated yeast, and infection is acquired from the environment. *Cryptococcus neoformans* var. *grubii*, *C. neoformans* var. *neoformans* and *C. gattii* are the causes of opportunistic infections which are classified as AIDS-defining illness [7]. Non-*Cryptococcus neoformans* species, including *C. laurentii* and *C. albidus*, have historically been classified as exclusively saprophytic. However, recent studies have increasingly implicated these organisms as the causative agent of opportunistic infections in humans [8].

The lipid-dependent *Malassezia furfur* complex causes pityriasis versicolor, whereas the non-lipophilic *M. pachydermatis* is occasionally responsible for invasive infections in humans. *Trichosporon beigelii* used to be known as the principal human pathogen of the genus *Trichosporon*. Four newly delineated taxa (*T. asahii* and less frequently *T. mucoides*, *T. inkin* and *T. louberi*) are associated with systemic infections in man. *T. mycotoxinivorans* has been described recently as the cause of fatal infections in patients suffering from cystic fibrosis [4].

Saprochaete and *Geotrichum* spp. are rare emerging fungi causing invasive fungal diseases in immunosuppressed patients, mainly in patients with haematological malignancies, but also other non-haematological diseases as underlying disease have been reported [9]. The most important risk factor is profound and prolonged neutropenia [10].

Saccharomyces cerevisiae is a common food organism and can be recovered from mucosal surfaces, gastrointestinal tract and female genital tract of healthy persons. Occasionally, it causes vaginal infections and on very rare occasions invasive infections in immunocompromised and critically ill patients [4].

Rhodotorula species have traditionally been considered as one of common non-virulent environmental inhabitant. They have emerged as an opportunistic pathogen, particularly in immunocompromised hosts, and most infections have been associated with intravenous catheters in these patients. *Rhodotorula* spp. have also been reported to cause localized infections including meningeal, skin, ocular, peritoneal and prosthetic joint infections; however, these are not necessarily linked to the use of central venous catheters or immunosuppression [11].

Pneumocystis jirovecii (formerly known as *P. carinii*) is a unicellular, eukaryotic organism occurring in lungs of many mammals. *P. jirovecii* is a causative agent of *Pneumocystis* pneumonia. Although the incidence of *Pneumocystis* pneumonia (PCP) has decreased since the introduction of combination antiretroviral therapy, it remains an important cause of disease in both HIV-infected and non-HIV-infected immunosuppressed populations. The epidemiology of PCP has shifted over the course of the HIV epidemic both from changes in HIV and PCP treatment and prevention and from changes in critical care medicine. Although less common in non-HIV-infected immunosuppressed patients, PCP is now more frequently seen due to the increasing numbers of organ transplants and development of novel immunotherapies [12].

1.1.2 Filamentous Fungi

Filamentous fungi form colonies of different colours with a more or less woolly surface formed by the filamentous hyphae that may carry conidia (spores) that are disseminated easily via the air (asexual propagation). These fungi are generally perceived as moulds.

Although a wide variety of pathogens are associated with invasive mould diseases, *Aspergillus* spp. are counted among the most common causative organisms. Overall, the genus *Aspergillus* contains about 250 species divided into subgenera, which in turn are subdivided into several sections or species complexes. Of these, 40 species are known to cause diseases in humans. Most invasive infections are caused by members of the *A. fumigatus* species complex, followed by *A. flavus*, *A. terreus* and *A. niger* species complexes [13]. The *Aspergillus fumigatus* species complex remains the most common one in all pulmonary syndromes, followed by *Aspergillus flavus* which is a common cause of allergic rhinosinusitis, postoperative aspergillosis and fungal keratitis. Lately, increased azole resistance in *A. fumigatus* has become a significant challenge in effective management of aspergillosis. The full extent of the problem is still unknown, but some studies suggest that resistance in *A. fumigatus* may be partially driven by the use of agricultural azoles, which protect grain from fungi [14]. Other species of *Aspergillus* may also be resistant to amphotericin B, including *A. lentulus*, *A. nidulans*, *A. ustus* and *A. versicolor*. Hence, the identification of unknown *Aspergillus* clinical isolates to species level may be important given that different species have variable susceptibilities to multiple antifungal drugs.

Mucormycosis is caused by fungi of the order *Mucorales*. Of fungi in the order *Mucorales*, species belonging to the family *Mucoraceae* are isolated more frequently from patients with mucormycosis than any other family. Among the *Mucoraceae*, *Rhizopus* is by far the most common genus causing infection, with *R. oryzae* (*R. arrhizus*) being the most common one [15, 16]. *Lichtheimia corymbifera*, *Rhizomucor* spp., *Mucor* spp. and *Cunninghamella* spp. are also known to cause jeopardizing infections. *Mucorales* are resistant to voriconazole and caspofungin in vitro and in vivo. The incidence of mucormycosis may be underestimated due to the low performance of diagnostic techniques based on conventional microbiological procedures, such as culture and microscopy. The most useful methods for detecting *Mucorales* are still microscopic examination of tissues and histopathology, which offer moderate sensitivity and specificity. Recent clinical studies have reported that mucormycosis is the cause of >10% of all invasive fungal infections when techniques based on DNA amplification by quantitative used to complement conventional methods [17].

Besides *Mucorales*, the emergence of other opportunistic pathogens, including *Fusarium* spp., *Paecilomyces* spp., *Scedosporium* spp. and the dematiaceous fungi (e.g. *Alternaria* spp.), became evident [5]. *Fusarium* spp., *Alternaria* spp. and *Scedosporium* spp. also account for mould infections among solid organ transplant recipients.

The genus *Fusarium* includes several fungal species complexes. These are ubiquitous soil saprophytes and pathogenic for plants [13]. Only a few species cause infections in humans [18]. Among these are the species complexes *F. solani*, *F. oxysporum*, *F. verticillioides* and *F. fujikuroi* [19]. *Fusarium* spp. have been involved in superficial and deep mycosis and are the leading causes of fungal keratitis in the world [18, 20]. Recently, these fungi have been identified as emerging and multiresistant pathogens causing opportunistic disseminated infections [21, 22].

The genus *Scedosporium* has undergone a taxonomic reclassification. According to the new classification, the most common *Scedosporium* spp. involved in human infections are *S. apiospermum* (telemorphic state, *Pseudallescheria apiosperma*), *S. boydii* (*Pseudallescheria boydii*), *S. aurantiacum* and *S. prolificans* (*Lomentospora prolificans*). Owing to epidemiological reasons, most recent reports divide human infections by these species into mycoses caused by the *S. apiospermum* complex (which includes *S. apiospermum*, *S. boydii* and *S. aurantiacum*) and by *S. prolificans* [13].

Species belonging to the *S. apiospermum* complex are cosmopolitan, being ubiquitously present in the environment, but predominantly in temperate areas. They are commonly isolated from soil, sewage and polluted waters, composts and the manure of horses, dogs, cattle and fowl [23]. *S. prolificans* appears to have a more restricted geographical distribution, being found largely in hot and semiarid soils in southern Europe, Australia and California [24].

Table 1.1 shows the most common yeasts and moulds causing IFI.

1.1.2.1 Relevant Diagnostic Material for Diagnosis of Clinical Mycoses

For definite diagnosis of proven invasive fungal infections, histological and cultural evidence from biopsies, resection material or other specimens obtained from normally sterile body sites is required.

Table 1.1 Spectrum of opportunistic yeasts and moulds (exemplary, without claiming completeness)

Yeasts		Moulds	
Candida	*C. albicans* *C. glabrata* *C. parapsilosis complex* *C. tropicalis* *C. guilliermondii* *C. auris*	*Aspergillus* species complex	*A. fumigatus* *A. flavus* *A. terreus* *A. niger*
Cryptococcus	*C. neoformans* var. neoformans *C. neoformans* var. grubii *C. gattii*	*Mucorales*	*Rhizopus* spp. *Rhizomucor* spp. *Mucor* spp. *Lichtheimia corymbifera* *Cunninghamella* spp.
Trichosporon	*T. asahii* *T. mucoides* *T. inkin* *T. louberi* *T. mycotoxinivorans*	*Fusarium* species complexes	*F. solani* *F. oxysporum* *F. verticillioides* *F. fujikuroi*
Malassezia	*M. furfur* species complex *M. pachydermatis*	*Scedosporium*	*S. apiospermum* *S. boydii* *S. aurantiacum* *S. prolificans* = *Lomentospora prolificans*
Geotrichum and *Saprochaete*	*G. candidum* *S. capitate* *S. clavata*	*Paecilomyces*	*P. variotii*
Saccharomyces	*S. cerevisiae*	*Scopulariopsis*	*S. brevicaulis*
Rhodotorula	*R. rubra* *R. mucilaginosa* *R. glutinis* *R. minuta*	*Alternaria*	

Superficial samples like swabs, respiratory secretion, sputum or stools are not helpful for the diagnosis of invasive fungal infection as both yeasts and filamentous fungi easily colonize body surfaces.

1.1.2.2 Currently Available Diagnostic Methods

Currently, available laboratory methods for diagnosing invasive fungal infections include microscopic detection, isolation of the fungus, serologic detection of antibodies and antigen or histopathologic evidence of invasion [25]. Because of the limited sensitivity of all these diagnostic procedures, and concerns about specificity of some of them, a combination of various testing strategies is the hallmark of IFI diagnosis [17, 25].

1.1.2.3 Histopathology

Histopathology of excised human tissue samples is the cornerstone for diagnosing and identifying fungal pathogens. Direct examination for the presence of mycelial elements using appropriate staining (e.g. Grocott-Gomori methenamine silver, periodic acid-Schiff, potassium hydroxide-calcofluor white) should be performed on all clinical specimens, including respiratory secretions or any tissue sample [17].

However, identifying the specific pathogen based solely on morphological characteristics can be difficult or impossible, because several different organisms may have similar histopathological characteristics, e.g. *Fusarium* spp., and other filamentous fungi are indistinguishable from *Aspergillus* in tissue biopsies [26]. As *Aspergillus* is far more commonly encountered than the other pathogens mentioned, a pathologist often may describe an organism as *Aspergillus* or *Aspergillus*-like based upon morphological features alone. This can hinder diagnosis and may entail inappropriate therapy [27].

1.1.2.4 Microscopy

Direct microscopy is most useful in the diagnosis of superficial and subcutaneous fungal infections and, in those settings, should always be performed together with culture.

Recognition of fungal elements can provide a reliable and rapid indication of the mycosis involved. Various methods can be used: unstained wet-mount preparations can be examined by light-field, dark-field or phase contrast illumination [28]. Because yeast and moulds can stain variably with the Gram stain, a more specific fungal stain is recommended [29].

Microscopy may help to discern whether an infection is caused by yeast or moulds. The presence of pseudohyphae and optionally blastoconidia indicates the presence of yeast, whereas moulds are most commonly seen as hyaline hyphomycetes, generally characterized by parallel cell walls, septation (cross wall formation in hyphae), lack of pigmentation and progressive dichotomous branching as in *Aspergillus*, *Fusarium* or *Scedosporium* species [30]. However, it is impossible to differentiate between the respective genera of the mentioned fungi. It is important to look for septate and nonseptate hyphae, thus allowing to distinguish between *Aspergillus* sp. and members of the *Mucorales*. Mucoraceous moulds have large ribbon-like, multinucleated hyphal cells with non-parallel walls and infrequent septa. The branching is irregular and sometimes at right angles. Hyphae can appear distorted with swollen cells, or compressed, twisted and folded [30]. Another group of moulds causing tissue invasion with a distinctive appearance is the agents of phaeohyphomycosis, such as *Alternaria* and *Curvularia*. These fungi have melanin in their cell walls and appear as pigmented, septate hyphae [31]. The detection of fungal hyphae and/or arthrospores in skin, nail or hair samples may indicate the presence of dermatophytes but give no special hint as to the species involved.

The most common direct microscopic procedure relies on the use of 10–20% potassium hydroxide (KOH), which degrades the proteinaceous components of specimens while leaving the fungal cell wall intact, thus allowing their visualization [30].

The visibility of fungi within clinical specimens can be further enhanced by the addition of calcofluor white or blankophores. These are fluorophores, which are members of a group of compounds known as fluorescent brighteners or optical brighteners or "whitening agents" and bind to beta 1–3 and beta 1–4 polysaccharides, such as found in cellulose and chitin. When excited with ultraviolet or violet radiation, these substances will fluoresce with an intense blueish/white colour [25]. Optical brightener methods have been shown to be more sensitive than KOH wet mount [31]. Filamentous fungi like aspergilli, which stain poorly by the Gram procedure, may be unveiled on gram-stained microscopic mounts after removal of immersion oil by subsequent Blankophor staining [32]. As optical brighteners provide a rapid and sensitive method for the detection of most fungi, their use is encouraged for respiratory samples, pus, tissue samples and fluids from sterile sites when a fluorescence microscope is available [33].

Also, lactophenol cotton blue is easy to handle and often used for the detection and identification of fungi. Other stains are frequently used in direct microscopy, such as the India ink wet mount, which is useful for visualization of encapsulated fungi, particularly *Cryptococcus neoformans*. Although a negative direct examination cannot rule out fungal disease, visualization of fungal elements in specimens can often secure initial information helpful in the selection of empirical antifungal therapy [32].

For detection of *P. jirovecii*, special staining as, for example, direct immunofluorescent staining is required. Sputum induction and BAL are the most commonly used, although non-HIV-infected patients with PCP may require lung biopsy for diagnosis. Standard staining methods include methenamine silver, toluidine blue-O or Giemsa stain. Monoclonal antibodies can be used to detect *Pneumocystis* with a rapid, sensitive and easy-to-perform immunofluorescence assay [12].

1.1.2.5 Culture

Culture remains one of the key methods for diagnosing fungal infection. Though often slow, sometimes insensitive and sometimes confusing with respect to contamination, culture may yield the specific aetiological agent and may allow susceptibility testing to be performed. Proper collection and transportation of the specimen is essential. Particularly, sterile materials are important for diagnosis of invasive fungal infections. Fungal selective media must be included, and it should be observed that some species take a certain period of time (5–21 days) to grow in culture. Negative culture results do not exclude fungal infection. Identification of the isolate to species level is mandatory [34].

Blood cultures (BC) are the first-line test and currently considered the "gold standard" in the event of any suspected case of systemic mycosis [35]. Several commercial blood culture systems are available. Lysis centrifugation was one of the first systems to detect fungi and became a gold standard [25]. However, the more commonly used automated blood culture systems appear to show the same sensitivity for the majority of invasive fungi [36].

The Bactec System (BD Diagnostic System, Sparks, Md., USA) and the BacT/Alert System (bioMérieux, Marcy l'Etoile, France) are widely used automated systems. The Bactec system proposes a specifically formulated medium for the isolation of fungi, called Mycosis IC/F medium. The recommended incubation period by the manufacturers for Bactec Mycosis IC/F and BacT/Alert FA vials is 14 and 5 days, respectively. In various studies, the vast majority of the *Candida* species were detected in 5 days [37, 38]. The main reason for 14 days of incubation for Bactec Mycosis IC/F vials is to detect the growth of filamentous fungi which may take longer as this is the case for *Histoplasma capsulatum*.

In 2012, recommendations concerning diagnostic procedures for detection of *Candida* diseases have been published by the ESCMID Fungal Infection Study Group [34]. Concerning candidaemia, the number of BC recommended in a single session is 3 [2–4], with a total volume varying according to the age of the patient, 40–60 mL for adults, 2–4 mL for children under 2 kg, 6 mL between 2 and 12 kg and 20 mL between 12 and 36 kg. The timing for obtaining the BC is one right after the other from different sites, and venipuncture remains the technique of choice. A BC set comprises of 60 mL blood for adults obtained in a single session within a 30-min period and divided in 10-mL aliquots among three aerobic and three anaerobic bottles. The frequency recommended is daily when candidaemia is suspected, and the incubation period must be at least 5 days.

When these recommendations have been followed, the sensitivity of BC to detect *Candida* is 50–75% although lower sensitivity rates in neutropenic patients and those undergoing antifungal treatment have been reported [39, 40].

Despite the advances in blood culture technology, the recovery of fungi from the blood remains an insensitive marker for invasive fungal infections. Filamentous fungi will be detected to a much lesser extent than yeasts, because most of them do not sporulate in the blood with the exception of *Fusarium* spp. [17, 41]. Concerning *Aspergillus*, only *A. terreus* has been described to be detected by blood cultures.

Cultures of lower respiratory secretions collected by bronchoscopy and bronchoalveolar lavage fluid (BALF) are part of the diagnostic work-up of invasive pulmonary mould infections. However, the yield of BALF culture is notoriously low, usually showing a sensitivity of 20–50% [17]. In addition, positive BALF culture may reflect colonization and not infection, particularly in lung transplant recipients or patients with chronic lung diseases. On the other hand, the ubiquitous nature of airborne conidia and the risk of accidental contamination with moulds may hamper the interpretation of a positive result. It has to be considered that the positive predictive value of culture depends on the prevalence of the infection and thus it is higher among immunocompromised patients [42]. One study suggests that positive BALF culture for *Aspergillus* spp. may be associated with IA in as many as 50% of ICU patients even in the absence of high-risk host conditions [43]. As a consequence, it is recommended that respiratory tract samples positive for *Aspergillus* spp. in the critically ill should always prompt further diagnostic assessment. Attention has to be paid that the absence of hyphal elements or a negative culture does not exclude a fungal infection.

Culture is highly sensitive (98%) in patients with Cryptococcus meningitis [44]. However, in central nervous system, aspergillosis or candidiasis cultures from cerebrospinal fluid (CSF) are less sensitive [45]. All yeasts and moulds obtained from sterile sites, including blood and continuous ambulatory peritoneal dialysis (CAPD) fluids, and intravenous-line tips should be identified to species level. This is also valid for bronchoscopically obtained specimens. When looking for dermatophytes, all samples are cultured on agar for identification, which takes at least 2 weeks. A negative culture result cannot be confirmed until plates have been incubated for 6 weeks. Treatment of clinically obvious or severe cases should not be delayed for culture results, although treatment may need to be altered according to the dermatophyte grown. The presence or absence of fungal elements on microscopy is not always predictive of positive culture results, and if a clinician is faced with unexpectedly negative results, investigations should be repeated, while alternative diagnoses are considered [46].

Yeasts are identified by their assimilation pattern and their microscopic morphology and moulds by their macroscopic and microscopic morphology. Commercially available biochemical test systems identify most of the commonly isolated species of yeast accurately, but it has to be kept in mind that no identification or misidentification of more unusual isolates might occur. Due to their slow growth, identification can take several days and in rare occasions even weeks. Certain *Candida* spp. can be identified more rapidly by using chromogenic media.

Chromogenic media have also been shown to allow easier differentiation of *Candida* species in mixed yeast populations than the traditional Sabouraud glucose agar [25].

Identifying filamentous fungi is much more cumbersome. Generally, macroscopic and microscopic morphology is the key to identification. The macroscopic examination of the colonies can reveal important characteristics concerning colour, texture, exudates, pigments, specific structures, growth rate and growth zones, and the texture of the aerial mycelium. The colour of the reverse of the colony must be recorded along with any pigment that diffuses into the medium. In addition, microscopic elements have to be evaluated for identification [30].

As an alternative to the conventional identification schemes, proteomic profiling by mass spectral analysis has recently emerged as a simple and reliable method to identify yeasts, moulds and dermatophytes [47]. Matrix-assisted laser desorption ionization-time of flight mass spectrometry (MALDI-TOF) is now commonly used in routine laboratories for yeast identification, while the identification of moulds and dermatophytes using this technique is still not as common as for yeasts.

Yeasts including *Candida*, *Pichia* and *Cryptococcus* genera are most easily processed and analysed. Furthermore, closely related yeast species which cannot be discriminated with common biochemical methods such as the *Candida ortho-/meta-/parapsilosis*, *Candida glabrata/bracarensis/nivariensis*, *Candida albicans/dubliniensis*, *Candida haemulonii* group I and II complexes or the phenotypically similar species *Candida palmioleophila*, *Candida famata* and *Candida guilliermondii* can be resolved without difficulty by MALDI-TOF MS [48]. Even *C. auris*, a recently described multiresistant *Candida* species being typically misidentified by commercial API-20C or Vitek-2 systems, is correctly identified by MALDI-TOF [49].

This technique has also been applied directly on positive blood cultures without the need for its prior culturing, and thus reducing the time required for microbiological diagnosis. Results are available in 30 min, suggesting that this approach is a reliable, time-saving tool for routine identification of *Candida* species causing bloodstream infection [25].

The differentiation of moulds like *Aspergillus* sp., *Penicillium* sp., *Fusarium* sp. and dermatophytes appears to be far more difficult. Reference databases and the database query methods (i.e. comparing and subsequent scoring of the similarity of an unknown spectrum to each database reference spectrum) may directly affect the performance of MALDI-TOF MS for the identification of fungi. While the reference database provided with each commercial MALDI-TOF

MS platform may not be sufficient for routine analyses, some authors noticed that increasing the number of mass spectra obtained from distinct subcultures of strains included in the reference spectrum library (i.e. the number of reference entries) would improve the accuracy of MALDI-TOF MS-based mould identification [50].

Normand et al. developed a free online application which seems to improve the rate of successful identifications [51]. Up to 92.61% of 501 fungal isolates derived from human samples were correctly identified. Only 5% of the identifications were unsatisfactory (i.e. correct at the genus level but not at the species level), and none of the identifications were false at the genus level. These results are better than those usually obtained via phenotypic identification and thus encourage the use of MALDI-TOF in a routine laboratory for mould identification.

1.1.2.6 Surrogate Markers: Biomarkers of Invasive Fungal Infections

Early and reliable diagnosis and rapid initiation of appropriate antifungal therapy has been shown to improve survival significantly. It has been demonstrated that surrogate markers of fungal infections are able to speed up diagnosis and thus further improve treatment and outcomes for patients with IFIs [52].

1.2 Antigen and Antibody Detection

Antibody and antigen detection often provides supplemental information for the diagnosis of invasive fungal infections. Antibody tests are often used in the diagnosis of endemic mycoses, which are often difficult to detect by traditional methods.

1.2.1 Candidiasis

In some cases, antibody tests are a supplemental test in the diagnosis of invasive candidiasis. Interestingly, serum immunoglobulin G (IgG) responses against specific antigens have generally performed better than IgM, suggesting that many patients mount amnestic responses or have ongoing, subclinical tissue invasion [52]. Patients infected with non-*C. albicans* species can be identified by responses against recombinant *C. albicans* antigens [53].

However, it has to be considered that the detection of anti-*Candida* antibodies fails to discriminate between disseminated and superficial infections and may also indicate colonization in uninfected patients. In immunocompromised patients not reliably producing antibodies, diagnosis based on antibody detection is rendered nearly impossible [25, 35]. A number of reports indicate substantial improvement of sensitivity and specificity of invasive candidiasis is when mannan antigen and anti-mannan antibody assays are used in combination. Mikulska et al. [54] reported a combined mannan/anti-mannan sensitivity and specificity for invasive candidiasis diagnosis of 83% and 86%, respectively (compared with separate sensitivities and specificities of 58% and 93% for mannan antigen alone and 59% and 83% for anti-mannan antibodies alone). Thus, detection of serum mannan and anti-mannan antibodies is turning out to be very interesting for earlier diagnosis of invasive candidiasis.

Serial determinations may be necessary. It shows also very high negative predictive value (>85%) and can be used to rule out infection [34].

1.2.2 Cryptococcosis

The detection of cryptococcal capsular polysaccharide is one of the most valuable rapid serodiagnostic tests for fungi performed on a routine basis. The cryptococcal antigen (CrAg) can be detected either by latex agglutination test (LA) or by ELISA. False-positive reactions have been reported in patients with disseminated trichosporonosis, *Capnocytophaga canimorsus* septicaemia, malignancy and positive rheumatoid factor when using the LA. Another assay format is the EIA, the PREMIER Cryptococcal antigen assay (Meridian Diagnostics, Inc.) utilizing a polyclonal capture system and a monoclonal detection system. The Premier EIA was reported to be as sensitive as the latex agglutination system for the detection of capsular polysaccharide in serum and cerebrospinal fluid. In addition, it does not react with rheumatoid factor and gives fewer false-positive results [25].

Since 2009, there is also lateral flow assay (LFA) for the detection of the CrAg available [55]. The CrAg LFA is a well-established point-of-care (POC) test and has an excellent test performance, it is easy to use, and test results are available in 10 min. Moreover, the CrAg LFA is temperature stable, and cross-reactions with other fungi are rare. Serum, plasma, urine and CSF specimens can be used and have shown an excellent sensitivity and specificity [56]. Importantly, CrAg LFA is not useful to check treatment response, as the clearance of CrAg is a slow and also independent process that devitalizes the yeast [57, 58]. Therefore, CrAg LFA titres may therefore remain elevated even if therapy is effective [55, 58].

1.2.3 Invasive Aspergillosis (IA)

Aspergillus antibodies are only infrequently detectable in immunocompromised patients but are often helpful in patients with aspergilloma, allergic bronchopulmonary aspergillosis and cystic fibrosis [59].

Significant advances to the field were brought by the introduction of noncultural diagnostic tests in blood and BALF, including galactomannan antigen (GM) testing for invasive aspergillosis and beta-D-glucan (BDG) testing in patients at risk [52]. When noncultural diagnostic tests were introduced, the rate of fungal infections diagnosed pre-mortem (versus postmortem) was shown to increase from 16 to 51% in a large autopsy study [60].

The most commonly used, commercially available antigen test for *Aspergillus* detection is the double-sandwich ELISA test Platelia Aspergillus® (Bio-Rad Laboratories, Marnes, France), which is validated for the use in serum and BALF [25, 52]. GM testing is currently considered the gold standard when it comes to biomarkers for IA diagnosis as sensitivity and specificity are generally high. Recently, it has been reported that this assay shows a good diagnostic performance when urine and CSF samples are used [52, 61, 62].

However, false-positive and false-negative results of GM have been described in certain patient groups by various authors [25, 42]. False-negative results occur in patients who are receiving antifungal agents other than fluconazole.7 False-positive results occur in patients who are colonized but not infected with *Aspergillus* species. As colonization is undesirable in solid organ transplant or haematology patients at high risk for invasive aspergillosis, results attributed to colonization should not be disregarded but rather should prompt additional investigation to exclude invasive disease or to assess the effectiveness of antifungal prophylaxis or therapy and follow-up evaluation for subsequent invasive disease [63].

Patients who have infection with *Fusarium* species, *Paecilomyces* spp., *Histoplasma capsulatum* and *Blastomyces dermatitidis* may also show positive results because these fungi have similar galactomannans in their cell walls. Cross-reactions may occur with non-pathogenic fungi that are closely related to *Aspergillus* spp., such as *Penicillium* spp. False-positive reactions may be due to the presence of GM in blood-derived products, sodium gluconate containing hydration solutions, antibiotics or food products [64–66].

False-positive reactions with piperacillin-tazobactam have been reported in the past, but manufacturing changes have eliminated this problem. Other reported causes of false-positive results include severe mucositis, severe gastrointestinal graft-versus-host disease, blood products collected in certain commercially available infusion bags, multiple myeloma (IgG type) and flavoured ice pops or frozen desserts containing sodium gluconate [67]. However, solely testing for antigenemia does not replace other tests for IA. To maximize sensitivity, testing should precede empiric antifungal therapy, and positive results should be confirmed on a new specimen [25].

1.2.4 Aspergillus-Specific Lateral Flow Device Test (LFD)

In 2012, Thornton et al. developed a new promising LFD for the detection of *Aspergillus* in patients suffering from haematological malignancies. The technology is based on the detection of *Aspergillus*-specific JF5 by MabJF5 monoclonal antibodies. The JF5 is an extracellular glycoprotein that is exclusively secreted during active growth of the fungus and represents a surrogate marker of *Aspergillus* infection [68]. Minimal required training, simple handling by using BALF samples without any pretreatment, no need for specially equipped laboratories, rapid availability of test results within 15 min and low costs are the major advantages of the LFD [52]. In case of serum testing, samples need to be pretreated by heating, centrifugation and adding a buffer solution according to the manufacturer's recommendations. Results are read by eye after 15-min incubation time and are interpreted depending on the intensity of the test line as negative (−) or weak (+) to strong (+++) positive. Cross-reactivities are rare with the LFD. It appears that only *Penicillium* spp. cause cross-reactions [55]. In clinical studies, sensitivity and specificity rates were acceptable; in particular in BALF samples, even during antimould prophylaxis/treatment, the overall sensitivity was 56% during antifungals versus 86% without [69]. The combination with other biomarkers is currently the most promising approach to indicate IPA [70–77]. Similar to other fungal diagnostics, sensitivity of the LFD is reduced in the presence of antifungal prophylaxis/treatment. Following extensive appraisal of the prototype LFD, the test has now been formatted for large-scale manufacture and CE marking as an in vitro diagnostic (IVD) device. It shows promising performance in a first clinical study [78].

1.3 1-3-β-D-Glucan (BDG) as a Marker for Invasive Fungal Infection

Whereas GM has the limitation of being able to detect only invasive aspergillosis, BDG as a cell wall component of many pathogenic fungi can be detected in a variety of invasive infections including *Aspergillus* spp., *Candida* spp., *Pneumocystis jirovecii*, *Fusarium* spp., *Trichosporon* spp. and *Saccharomyces* spp. but does not allow differentiation of yeast from mould infections [79]. However, it is absent in mucormycosis and at least according to most authors in cryptococcosis. BDG is a major component of the fungal cell wall. It can be detected by the activation of the coagulation cascade in an amoebocyte lysate of horseshoe crabs (*Limulus polyphemus* or *Tachypleus tridentatus*). Various tests are commercially available. The Fungitell assay (Associates of Cape Cod, Falmouth, MA, USA) has been approved by US FDA and is widely used in Europe, while other assays (Fungitec-G, Seikagaku Corporation; Wako Pure Chemicals Industries Ltd.; Maruha-Nichiro Foods Inc.; Tokyo, Japan) have been commercialized in Asia [17]. The role of serum BDG testing to diagnose IFI has been well documented, but other samples, including BALF and CSF fluid, might work as well [80].

Similar to GM, BDG is included as mycological criterion in the revised definitions of IFI from the EORTC/MSG consensus group [81]. This test is considered to be a useful adjunct, especially for patients with intra-abdominal infections, where the sensitivity of cultures is decreased [81]. Studies in adults suggest that monitoring of BDG might be a useful method to exclude IFI in clinical environment with low to moderate prevalence of IFI. Many potential sources for contamination have been demonstrated and may lead to false-positive results [17]. It has also been reported that dialysis filters made from cellulose significantly increase serum-glucan concentrations and thus may lead to false-positive test results [82]. In addition, patients likely to be colonized with fungi may show false-positive results. Therefore, this test has been recommended for exclusion of fungal infection in case of negative results and can be used in the sense of antifungal stewardship. It is crucial for clinicians to know that the BDG assays should always be interpreted in the context of clinical, radiographic and microbiological findings [35].

A more recent approach is the combined use of BDG and procalcitonin for the differential diagnosis of candidaemia and bacteraemia, which is an important issue in intensive care patients [83].

In children and neonates, the diagnostic role of BDG is unclear. Children have shown higher mean BDG levels than in adults [84]. However, very high levels of BDG exist in neonates and children with proven IFI [85] so that the diagnostic cut-off may be increased to 125 pg/ml in neonates with invasive candidiasis (and not 80 pg/ml as suggested for adults) [86]. Due to a high number of false-positive and false-negative results in paediatric patients with hematologic disorders and HSCT recipients BDG is not considered a reliable efficient diagnostic tool in this population [87].

Concerning cryptococcal meningitis, the role of BDG testing has been debated controversially. Though it was once believed that *C. neoformans* does not contain BDG in its cell wall, detectable levels of BDG in CSF were found to correlate with quantitative fungal cultures, and high CSF BDG levels (>500 pg/mL) and were associated with a three times higher risk of 10-week mortality. Although CSF BDG levels do not have adequate sensitivity or specificity to make this assay the preferred cryptococcal diagnostic test, positive results should warrant further diagnostic testing, especially in high-risk, immunocompromised patients [88]. Nucleic acid amplification tests for direct detection of fungi.

Molecular amplification techniques enable the fast and sensitive detection and identification at a species level by direct detecting and analysing tiny amounts of fungal DNA present in serum and blood without the need of prior cultivation [89]. Multiple in-house PCR assays targeting various genetic sequences (18S rDNA, 28S rDNA, 5.8S rDNA, internal transcribed spacer region, mitochondrial DNA) have been developed for the detection of a broad range of fungi in different specimens such as blood, serum, plasma, BAL, sterile fluids and tissues though only a few of these techniques have been standardized so far. Depending on the primers used, fungal pathogens can be detected generally or more specifically, including rapid identification of particular fungal pathogenic species with suitable primers and assays like real-time PCR [90]. The sensitivity and specificity results of the various techniques are variable, but mostly there is an improved sensitivity observed when compared to classical cultural-based methods [25].

The use of PCR to diagnose medical mycoses has been challenging, however, because fungi have cell walls that impede the efficient lysis of organisms and liberation of DNA, thus leading to false-negative PCR results. On the other hand, some human pathogens are also ubiquitous in the environment and may therefore cause false-positive results [91]. A crucial distinction must be made between identification and detection of fungal pathogens using PCR: identification from culture or biopsies requires specific DNA extraction procedures, since the fungal wall has to be broken to avoid false negatives. By contrast, in serum or plasma, fungal DNA is already free and may be more easily detected. Recent technological advancements such as microarray, multiplex PCR with magnetic resonance and others have mitigated the technical difficulty of performing nucleic amplification in both yeast and mould and as a consequence improved the sensitivity and specificity of PCR-based assays for the identification of human fungal pathogens [92, 93].

Several *Candida*-PCR assays have been developed and evaluated and have shown benefit concerning the enhancement of rapid diagnosis. It has been demonstrated that the use of direct PCR is associated with good sensitivity and specificity for rapid diagnosis when using blood samples [35, 94, 95].

A recently developed and already commercially launched diagnostic test detecting *Candida* bloodstream infections is T2Candida panel [93, 96]. The T2Candida panel in combination with the T2Dx instrument (both T2 Biosystems) forms a fully automated and rapid diagnostic tool for early detection of yeasts. This method is magnetic resonance-based and allows highly sensitive detection directly in complex samples, such as whole blood, and is able to detect five *Candida* spp., namely, *C. albicans*, *C. tropicalis*, *C. parapsilosis*, *C. krusei* and *C. glabrata*. The technology allows for the lysis of yeast cells, releasing fungal DNA, then makes copies of the target DNA using PCR and detects the amplified nucleic acids in aqueous solution using magnetic resonance. The platform can use a single blood sample to identify candidaemia within 3 to 5 hours, whereas traditional testing methods can take 6 days or more. This is a magnetic resonance-based diagnostic approach that measures how water molecules react in the presence of magnetic fields

[17, 96]. When particles coated with target-specific-binding agents are added to a sample containing the target, the particles bind and cluster around the target. This clustering changes the microscopic environment of water in the sample, which in turn alters the T2 magnetic resonance signal or the T2 relaxation signal, indicating the presence of the target. This method differs from traditional PCR, where as much as 99% of the fungal DNA target can be lost. T2Candida can detect microbes at a density as low as 1 colony-forming unit (CFU) per ml of whole blood, compared with the 100–1000 CFU/ml typically required for conventional PCR-based methods. Sensitivity of 91.0% and specificity of 98.1% have been reported to be higher than 90% in several studies with PPV 71.6% to 84.2% and NPV ranging from 99.5% to 99.0% [95]. Paediatric patient studies revealed a 100% concordance with blood culture results and T2MR [97].

The speed and sensitivity of T2Candida give it the potential to improve patient care, but the reagents and instrumentation are expensive. A more recent regulatory decision by the FDA gave the superiority claim of T2Candida over blood culture systems. As data is scarce, it is currently under investigation for use in clinical practice [98].

PCR for invasive aspergillosis has been established for whole blood, serum, plasma and other specimens but is very challenging because of the very low amount of DNA in samples [17, 25, 35, 42, 69, 99]. In 2006, the European Aspergillus PCR Initiative (EAPCRI) was launched to seek proposals for a technical consensus. This consensus was possible, thanks to the generalization of real-time quantitative PCR (qPCR), which dramatically reduces the risk of contamination from environmental amplicons and allows quantitative management of the amplification reaction to detect inhibition [100]. Because whole blood is technically more demanding for the extraction steps, serum appears to be a better specimen [101]. However, plasma is now preferred to serum as it shows a better sensitivity [102].

For the time being, the combination of PCR and other biomarkers such as GM or BDG seems to be the most forward strategy. Studies comparing the performance of PCR and fungal biomarkers in serum (GM or BDG) or BAL (GM) have yielded encouraging results, suggesting optimal diagnostic accuracy when combined [17, 103].

A recent meta-analysis showed that the association of GM and PCR tests is highly suggestive of an active infection with a positive predictive value of 88% [104]. However, the combined use of LFD, instead of GM, and qPCR could be a better strategy [99].

Multiplex PCR assays targeting the most clinically relevant *Mucorales* in serum or BAL have also been developed and show promising results for the early diagnosis of mucormycosis but have to be further evaluated and standardized [17].

Panfungal PCR A different method used in molecular diagnostics of fungal infections is the use of a PCR that can detect a wide variety of fungi at once in the same specimen. The technique is fairly simple and is based on the use of primers specifically designed to amplify a region that is conserved among different fungal genera. Nevertheless, limitations should also be considered, such as the facts that panfungal PCR could be less sensitive in case of some fungi, e.g. interference of melanin with the amplification in case of dematiaceous hyphomycetes. Furthermore, presence of a mixed fungal infection or the presence of the microorganism due to colonization or accidental contamination needs to be taken into account when interpreting the results. However, several studies have shown the utility of panfungal PCRs, but still clinical evaluation is needed [91, 105, 106].

When performing panfungal PCR assays, DNA sequence analysis is often required when obtaining the amplification product. For DNA sequence analysis, the results must be compared with those deposited in databases from known organisms in order for an identity to be obtained. Publically available databases for DNA fungal sequence comparisons are available, including those at the National Center for Biotechnology Information (GenBank; www.ncbi.nlm.nih.gov/genbank/), the Centraalbureau voor Schimmelcultures Fungal Biodiversity Center in the Netherlands (CBS-KNAW; www.cbs.knaw.nl), the International Society of Human and Animal Mycology ITS Database (ISHAM; its.mycologylab.org) and the Fusarium-ID database (http://isolate.fusariumdb.org). The use of sequence results can be extremely useful when compared with credible deposits.

Not all fungal deposits within databases, however, have been confirmed to be from accurately identified organisms [107]. This can lead to erroneous results and the misidentification of the cultured specimen. In addition, the choice of the proper target sequence can be critical for the identification of fungi. Although the internal transcribed spacer (ITS) region has been put forth as a universal barcode for the identification of fungi [108], this target cannot always be used alone to discriminate between closely related fungi. Several other DNA targets may be required to identify fungi in the clinical setting, and the choice of targets depends on the suspected genus [109].

The commercially available PCR kit the LightCycler® SeptiFast Test MGRADE, designed to detect the 25 most prevalent microorganisms in blood culture (also comprising 5 *Candida* spp., as well as *Aspergillus fumigatus*) is based on real-time PCR targeting species-specific ITS regions and has been evaluated for a few years now in Europe (Roche Diagnostics GmbH, Mannheim, Germany). The complete test procedure is validated by detection of positive signals generated by an integrated internal control DNA in order to reassure an uninhibited amplification and detection within the test specimen. In case of *Candida* spp. and *A. fumigatus*, the SeptiFast test turned out to be more sensitive than conventional BC and was not affected by the administration of antimicrobial therapy [25, 89, 110].

PCR has been shown to work well in the paediatric population. A potential drawback of PCR testing in these patients is the amount of specimen needed to perform valid testing (about 2 ml), which is markedly more material than that needed for the GM, BDG and LFD tests [80]. Advantages and disadvantages of the various test assays are listed in Table 1.2.

Table 1.2 Current approaches to laboratory diagnosis

Test	Specimen	Advantage	Disadvantage	Recommendation
Histopathology	Tissue	Enables proven diagnosis	Requires biopsy, no identification to genus and species	
Direct microscopy	Any	Low cost	Labour intensive, no identification to genus and species	Better sensitivity when using calcofluor white
Culture	Any	Allows exact identification and susceptibility testing	Slow, dependent on viable organisms	Use of specific media
Galactomannan	Serum, BAL; investigational: CSF, urine	Sensitive, specimens easy to obtain, rapid results	Decreased sensitivity when patient is on antifungals	Useful for monitoring therapeutic response, useful for diagnosing IA when using BAL
Beta-D-glucan	Serum; investigational: BAL, CSF	Sensitive, specimens easy to obtain, rapid results	Lacks specificity, high rate of false-positive results	Especially for exclusion of fungal infections; could be useful as a screening technique when doing serial determinations in haematological patients at high risk
Lateral flow test	Serum, BAL	Sensitive, rapid results Very reliable for detection of cryptococcosis	Performance derived from small studies (IA)	Useful technique in combination with other tests for IA (GM, PCR)
DNA detection	Any	Sensitive, results within several hours	Labour intensive, expensive, only little standardization, may have low	Could be useful as a screening technique when doing serial determinations in haematological

Threshold for patients at high contamination risk

1.4 Antifungal Susceptibility Testing (AST)

Antifungal drug resistance can occur with all drug classes and involves strains with acquired resistance and inherently less susceptible species. In vitro susceptibility testing is often used to select agents with likely activity for a given infection, but perhaps its most important use is in identifying agents that will not work, i.e. to detect resistance. Thus, it is a useful tool to provide information to clinicians to help to guide therapy [109, 111].

AST may be used for the assessment of the in vitro activity. As elevated antifungal minimum inhibitory concentration (MIC) values represent decreased vitro activity and are associated with poor outcomes and breakthrough infections, this may be used for therapeutic management. Secondly, AST is also used as a means to survey the development of resistance and to predict the therapeutic potential and spectrum of activity of investigational agents. In any case, AST should be clinically useful; thus, it must reliably predict the likelihood of clinical success. There are several factors that also influence outcomes in patients with fungal infections other than antifungal susceptibility. These include (1) the host's immune response, (2) the severity of the underlying disease and other comorbidities, (3) drug interactions and (4) the pharmacokinetics of the agents and concentrations achieved at the site of infection [109].

Currently, there are two independent standards for broth microdilution (BMD) susceptibility testing of *Candida* and filamentous fungi: the Clinical and Laboratory Standards Institute (CLSI) methods and the European Committee on Antimicrobial Susceptibility Testing (EUCAST) methods [112, 113] (http://www.eucast.org/ast_of_fungi/). Both of these methods use BMD, although there are some differences in inoculum size and MIC endpoint determination results obtained when testing azoles and echinocandins against *Candida* and azoles against *Aspergillus* species are in close agreement [114]. CLSI also established disk diffusion assays for *Candida* (fluconazole, voriconazole, echinocandins) and *Aspergillus* [115]. Also, interpretative breakpoints have been provided for azoles, caspofungin and micafungin.

Over the past several years, there have been efforts to harmonize the methods and clinical breakpoints (CBP) for antifungal susceptibility testing between these two groups. Some differences do exist, but the results are comparable [116, 117]. One issue with both the CLSI and EUCAST broth microdilution susceptibility testing that has been identified is the problem of interlaboratory variability for caspofungin MICs, with some laboratories reporting low values, whereas others report high values for this echinocandin [118]. This variability seems to be greatest for *C. glabrata* and *C. krusei* and may lead to falsely classifying susceptible isolates as resistant to the echinocandins. Because of this, EUCAST does not recommend susceptibility testing with caspofungin but instead recommends the use of micafungin or anidulafungin MICs as surrogate markers for caspofungin susceptibility or resistance [117]. Studies have clearly demonstrated high concordance rates for anidulafungin and micafungin MICs in detecting mutations within the *FKS* gene that confer echinocandin resistance in multiple *Candida* species [119, 120].

There are also differences in the CBP that define resistance as set by CLSI and EUCAST. Despite the differences in methods, the categorical agreement that is obtained is comparable although some differences have been reported. CBP have not been set for each antifungal agent against each type of fungus. The CLSI has only established breakpoints for fluconazole, voriconazole and the echinocandins against certain *Candida* species, and no breakpoints have been set against moulds or endemic fungi. In contrast, EUCAST has established breakpoints for certain antifungals against yeast and some moulds, including *Aspergillus* species [109].

As these methods are time-consuming and commercially available, test kits for MIC determination are a good alternative. These include gradient diffusions assays, colorimetric assays and automated tests. The antifungal MIC agar-based assay Etest® (bioMérieux) directly quantifies antifungal susceptibility in terms of discrete

MIC values. This method is commonly used for susceptibility testing against various *Candida* species and is also considered a sensitive and reliable method for detecting decreased susceptibility to amphotericin B among *Candida* isolates and *Cryptococcus neoformans* [109]. Several studies have reported very good essential agreement (>90%) between the Etest assay and the CLSI and EUCAST broth microdilution reference methods [121, 122]. A clear benefit of utilizing Etest is assessing the susceptibility to amphotericin B, as this method gives much broader MIC ranges than BMD. Etest is also highly suitable for determining the activity of echinocandins against yeasts as it produces easy to read, sharp zones of inhibition. However, for echinocandins, the paradoxical effect has been observed for *Candida* and *Aspergillus* in vitro. The paradoxical effect refers to an attenuation of echinocandin activity at higher concentrations despite an inhibitory effect at lower drug levels. It appears to be species-related and varies with the echinocandin. The effect has been noted most often for caspofungin and is not related to FKS1 mutations or upregulation of echinocandin sensitivity of the glucan synthase complex in the presence of drug. The clinical relevance of this in vitro effect is uncertain [123, 124].

Others have reported less than optimal categorical agreement between the Etest assay and the CLSI broth microdilution method for caspofungin against *C. glabrata* and *C. krusei* based on the revised CLSI echinocandin clinical breakpoints [125–127]. In addition, a recent study reported poor overall agreement between Etest and EUCAST MICs for amphotericin B and posaconazole (75.1%) when used to measure activity against members of the order *Mucorales* and recommended that the Etest assay should not be used when testing these fungi [128].

The YeastOne Sensititre test (Thermo Scientific, Waltham, MA, USA formerly TREK Diagnostic Systems) is a broth microdilution assay format that uses the blue colorimetric dye resazurin (alamarBlue) that is converted to by metabolically active cells to resorufin. Several studies of the YeastOne assay, including multicentre evaluations, have demonstrated excellent reproducibility and very good agreement with the broth microdilution reference methods.

Overall categorical agreement, however, was somewhat lower for caspofungin than micafungin (93.6 vs 99.6%) between the YeastOne assay and the CLSI broth microdilution method, and this was due to the low categorical agreement for caspofungin against *C. glabrata* and *C. krusei* (69.1%) between the two methods [109].

The yeast susceptibility test, Vitek 2 (bioMérieux, France), is a fully automated assay for performing antifungal susceptibility testing. Several studies have reported reproducible and accurate results compared with the CLSI broth microdilution method. One of the limitations of this system for caspofungin is that a correct discrimination between susceptible and intermediate categories for *C. glabrata* isolates is impossible as the lower end of the concentration range is 0.25 μg/mL [109, 122]. In addition, it was reported that 19.4% of caspofungin-resistant *Candida* isolates with known mechanisms of resistance (mutations in *FKS* hotspot regions) were misclassified as susceptible to caspofungin [129].

As azole-resistant *Aspergillus fumigatus* is emerging worldwide, easy test formats are urgently needed. Therefore, a screening method based on an agar-based test has been developed and commercialized (VIP CheckTM, Beneden-Leeuwen, the Netherlands). Multiple colonies are sub-cultured on a four-well plate with a growth control and itraconazole, voriconazole and posaconazole added to the agar. This approach detects with high sensitivity and specificity potential resistance in the isolates in a simplified way, i.e. isolates growing only on the growth-control well excludes resistance [130]. The overall performance of the four-well screening plates was evaluated with respect to the sensitivity and specificity to differentiate between different mutant and WT isolates. The overall sensitivity and specificity for the four-well plate (no growth versus growth) was 99% (range 97%–100%) and 99% (95%–100%), respectively [131]. Sensititre YeastOne can also be used for *Aspergillus*, and some studies have shown that this assay might be useful in detecting resistance to itraconazole and voriconazole [132].

In recent years, progress has been made towards the description of resistance mechanisms at molecular level. There are methods of detection that can be useful for clinical laboratories, but lack of standardization precludes their integration in the routine daily practice. The molecular detection of *Candida* resistance to azoles and to echinocandins and of *Aspergillus* resistance to triazoles can be clinically relevant and could help to design more efficient prevention and control strategies. However, multicentre studies including third-party validation and reproducibility assessment are needed for further acceptance and standardization. New automated and massive sequencing technique could change AST procedures in the upcoming years [45].

Susceptibility testing is indicated to provide the basis for selection of appropriate antifungal treatment in individual patient cases and for epidemiological reasons in order to continuously follow susceptibility patterns and thereby detect any emergence of resistance at an early stage. Recommendations for AST are displayed in Table 1.4. However, for individual patient care, the isolate should be identified to species level to predict the susceptibility pattern. Important examples of fungi that have low susceptibility to antifungal agents include *C. krusei*, which is intrinsically resistant to fluconazole and less susceptible to amphotericin B than other *Candida* spp.; *Aspergillus* spp., *Scedosporium apiospermum*, *Trichosporon* spp. and *Scopulariopsis* spp. which are resistant to amphotericin B; *Mucorales* which are resistant to all licensed azoles; and *C. glabrata* which is frequently less susceptible to fluconazole than other *Candida* spp. For better illustration, Table 1.3 shows the susceptibility pattern of the most common *Candida* spp. In cases where the susceptibility pattern cannot be reliably predicted based on the species identification alone, antifungal susceptibility testing should be performed [111, 133].

Attention has to be paid that for emerging fungal pathogens, such as *Mucorales*, dematiaceous moulds and *Fusarium*, no standardized breakpoints are available as of yet. Species belonging to the order *Mucorales* are more resistant to antifungal agents than *Aspergillus* spp. All species of *Mucorales* are unaffected by voriconazole, and most show moderate resistance in vitro to echinocandins; use of voriconazole as first-line treatment for aspergillosis and use of echinocandins as empirical treatment for febrile neutropenia and disseminated candidiasis have been blamed for the increased incidence of mucormycosis. Amphotericin B and posaconazole show the most potent activity in vitro against the *Mucorales* [13]. Table 1.4 shows the susceptibility pattern of common opportunistic moulds.

In recent years, progress has been made towards the description of resistance mechanisms at molecular level. There are methods of detection that can be useful for clinical laboratories, but lack of standardization precludes their integration in the routine daily practice. The molecular detection of *Candida* resistance to azoles and echinocandins and of *Aspergillus* resistance to triazoles can be clinically relevant and could help to design

Table 1.3 General susceptibility patterns of certain yeasts and moulds

Fungus	AmB	FLU	ITRA	VOR	POS	EC
C. albicans	S	S	S	S	S	S
C. tropicalis	S	S	S	S	S	S
C. parapsilosis	S	S	S	S	S	I
C. glabrata	S	I	I	I	I	S
C. krusei	S	R	S-I-R	S-I-R	S-I-R	S
C. lusitaniae	S to R	S	S	S	S	S
C. guilliermondii	S	R	R	R	R	R
C. auris	X	R				X

AmB amphotericin B, *FLU* fluconazole, *ITRA* itraconazole, *VOR* voriconazole, *POS* posaconazole, *EC* echinocandins, *S* susceptible, *SDD* susceptible dose dependent, *I* intermediate, *R* resistant

"X" denotes that the MICs for the antifungal compound are elevated compared to those for *C. albicans*

more efficient prevention and control strategies [133]. The commercially developed AsperGenius species assay (PathoNostics, Maastricht, the Netherlands) is a multiplex real-time PCR capable of detecting aspergillosis and genetic markers associated with azole resistance [134]. The assay is validated for testing bronchoalveolar lavage (BAL) fluids, replacing the requirement for culture to differentiate susceptible from resistant *A. fumigatus* strains [135, 136]. A novel and highly accurate diagnostic platform has been developed for rapid identification of FKS mutations associated with echinocandin resistance in *C. glabrata* which needs evaluation, and further development to cover the entire FKS mutation spectrum would enhance its appeal as a diagnostic platform [137]. Recommendations for the antifungal susceptibility testing are presented in Table 1.5.

Table 1.4 General susceptibility patterns of selected moulds

Fungus	AmB	ITRA	VOR	POS	ISA	EC
A. fumigatus	S	S	S	S	S	S
A. flavus	S/R	S	S/R	S	S	S
A. terreus	R	S	S	S	S	S
A. lentulus	R	R	R	S/R	S/R	R
Rhizopus spp.	S	S/R	R	S/R	S/R	R
Mucor spp.	S/R	R	R	S/R	S/R	R
Fusarium spp.	S/R	R	S/R	S/R	S/R	R
Scedosporium spp.	S/R	R	S/R	S/R	R	R

AmB amphotericin B, *ITRA* itraconazole, *VOR* voriconazole, *POS* posaconazole, *ISA* isavuconazole, *EC* echinocandins, *S* susceptible, *R* resistant

Table 1.5 Antifungal susceptibility testing: when and how to test

When to test?
Routine antifungal testing of fluconazole and an echinocandin against *C. glabrata* from deep sites Consider cross-resistance between fluconazole and all other azoles to be complete for *C. glabrata* In invasive fungal infections In invasive and mucosal infections failing therapy For yeasts and moulds from sterile sites For isolates considered clinically relevant particularly in patients exposed to antifungals
How to test?
Identification to species level For *Candida* spp. perform routine susceptibility testing for fluconazole and according to the local epidemiology include other azoles Selection of susceptibility testing methods: standardized methods • CLSI methods • EUCAST EDef 7.1 – Broth based, M27-A3 – Agar based, M44-A2 Commercial methods • Etest • Sensititre YeastOne • Vitek 2 • Molecular assays Aspergillus—azoles (available) Candida—echinocandins, azoles (in progress) No testing of isolates with a high rate of intrinsic resistance: • *C. lusitaniae* and amphotericin • *C. krusei* and fluconazole, flucytosine • *C. guilliermondii* and echinocandins • *A. terreus* and amphotericin B

However, multicentre studies including third-party validation and reproducibility assessment are needed for further acceptance and standardization. New automated and massive sequencing technique could change AST procedures in the upcoming years [133].

References

1. Spellberg B, Edwards J Jr, Ibrahim A (2005) Novel perspectives on mucormycosis: pathophysiology, presentation, and management. Clin Microbiol Rev 18(3):556–569
2. Benedict K, Richardson M, Vallabhaneni S, Jackson BR, Chiller T (2017) Emerging issues, challenges, and changing epidemiology of fungal disease outbreaks. Lancet Infect Dis 17:e403–e411
3. Kronen R, Liang SY, Bochicchio G, Bochicchio K, Powderly WG, Spec A (2017) Invasive fungal infections secondary to traumatic injury. Int J Infect Dis 62:102–111
4. Campell CK, Johnson EM, Warnock DW (2013) Identification of pathogenic fungi, 2nd edn. Wiley-Blackwell, West Sussex, pp 263–304
5. Richardson M, Lass-Flörl C (2008) Changing epidemiology of systemic fungal infections. Clin Microbiol Infect 14(Suppl 4):5–24
6. Sears D, Schwartz BS (2017) Candida auris: an emerging multidrug-resistant pathogen. Int J Infect Dis 63:95–98
7. Limper AH, Adenis A, Le T et al (2017) Fungal infections in HIV/AIDS. Lancet Infect Dis 17:e334–e343
8. Smith N, Sehring M, Chambers J et al (2017) Perspectives on non-*neoformans* cryptococcal opportunistic infections. J Community Hosp Intern Med Perspect 7:214–217
9. Mazzacato S, Marchionni E, Fothergill AW et al (2015) Epidemiology and outcome of systemic infections due to Saprochaete capitate: case report and review of the literature. Infection 43:211–215
10. Graeff l D, Seidel D, Vehreschild MJ et al (2017) Invasive infections due to Saprochaete and Geotrichum species: report of 23 cases from the FungiScope Registry. Mycoses 60:273–279
11. Wirth F, Goldani LZ (2012) Epidemiology of *Rhodotorula*: an emerging pathogen. Interdiscip Perspect Infect Dis 2012:465717
12. Morris A, Norris KA (2012) Colonization by pneumocystis jirovecii and its role in disease. Clin Microbiol Rev 25:297–317
13. Lass-Flörl C, Cuenca-Estrella M (2017) Changes in the epidemiological landscape of invasive mould infections and disease. J Antimicrob Chemother 72(suppl_1):i5–i11
14. Meis JF, Chowdhary A, Rhodes JL, Fisher MC, Verweij PE (2016) Clinical implications of globally emerging azole resistance in Aspergillus fumigatus. Philos Trans R Soc B 371:20150460
15. Quan C, Spellberg B (2010) Mucormycosis, pseudallescheriasis, and other uncommon mold infections. Proc Am Thorac Soc 7:210–215
16. Mendoza L, Vilela R, Voelz K et al (2015) Human fungal pathogens of mucorales and entomophthorales. Cold Spring Harb Perspect Med 5(4):a019562
17. Lamoth F, Calandra T (2017) Early diagnosis of invasive mould infections and disease. J Antimicrob Chemother 72(suppl_1):i19–i28
18. Tortorano AM, Richardson M, Roilides E et al (2014) ESCMID & ECMM Joint Guidelines on diagnosis and management of hyalohyphomycosis: Fusarium spp, Scedosporium spp, and others. Clin Microbiol Infect 20(Suppl 3):27–46
19. Al-Hatmi AMS, Hagen F, Menken SBJ et al (2016) Global molecular epidemiology and genetic diversity of Fusarium, a significant emerging group of human opportunists from 1958 to 2015. Emerg Microbes Infect 5:e124
20. Gavalda J, Meije Y, Fortun J et al (2014) Invasive fungal infections in SOT recipients. Clin Microbiol Infect 20(Suppl 7):27–48
21. Atalla A, Garnica M, Maiolino A et al (2015) Risk factors for invasive mold diseases in allogeneic hematopoietic cell transplant recipients. Transpl Infect Dis 17:7–13
22. Garnica M, daCunha MO, Portugal R et al (2015) Risk factors for invasive fusariosis in patients with acute myeloid leukemia and in hematopoietic cell transplant recipients. Clin Infect Dis 60:875–880
23. Guarro J, Kantarcioglu AS, Horre R et al (2006) Scedosporium apiospermum: changing clinical spectrum of a therapy-refractory opportunist. Med Mycol 44:295–327
24. Rodriguez-Tudela JL, Berenguer J, Guarro J et al (2009) Epidemiology and outcome of Scedosporium prolificans infection, a review of 162 cases. Med Mycol 47:359–370
25. Willinger B, Kienzl D, Kurzai O (2014) Diagnostics in fungal infections. In: Kurzai O (ed) Human fungal pathogens, vol XII, 2nd edn. Springer, Berlin, pp 229–259
26. Alexander B, Pfaller M (2006) Contemporary tools for the diagnosis and management of invasive mycoses. Clin Infect Dis 43:S15–S27
27. Chandrasekar P (2009) Diagnostic challenges and recent advances in the early management of invasive fungal infections. Eur J Haematol 84:281–290
28. Richardson MD, Warnock DW (2012) Fungal Infection. Diagnosis and Management. Blackwell Publishing, Inc, Maiden
29. Clinical and Laboratory Standards Institute (2012) Principles and procedures for detection of fungi in clinical specimens—direct examination and culture; approved guideline, CLSI document M54-A. Clinical and Laboratory Standards Institute, Villanova
30. Vyzantiadil TA, Johnson EM, Kibbler CC (2012) From the patient to the clinical mycology labora-

tory: how can we optimise microscopy and culture methods for mould identification? J Clin Pathol 65:475–483
31. Revankar SG (2007) Dematiaceous fungi. Mycoses 50:91–101
32. Lease E, Alexander B (2011) Fungal diagnostics in pneumonia. Semin Respir Crit Care Med 32:663–672
33. Rüchel R, Schaffrinski M (1999) Versatile fluorescent staining of fungi in clinical specimens by using the optical brightener Blankophor. J Clin Microbiol 37:2694–2696
34. Cuenca-Estrella M, Verweij PE, Arendrup MC et al (2012) ESCMID* guideline for the diagnosis and management of *Candida* diseases 2012: diagnostic procedures. Clin Microbiol Infect 18:9–18
35. Ostrosky-Zeichner L (2012) Invasive mycoses: diagnostic challenges. Am J Med 125(Suppl):S14–S24
36. Arendrup MC, Bergmann OJ, Larsson L, Nielsen HV, Jarløv JO, Christensson B (2010) Detection of candidaemia in patients with and without underlying haematological disease. Clin Microbiol Infect 16:855–862
37. Ericson EL, Klingspor L, Ullberg M, Özenci V (2012) Clinical comparison of the Bactec Mycosis IC/F, BacT/Alert FA, and BacT/Alert FN blood culture vials for the detection of candidemia. Diagn Microbiol Infect Dis 73:153–156
38. Meyer MH, Letscher-Bru V, Jaulhac B, Waller J, Candolfi E (2004) Comparison of Mycosis IC/F and plus Aerobic/F media for diagnosis of fungemia by the Bactec 9240 system. J Clin Microbiol 42:773–777
39. Arendrup MC, Fuursted K, Gahrn-Hansen B et al (2008) Semi-national surveillance of fungaemia in Denmark 2004-2006: increasing incidence of fungaemia and numbers of isolates with reduced azole susceptibility. Clin Microbiol Infect 14:487–494
40. Arendrup MC, Bruun B, Christensen JJ et al (2011) National surveillance of fungemia in Denmark (2004 to 2009). J Clin Microbiol 49:325–334
41. Nucci M, Anaissie E (2007) Fusarium infections in immunocompromised patients. Clin Microbiol Rev 20:695–704
42. Bernal-Martínez L, Alastruey-Izquierdo A, Cuenca-Estrella M (2016) Diagnostics and susceptibility testing in *Aspergillus*. Future Microbiol 11:315–328
43. Vandewoude KH, Blot SI, Depuydt P et al (2006) Clinical relevance of Aspergillus isolation from respiratory tract samples in critically ill patients. Crit Care 10:R31
44. Denning DW, Kibbler CC, Barnes RA (2003) British society for medical mycology proposed standards of care for patients with invasive fungal infections. Lancet Infect Dis 3:230–240
45. Arendrup MC, Bille J, Dannaoui E et al (2012) ECIL-3 classical diagnostic procedures for the diagnosis of invasive fungal diseases in patients with leukaemia. Bone Marrow Transplant 47:1030–1045
46. Moriarty B, Hay R, Morris-Jones R (2012) The diagnosis and management of tinea. BMJ 345:e4380
47. Cassagne C, Normand AC, L'Ollivier C et al (2016) Performance of MALDI-TOF MS platforms for fungal identification. Mycoses 59:678–690
48. Bader O (2013) MALDI-TOF-MS-based species identification and typing approaches in medical mycology. Proteomics 13:788–799
49. Kathuria S, Singh PK, Sharma C et al (2015) Multidrug-resistant Candida auris misidentified as Candida haemulonii: characterization by matrix-assisted laser desorption ionization-time of flight mass spectrometry and DNA sequencing and its antifungal susceptibility profile variability by vitek 2, CLSI Broth microdilution, and etest method. J Clin Microbiol 53:1823–1830
50. Sanguinetti M, Posteraro B (2017) Identification of molds by matrix- assisted laser desorption ionization-time of flight mass spectrometry. J Clin Microbiol 55:369–379
51. Normand AC, Becker P, Gabriel F et al (2017) Validation of a new web application for identification of fungi by use of matrix-assisted laser desorption ionization-time of flight mass spectrometry. J Clin Microbiol 55:2661–2670
52. Heldt S, Hoenigl M (2017) Lateral flow assays for the diagnosis of invasive aspergillosis: current status. Curr Fungal Infect Rep 11:45–51
53. Clancy CJ, Nguyen MH (2013) Finding the "missing 50%" of invasive candidiasis: how nonculture diagnostics will improve understanding of disease spectrum and transform patient care. Clin Infect Dis 56:1284–1292
54. Mikulska M, Calandra T, Sanguinetti M et al (2010) The use of mannan antigen and anti-mannan antibodies in the diagnosis of invasive candidiasis: recommendations from the Third European Conference on Infections in Leukemia. Crit Care 14:R222
55. Prattes J, Heldt S, Eigl S et al (2016) Point of care testing for the diagnosis of fungal infections: are we there yet? Curr Fungal Infect Rep 10:43–50
56. Jarvis JN, Percival A, Bauman S et al (2011) Evaluation of a novel point-of-care cryptococcal antigen test on serum, plasma, and urine from patients with HIV-associated cryptococcal meningitis. Clin Infect Dis 53:1019–1023
57. Brouwer AE, Teparrukkul P, Pinpraphaporn S et al (2005) Baseline correlation and comparative kinetics of cerebrospinal fluid colony-forming unit counts and antigen titers in cryptococcal meningitis. J Infect Dis 192:681–684
58. Aberg JA, Watson J, Segal M et al (2000) Clinical utility of monitoring serum cryptococcal antigen (sCRAG) titers in patients with AIDS-related cryptococcal disease. HIV Clin Trials 1:1–6
59. Kappe R, Rimek D (2010) Mycoserology-did we move on? *Aspergillus*. Mycoses 53(Suppl 1):26–29
60. Lewis RE, Cahyame-Zuniga L, Leventakos K et al (2013) Epidemiology and sites of involvement of invasive fungal infections in patients with haematological malignancies: a 20-year autopsy study. Mycoses 56:638–645

61. Reischies FMJ, Raggam RB, Prattes J et al (2016) Urine galactomannan-to- creatinine ratio for detection of invasive aspergillosis in patients with hematological malignancies. J Clin Microbiol 54:771–774
62. Chong GM, Maertens JA, Lagrou K et al (2016) Diagnostic performance of galactomannan antigen testing in cerebrospinal fluid. J Clin Microbiol 54:428–431
63. Hage CA, Knox KS, Davis TE et al (2011) Antigen detection in bronchoalveolar lavage fluid for diagnosis of fungal pneumonia. Curr Opin Pulm Med 17:167–171
64. Ansorg R, van den Boom R, Rath PM (1997) Detection of Aspergillus galacto-mannan antigen in foods and antibiotics. Mycoses 40:353–357
65. Martin-Rabadan P, Gijon P, Alonso Fernandez R et al (2012) False-positive Aspergillus antigenemia due to blood product conditioning fluids. Clin Infect Dis 55:e22–e27
66. Petraitiene R, Petraitis V, Witt JR et al (2011) Galactomannan antigenemia after infusion of gluconate-containing Plasma-Lyte. J Clin Microbiol 49:4330–4332
67. Miceli MH, Kauffman CA (2017) *Aspergillus* galactomannan for diagnosing invasive aspergillosis. JAMA 318:1175–1176
68. Thornton C, Johnson G, Agrawal S (2012) Detection of invasive pulmonary aspergillosis in haematological malignancy patients by using lateral-flow technology. J Vis Exp 61:3721
69. Buchheidt D, Reinwald M, Hönigl M et al (2017) The evolving landscape of new diagnostic tests for invasive aspergillosis in hematology patients: strengths and weaknesses. Curr Opin Infect Dis 30(6):539–544
70. Hoenigl M, Koidl C, Duettmann W et al (2012) Bronchoalveolar lavage lateral-flow device test for invasive pulmonary aspergillosis diagnosis in haematological malignancy and solid organ transplant patients. J Infect 65:588–591
71. Prattes J, Lackner M, Eigl S et al (2015) Diagnostic accuracy of the Aspergillus specific bronchoalveolar lavage lateral-flow assay in haematological malignancy patients. Mycoses 58:461–469
72. Eigl S, Prattes J, Reinwald M et al (2015) Influence of mould-active antifungal treatment on the performance of the Aspergillus-specific bronchoalveolar lavage fluid lateral-flow device test. Int J Antimicrob Agents 46:401–405
73. White PL, Parr C, Thornton C, Barnes RA (2013) Evaluation of real-time PCR, galactomannan enzyme-linked immunosorbent assay (ELISA), and a novel lateral-flow device for diagnosis of invasive aspergillosis. J Clin Microbiol 51:1510–1516
74. Held J, Schmidt T, Thornton CR et al (2013) Comparison of a novel Aspergillus lateral-flow device and the Platelia(R) galactomannan assay for the diagnosis of invasive aspergillosis following haematopoietic stem cell transplantation. Infection 41:1163–1169
75. Johnson GL, Sarker SJ, Nannini F et al (2015) Aspergillus-specific lateral-flow device and real-time PCR testing of bronchoalveolar lavage fluid: a combination biomarker approach for clinical diagnosis of invasive pulmonary Aspergillosis. J Clin Microbiol 53:2103–2108
76. Hoenigl M, Prattes J, Spiess B et al (2014) Performance of galactomannan, beta-d-glucan, Aspergillus lateral-flow device (LFD), conventional culture, and PCR tests with bronchoalveolar lavage fluid for diagnosis of invasive pulmonary aspergillosis. J Clin Microbiol 52:2039–2045
77. Miceli MH, Goggins MI, Chander P et al (2015) Performance of lateral flow device and galactomannan for the detection of Aspergillus species in bronchoalveolar fluid of patients at risk for invasive pulmonary aspergillosis. Mycoses 58:368–374
78. Hoenigl M, Eigl S, Heldt S et al (2017) Clinical evaluation of the newly formatted lateral-flow device for invasive pulmonary aspergillosis. Mycoses 00:1–4
79. McCarthy MW, Petraitiene R, Walsh TJ (2017) Translational development and application of (1→3)-β-d-glucan for diagnosis and therapeutic monitoring of invasive mycoses. Int J Mol Sci 18:1124
80. Warris A, Lehrnbecher T (2017) Progress in the diagnosis of invasive fungal disease in children. Curr Fungal Infect Rep 11:35–44
81. De Pauw B, Walsh TJ, Donnelly JP et al (2008) Revised definitions of invasive fungal disease from the European Organization for Research and Treatment of Cancer/invasive fungal infections cooperative group and the National Institute of Allergy and Infectious Diseases mycoses study group (EORTC/MSG) consensus group. Clin Infect Dis 46:1813–1821
82. Giacobbe DR, Mikulska M, Tumbarello M et al (2017) Combined use of serum (1,3)-β-d-glucan and procalcitonin for the early differential diagnosis between candidaemia and bacteraemia in intensive care units. Crit Care 21:176
83. Karageorgopoulos DE, Vouloumanou EK, Ntziora F et al (2011) b-D-glucan assay for the diagnosis of invasive fungal infections: a meta-analysis. Clin Infect Dis 52:750–770
84. Smith PB, Benjamin DK Jr, Alexander BD et al (2007) Quantification of 1,3-beta-D-glucan levels in children: preliminary data for diagnostic use of the beta-glucan assay in a pediatric setting. Clin Vaccine Immunol 14:924–925
85. Mularoni A, Furfaro E, Faraci M et al (2010) High levels of beta-D-glucan in immunocompromised children with proven invasive fungal disease. Clin Vaccine Immunol 17:882–883
86. Goudjil S, Kongolo G, Dusol L et al (2013) (1-3)-beta-D-glucan levels in candidiasis infections in the critically ill neonate. J Matern Fetal Neonatal Med 26:44–48
87. Koltze A, Rath P, Schoning SP et al (2015) Beta-D-glucan screening for detection of invasive fungal disease in children undergoing allogeneic hemato-

poietic stem cell transplantation. J Clin Microbiol 53:2605–2610
88. Rhein J, Boulware DR, Bahr NC (2015) 1,3-beta-D-glucan in cryptococcal meningitis. Lancet Infect Dis 15:1136–1137
89. Willinger B, Haase G (2013) State-of-the-art procedures and quality management in diagnostic medical mycology. Curr Fungal Infect Rep 7:260–272
90. Perfect JR (2013) Fungal diagnosis: how do we do it and can we do better? Curr Med Res Opin 29(suppl 4):3–11
91. McCarthy MW, Walsh TJ (2016) Molecular diagnosis of invasive mycoses of the central nervous system. Expert Rev Mol Diagn 17:129–139
92. Boch T, Reinwald M, Postina P et al (2015) Identification of invasive fungal diseases in immunocompromised patients by combining an Aspergillus specific PCR with a multifungal DNA-microarray from primary clinical samples. Mycoses 58:735–745
93. Mylonakis E, Clancy CJ, Ostrosky-Zeichner L et al (2015) T2 magnetic resonance assay for the rapid diagnosis of candidemia in whole blood: a clinical trial. Clin Infect Dis 60:892–899
94. Avni T, Leibovici L, Paul M (2011) PCR diagnosis of invasive candidiasis: systematic review and meta-analysis. J Clin Microbiol 49:665–670
95. Posch W, Heimdörfer D, Wilflingseder D et al (2017) Invasive candidiasis: future directions in non-culture based diagnosis. Expert Rev Anti-Infect Ther 15:829–838
96. Pfaller MA, Wolk DM, Lowery TJ (2015) T2MR and T2Candida: novel technology for the rapid diagnosis of candidemia and invasive candidiasis. Future Microbiol 11:103–117
97. Neely LA, Audeh M, Phung NA et al (2013) T2 magnetic resonance enables nanoparticle mediated rapid detection of candidemia in whole blood. Sci Transl Med 5:182ra154
98. Hamula CL, Hughes K, Fisher BT et al (2016) T2Candida provides rapid and accurate species identification in pediatric cases of candidemia. Am J Clin Pathol 145:858–861
99. Alanio A, Bretagne S (2017) Challenges in microbiological diagnosis of invasive *Aspergillus* infections. F1000Research 6:157
100. Alanio A, Bretagne S (2014) Difficulties with molecular diagnostic tests for mould and yeast infections: where do we stand? Clin Microbiol Infect 20(Suppl 6):36–41
101. White PL, Mengoli C, Bretagne S et al (2011) Evaluation of Aspergillus PCR protocols for testing serum specimens. J Clin Microbiol 49:3842–3848
102. White PL, Barnes RA, Springer J et al (2015) Clinical performance of Aspergillus PCR for testing serum and plasma: a study by the European Aspergillus PCR initiative. J Clin Microbiol 53:2832–2837
103. White PL, Wingard JR, Bretagne S et al (2015) Aspergillus polymerase chain reaction: systematic review of evidence for clinical use in comparison with antigen testing. Clin Infect Dis 61:1293–1303
104. Arvanitis M, Anagnostou T, Mylonakis E (2015) Galactomannan and polymerase chain reaction-based screening for invasive aspergillosis among high-risk hematology patients: a diagnostic meta-analysis. Clin Infect Dis 61:1263–1272
105. Zeller I, Schabereiter-Gurtner C, Mihalits V et al (2017) Detection of fungal pathogens by a new broad range real-time PCR assay targeting the fungal ITS2 region. J Med Microbiol 66(10):1383–1392
106. Ala-Houhala M, Koukila-Kähkölä P, Antikainen J et al (2017) Clinical use of fungal PCR from deep tissue samples in the diagnosis of invasive fungal diseases: a retrospective observational study. Clin Microbiol Infect 24(3):301–305
107. Bridge PD, Roberts PJ, Spooner BM et al (2003) On the unreliability of published DNA sequences. New Phytol 160:43–48
108. Seifert KA (2009) Progress towards DNA barcoding of fungi. Mol Ecol Resour 9:83–89
109. Albataineh MT, Sutton DA, Fothergill AW et al (2017) Update from the laboratory. Infect Dis Clin 30:13–35
110. Elges S, Arnold R, Liesenfeld O et al (2017) Prospective evaluation of the SeptiFAST multiplex real-time PCR assay for surveillance and diagnosis of infections in haematological patients after allogeneic stem cell transplantation compared to routine microbiological assays and an in-house real-time PCR method. Mycoses 60(12):781–788
111. Pfaller MA, Diekema DJ (2012) Progress in antifungal susceptibility testing of Candida spp. by use of Clinical and Laboratory Standards Institute broth microdilution methods, 2010 to 2012. J Clin Microbiol 50:2846–2856
112. Clinical and Laboratory Standards Institute, Clinical and Laboratory Standards Institute (2004) Method for antifungal disk diffusion suceptibility testing of yeasts: approved guideline. CLSI document M44-A2. Clinical and Laboratory Standards Institute, Wayne
113. Clinical and Laboratory Standards Institute (2009) Zone diameter interpretative standards, corresponding minimal inhibitory concentration (MIC) interpretative breakpoints, and quality control limits for anti-fungal disk diffusion suceptibility testing of yeasts; informational supplement, CLSI document M44-S3, 3rd ed. Clinical and Laboratory Standards Institute, Villanova
114. Pfaller MA, Espinel-Ingroff A, Boyken L, Hollis RJ, Kroeger J, Messer SA, Tendolkar S, Diekema DJ (2011) Comparison of the broth microdilution (BMD) method of the European Committee on antimicrobial susceptibility testing with the 24-hour CLSI BMD method for testing susceptibility of Candida species to fluconazole, posaconazole, and voriconazole by use of epidemiological cutoff values. J Clin Microbiol 49(3):845–850. https://doi.org/10.1128/JCM.02441-10
115. Clinical and Laboratory Standards Institute (2010) Reference method for antifungal disk diffusion test-

ing of non-dermatophyte filamentous fungi; approved guideline. CLSI document M51-A. Clinical and Laboratory Standards Institute, Villanova
116. Pfaller MA, Andes D, Diekema DJ et al (2010) Wild-type MIC distributions, epidemiological cutoff values and species-specific clinical breakpoints for fluconazole and *Candida*: time for harmonization of CLSI and EUCAST broth microdilution methods. Drug Resist Updat 13:180–195
117. Arendrup MC, Garcia-Effron G, Lass-Florl C et al (2010) Echinocandin susceptibility testing of *Candida* species: comparison of EUCAST EDef 7.1, CLSI M27-A3, Etest, disk diffusion, and agar dilution methods with RPMI and isosensitest media. Antimicrob Agents Chemother 54:426–439
118. Espinel-Ingroff A, Arendrup MC, Pfaller MA et al (2013) Interlaboratory variability of Caspofungin MICs for Candida spp. Using CLSI and EUCAST methods: should the clinical laboratory be testing this agent? Antimicrob Agents Chemother 57:5836–5842
119. Pfaller MA, Diekema DJ, Jones RN et al (2014) Use of anidulafungin as a surrogate marker to predict susceptibility and resistance to caspofungin among 4,290 clinical isolates of *Candida* by using CLSI methods and interpretive criteria. J Clin Microbiol 52:3223–3229
120. Pfaller MA, Messer SA, Diekema DJ et al (2014) Use of micafungin as a surrogate marker to predict susceptibility and resistance to caspofungin among 3,764 clinical isolates of *Candida* by use of CLSI methods and interpretive criteria. J Clin Microbiol 52:108–114
121. Alexander BD, Byrne TC, Smith KL et al (2007) Comparative evaluation of etest and sensititre YeastOne panels against the clinical and laboratory standards institute M27-A2 reference broth microdilution method for testing *Candida* susceptibility to seven antifungal agents. J Clin Microbiol 45:698–706
122. Cuenca-Estrella M, Gomez-Lopez A, Alastruey-Izquierdo A et al (2010) Comparison of the Vitek 2 antifungal susceptibility system with the clinical and laboratory standards institute (CLSI) and European Committee on Antimicrobial Susceptibility Testing (EUCAST) Broth Microdilution Reference Methods and with the Sensititre YeastOne and Etest techniques for in vitro detection of antifungal resistance in yeast isolates. J Clin Microbiol 48:1782–1786
123. Chen SC-A, Slavin MA, Sorrell TA (2011) Echinocandin antifungal drugs in fungal infections a comparison. Drugs 71:11–41
124. Wiederhold NP (2009) Paradoxical echinocandin activity: a limited in vitro phenomenon? Med Mycol 47(Suppl 1):S369–S375
125. Arendrup MC, Pfaller M, Danish Fungaemia Study Group (2012) Caspofungin Etest susceptibility testing of Candida species: risk of misclassification of susceptible isolates of *C. glabrata* and *C. krusei* when adopting the revised CLSI caspofungin breakpoints. Antimicrob Agents Chemother 56:3965–3968
126. Bourgeois N, Laurens C, Bertout S et al (2014) Assessment of caspofungin susceptibility of *Candida glabrata* by the Etest(R), CLSI, and EUCAST methods, and detection of FKS1 and FKS2 mutations. Eur J Clin Microbiol Infect Dis 33:1247–1252
127. Aigner M, Erbeznik T, Gschwentner M et al (2017) Etest and sensititre YeastOne susceptibility testing of echinocandins against Candida species from a single center in Austria. Antimicrob Agents Chemother 61(8):e00512–e00517
128. Caramalho R, Maurer E, Binder U et al (2015) Etest cannot be recommended for in vitro susceptibility testing of mucorales. Antimicrob Agents Chemother 59:3663–3665
129. Astvad KM, Perlin DS, Johansen HK et al (2013) Evaluation of Caspofungin susceptibility testing by the new Vitek 2 AST-YS06 yeast card using a unique collection of FKS wild-type and hot spot mutant isolates, including the five most common Candida Species. Antimicrob Agents Chemother 57:177–182
130. Meis JF, Chowdhary A, Rhodes JL et al (2016) Clinical implications of globally emerging azole resistance in Aspergillus fumigatus. Philos Trans R Soc Lond Ser B Biol Sci 371:1709
131. Arendrup MC, Verweij PE, Mouton JW et al (2017) Multicentre validation of 4- well azole agar plates as a screening method for detection of clinically relevant azole- resistant Aspergillus fumigatus. J Antimicrob Chemother 72:3325–3333
132. Lass-Flörl C, Perkhofer S (2008) *In vitro* susceptibility-testing in *Aspergillus* species. Mycoses 51:437–446
133. Cuenca-Estrella M (2014) Antifungal drug resistance mechanisms in pathogenic fungi: from bench to bedside. Clin Microbiol Infect 7:46–53
134. McCarthy MW, Denning DW, Walsh TJ (2017) Future research priorities in fungal resistance. J Infect Dis 216(suppl_3):S484–S492
135. White PL, Posso RB, Barnes RA (2015) Analytical and clinical evaluation of the PathoNostics AsperGenius assay for detection of invasive aspergillosis and resistance to azole antifungal drugs during testing of serum samples. J Clin Microbiol 53:2115–2121
136. Chong GL, van de Sande WW, Dingemans GJ et al (2015) Validation of a new Aspergillus real-time PCR assay for direct detection of Aspergillus and azole resistance of Aspergillus fumigatus on bronchoalveolar lavage fluid. J Clin Microbiol 53:868–874
137. Zhao Y, Nagasaki Y, Kordalewska M et al (2016) Rapid detection of FKS- associated echinocandin resistance in Candida glabrata. Antimicrob Agents Chemother 60:6573–6577

2 Immune System and Pathogenesis

Christina Forstner

Abbreviation

AIDS	Acquired immunodeficiency syndrome
CLRs	C-type lectin receptors
DCs	Dendritic cells
HIV	Human immunodeficiency virus
IFIs	Invasive fungal infections
Ig	Immunoglobulin
IL	Interleukin
ILCs	Innate lymphoid cells
NK cells	Natural killer cells
PAMPs	Pathogen-associated molecular patterns
PRRs	Pattern recognition receptors
PTX-3	Pentraxin-3
T_H cells	T helper cells
TLRs	Toll-like receptors
T_{reg} cells	Regulatory T cells

2.1 Introduction

Humans are constantly exposed to fungi, but only a limited number of fungi can cause infection, and clinical disease is rare in non-immunocompromised or noncritically ill patients [1, 2]. The development and severity of invasive fungal infections (IFIs) are closely related to the dysfunction of the patient's immune system. As the world population is changing and with the development of new treatments for patients with haematological malignancy and cancer, haematopoietic stem cell or solid organ transplantation and acquired immunodeficiency syndrome (AIDS), the number of immunocompromised patients has increased over the past two decades and will further increase in the future. As a consequence, the incidence of IFIs will also continue to rise [3].

The host defence mechanisms against fungi are numerous and range from protective mechanisms that were present early in the evolution of multicellular organisms ("innate immunity") to sophisticated adaptive mechanisms, which are specifically induced during infection and disease ("adaptive immunity") [1, 4].

2.2 Pathogenesis

Fungal infections can originate from exogenous source by inhalation of fungal conidia (such as *Aspergillus* sp., *Fusarium* sp., *Mucorales* or pathogens of endemic mycoses) or inhalation of aerosolized basidiospores (*Cryptococcus neoformans*), from endogen source mainly the gastro-intestinal tract for commensals (*Candida* sp.) or reactivation of a latent infection. The pathogenicity of the clinically important fungi is mediated

C. Forstner
Institute for Infectious Diseases and Infection Control, Jena University Hospital, Jena, Germany

Department of Medicine I, Division of Infectious Diseases and Tropical Medicine, Medical University of Vienna, Vienna, Austria
e-mail: christina.forstner@med.uni-jena.de

E. Presterl (ed.), *Clinically Relevant Mycoses*, https://doi.org/10.1007/978-3-319-92300-0_2

by a number of virulence factors that facilitate adherence to mucosa and promote formation of biofilms [2], the ability to acquire iron from intracellular host sources [5], the ability to evade host defences (escape from phagocytosis), the production of tissue-damaging hydrolytic enzymes (such as secreted proteases, hydrolyses, elastases, phospholipases and haemolysins) [2], the ability to grow at 37 °C (thermotolerance) [1], the ability to adapt to oxygen-limited microenvironments [6] and the ability to exist in different forms (yeast and hyphal growth forms) and to reversibly switch from one to the other during infection [1]. In particular, dimorphic fungi transform from saprobic filamentous moulds to unicellular yeasts in the host [1]. Some species of *Candida* can grow in different forms (yeasts, blastospores, pseudohyphae and hyphae) depending on infections sites [7]. Also filamentous fungi such as *Aspergillus* sp., inhaled as unicellular conidia, can germinate and transform into branching hyphae (the invasive form of filamentous fungi), in the lungs of an immunosuppressed patient [1, 2].

2.3 Host Immune System Response to Fungal Infection

Figure 2.1 summarizes the host innate and adaptive immune responses that cooperate with one another to eliminate the fungal pathogens. Cell-mediated immunity is the main mechanism of defence, but certain types of antibody response are also protective against fungal infection [4].

2.3.1 Innate Immune System Response to Fungal Infection

The physical barrier of body surfaces and the mucosal epithelial surfaces of the respiratory, gastrointestinal and genitourinary tract are the first line of defence [1, 2]. The skin und mucous membranes have antimicrobial substances on their surface, some of them synthesized by the epithelial and endothelial cells [4]. Furthermore, they have a commensal microflora of saprophytic microorganisms that impede colonization by pathogenic fungi [1]. Most of the inhaled fungal conidia, as well as most of the inspired particles, are eliminated by the action of the cilia of the epithelium of the upper part of the tracheobronchial tree (mucociliary clearance). But fungi, such as *Aspergillus fumigatus*, synthesize toxins that are able to inhibit this ciliary movement [4].

Once fungi invade the mucosa, the host response is mediated by innate immune cells with phagocytes consisting of polymorphonuclear neutrophils, mononuclear leukocytes (monocytes and macrophages), dendritic cells (DCs) and natural killer (NK) cells and by soluble mediators such as complement or different peptides [2]. The response to fungi is activated by soluble and innate cell-associated pattern recognition receptors (PRRs) which are able to recognize conserved structures of microorganisms called pathogen-associated molecular patterns (PAMPs) [2]. Well-known fungal PAMPs include proteins and polysaccharides such as mannan, galactomannan, α- and β-glucan and chitin [2, 8]. Recognition of fungi by the many PRRs is a highly complex and dynamic process. The most important soluble PRRs in the immune response against *Candida* sp. are C-type lectin receptors (CLRs), and against *Aspergillus* infection, opsonization with pentraxin-3 (PTX-3) is also critical [2]. The most important cell-associated PRRs against *Candida* and *Aspergillus* are CLRs, Toll-like receptors (TLRs) and NOD-like receptors [8, 9]. Among the PRRs, the (transmembrane and soluble) CLR receptors mainly recognize β-glucan and mannan. Dectin-1 is the most important CLR. Dectin-1 signalling is crucial for triggering phagocytosis and antifungal activity [10] and plays a key role in balancing T helper type 1/T helper type 17 response [11]. Polymorphisms in dectin-1 are associated with colonization of the genitourinary tract by *Candida* species, recurrent vulvovaginal candidiasis and aspergillosis [9, 12].

PTX-3, secreted by macrophages and epithelial cells during *Aspergillus* infection, binds galactomannan and coated conidia. This step is important because neutrophils take up PTX-3-coated spores much more efficiently than uncoated spores [13]. TLRs are a protein family of cellular receptors that mediate recognition of fungal pathogens

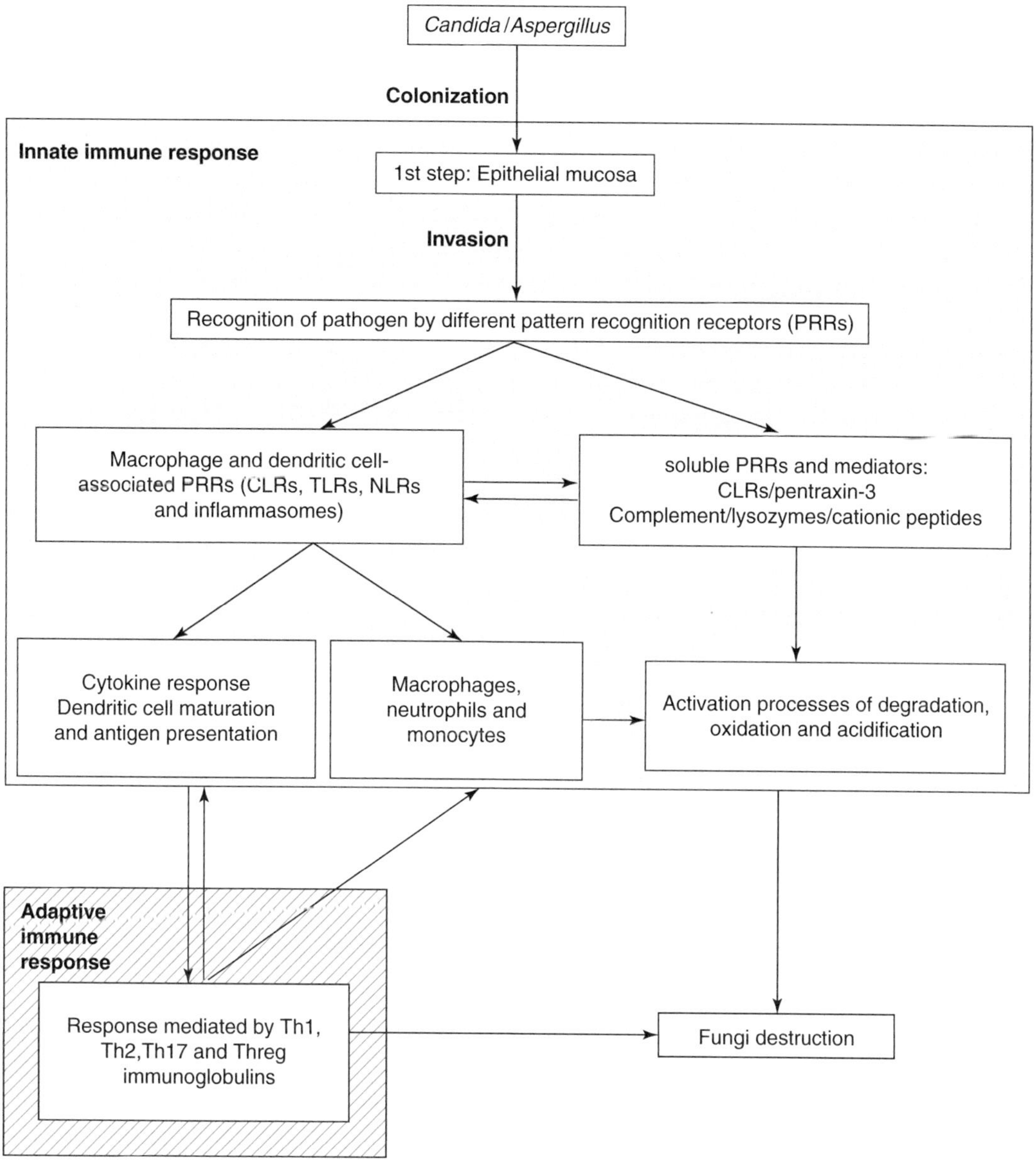

Fig. 2.1 Outline of the host immune response to fungal infections. *CLRs* C-type lectin receptors, *NLRs* NOD-like receptors, *TLRs* Toll-like receptors [2]

and subsequent inflammatory response. Some genetic polymorphisms such as polymorphisms with TLR3, TLR4 or TLR9 have been related to a higher risk of invasive aspergillosis [14, 15]. TLR1 polymorphisms have been also associated with an increased susceptibility to candidemia [16].

A critical point in the defence is the production of chemotactic factors at the site of fungal infection for effective recruitment of leukocytes at that site. These chemotactic factors include chemokines, produced by a variety of cells (including leukocytes, epithelial cells, endothelial cells, fibroblasts and smooth muscle cells), peptides derived from activation of complement pathway, leukotrienes and products synthesized by the fungi [4].

2.3.2 Innate Immune Cells and the Link with Adaptive Response

Polymorphonuclear neutrophils, mononuclear leukocytes and DCs have a different capacity of killing fungal cells depending on the species [1, 4, 17]. For example, macrophages are the primary cells involved in fungal killing during infection with *Cryptococcus* and *Pneumocystis*, whereas neutrophils are the primary effector cells in preventing infection by *Candida albicans* and *Aspergillus fumigatus*. Polymorphonuclear neutrophils are responsible for the destruction of hyphae of *Aspergillus fumigatus*, and they are able to kill the conidia that escape destruction of macrophages [1]. In neutropenic patients, NK cells play an important role in host defence against invasive aspergillosis by secreting IFN-γ, and IFN-γ is crucial for controlling *Aspergillus* infection. In an antigen-independent manner, NK cells induce cell death of the infected cells [8].

Furthermore, DCs can phagocytose both growth forms of *Aspergillus* sp., conidia and hyphae, via two different phagocytic mechanisms [4]. DCs also show greater fungicidal activity compared to macrophages or neutrophils in respect of *Histoplasma capsulatum* [4, 17].

But most important, the antigen-presenting DCs play a vital role in linking innate and acquired immunity against fungi [1, 2]. DCs sample fungi at the site of infection, transport them to the draining lymph nodes and initiate a T-cell response [1] via the secretion of cytokines by promoting the differentiation of naive CD4$^+$ T cells into effector T helper (T_H) cell subtypes: T_H1, T_H2, T_H17 or regulatory T (T_{reg}) cells [2]. The cytokines that drive the differentiation of each particular T_H phenotype are inhibitory to the development of the others, thereby maximizing the potential that only one type of T_H response is initiated at any one time [18].

T_H1 response leads to the production of protective pro-inflammatory cytokines such as IFN-gamma, interleukin (IL)-6 and IL-12, which are essential for clearance of a fungal infection by promoting cell-mediated immunity and phagocyte activation. The T_H2 response is associated with the production of IL-3, IL-4, IL-5 and IL-10 [2] and usually results in susceptibility to invasive fungal infection or allergic responses [4]. The T_H1/T_H2 response is a dynamic process that primarily has an antifungal effect but also plays a key part in balancing pro-inflammatory and anti-inflammatory signals.

IL-17 secreting T lymphocytes (T_H17 cells) are another subset of CD4$^+$ T_H cells. T_H17 cellular response is found early during an immune response and is associated with production of IL-17A, IL-17F and IL-22 [2, 18]. Differentiation of naive CD4$^+$ T cells to the T_H17 phenotype is driven initially by IL-1β, while maturation and terminal differentiation are dependent upon IL-23 signalling. IL-17A and IL-17F are involved in neutrophil recruitment and granulopoiesis. IL-22 is involved in the control of fungal growth at mucosal and non-mucosal sites [19].

T_{reg} cells, also known as suppressor T cells, suppress activation of immune system and maintain immune system homeostasis [19].

To a smaller extent, CD8$^+$ (cytotoxic) T cells and also B lymphocytes, which are cells that secrete antibodies—immunoglobulins (Ig)—principally of IgG type, are also involved in the immunological response to fungal pathogens [17]. In a CD4-deficient host, CD8$^+$ cells may come into play. DCs also activate CD8$^+$ cells by antigen presentation. In contrast, B cells directly react to fungal antigens. Although the role of acquired humoral-mediated immunity against IFIs was uncertain in the past, it has been shown that humoral immunity can protect against fungal infections if certain types of protective antibodies are available in sufficient quantity [4]. The main recognized functions of such antibodies include prevention of adherence, toxin neutralization, antibody opsonization and antibody-dependent cellular cytotoxicity. However, it appears that humoral factors by themselves are unable to prevent fungal development and they are not important in the first stage of infection [4].

Recently, a novel population of innate lymphocytes called innate lymphoid cells (ILCs) has been identified. ILCs differ from T cells because they lack a T-cell receptor. IL-17-producing ILCs have been described as being important in the defence against and the control of fungal pathogens at the mucosal barrier [8].

2.4 Link Between Immunopathogenesis and Clinical Risk Factors for Most Common Invasive Fungal Infections

Patients with high risk for invasive candidiasis include critically ill and severely immunocompromised patients. Factors associated with higher risk of candidiasis in patients admitted to an intensive care unit are mainly associated with mucosa disruption caused by surgery or catheters and *Candida* overgrowth due to antibiotic pressure. In contrast, in severely compromised patients, factors predisposing for candidiasis are similar to those that predispose to aspergillosis [2].

Predisposition to invasive aspergillosis includes cytopenia of all cells of innate immune response with prolonged neutropenia being the most important. Other risk factors for aspergillosis are defective neutrophil function (such as that seen in patients with chronic granulomatous disease), presence of graft-versus-host disease, receipt of corticosteroid therapy or immunosuppressive agents, cytomegalovirus disease and iron overload [2, 20].

The risk factors for mucormycosis are also similar to those of aspergillosis, but diabetes mellitus with poor metabolic control and the use of deferoxamine and voriconazole prophylaxis should also be taken into account [20].

Low CD4 levels, particularly found in HIV-infected/AIDS patients, are the main risk factors for developing fungal diseases with pathogens such as *Pneumocystis jirovecii* or *Cryptococcus neoformans* [20, 21].

References

1. Romani L (2004) Immunity to fungal infections. Nat Rev 4:1–13
2. Garcia-Vidal C, Viasus D, Carratala J (2013) Pathogenesis of invasive fungal infections. Curr Opin Infect Dis 26:270–276
3. Medici NP, Del Poeta M (2015) New insights on the development of fungal vaccines: from immunity to recent challenges. Mem Inst Oswaldo Cruz 110:966–973
4. Blanco JL, Garcia ME (2008) Immune response to fungal infections. Veterin Immunol Imnunopathol 125:47–70
5. Haas H (2012) Iron: a key nexus in the virulence of Aspergillus fumigatus. Front Microbiol 3:28
6. Grahl N, Shepardson K, Chung D, Cramer RA (2012) Hypoxia and fungal pathogenesis: to air or not to air? Eukaryot Cell 11:560–570
7. Jacobsen ID, Wilson D, Wächtler B, Brunke S, Naglik JR, Hube B (2012) Candida albicans dimorphism as a therapeutic target. Exp Rev Anti Ther 10:85–93
8. Becker KL, Ifrim DC, Quintin J, Netea MG, van de Veerdonk FL (2015) Antifungal innate immunity: recognition and inflammatory networks. Semin Immunpathol 37:107–116
9. Netea MG, Joosten LA, van der Meer JWM, Kullberg BJ, van de Veerdonk FL (2015) Immune defence against Candida fungal infections. Nat Rev Immunol 15:630–642
10. Goodridge HS, Reyes CN, Becker CA, Katsumoto TR, Ma J, Wolf AJ, Bose N, Chan AS, Magee AS, Danielson ME, Weiss A, Vasilakos JP, Underhill DM (2011) Activation of the innate immune receptor Dectin-1 upon formation of a 'phagocytic synapse'. Nature 472:471–475
11. Rivera A, Hohl TM, Collins N, Leiner I, Gallegos A, Saijo S, Coward JW, Iwakura Y, Pamer EG (2011) Dectin-1 diversifies Aspergillus fumigatus-specific T cell responses by inhibiting T helper type 1 CD4 T cell differentiation. J Exp Med 208:369–381
12. Ferwerda B, Ferwerda G, Plantinga TS, Willment JA, van Spriel AB, Venselaar H, Elbers CC, Johnson MD, Cambi A, Huysamen C, Jacobs L, Jansen T, Verheijen K, Masthoff L, Morré SA, Vriend G, Williams DL, Perfect JR, Joosten LA, Wijmenga C, van der Meer JW, Adema GJ, Kullberg BJ, Brown GD, Netea MG (2009) Human dectin-1 deficiency and mucocutaneous fungal infections. New Engl J Med 361:1760–1767
13. Moalli F, Doni A, Deban L, Zelante T, Zagarella S, Bottazzi B, Romani L, Mantovani A, Garlanda C (2010) Role of complement and Fc gamma receptors in the protective activity of the long pentraxin-3 against Aspergillus fumigatus. Blood 116:5170–5180
14. Carvalho A, Pasqualotto AC, Pitzurra L, Romani L, Denning DW, Rodrigues F (2008) Polymorphisms in toll-like receptor genes and susceptibility to pulmonary aspergillosis. J Infect Dis 197:618–621
15. Bouchd PY, Chien JW, Marr KA et al (2008) Toll-like receptor 4 polymorphisms and aspergillosis in stem-cell transplantation. N Engl J Med 359:1766–1777
16. Plantinga TS, Johnson MD, Scott WK, van de Vosse E, Velez Edwards DR, Smith PB, Alexander BD, Yang JC, Kremer D, Laird GM, Oosting M, Joosten LA, van der Meer JW, van Dissel JT, Walsh TJ, Perfect JR, Kullberg BJ, Netea MG (2012) Toll-like receptor 1 polymorphisms increase susceptibility to candidemia. J Infect Dis 205:934–943
17. Trzeciak-Ryczek A, Tokarz-Deptula N, Deptula W (2015) Antifungal immunity in selected fungal infections. Postepy Hig Med Dosw 69:469–473

18. Richardson JP, Moyes DL (2015) Adaptive immune responses to Candida albicans infection. Virulence 6:327–337
19. Casadevall A, Pirofski L (2012) Immunoglobulins in defense, pathogenesis, and therapy of fungal diseases. Cell Host Microb Rev 11:447–456
20. Curbelo J, Galvan JM, Aspa J (2015) Updates on Aspergillus, Pneumocystis and other opportunistic pulmonary mycoses. Arch Bronconeumol 51:647–653
21. Hole C, Wormley FL (2016) Innate host defenses against Cryptococcus neoformans. J Microbiol 54:202–211

3 Antifungal Agents

Wolfgang Graninger, Magda Diab-Elschahawi, and Elisabeth Presterl

3.1 Introduction

About 50 years after the first application of amphotericin B for the treatment of meningitis caused by *Coccidioides immitis* B, the era of new antifungals began with the development of new antifungal, e.g. broad-spectrum triazoles and the echinocandins (Table 3.1). Antifungal agents differ not only in their spectrum (Table 3.2) and their mechanism of action (Fig. 3.1) but also in terms of pharmacology and interactions with other pharmaceuticals.

3.2 Polyenes (Amphotericin B)

Polyenes include amphotericin B (AMB) and nystatin. Nystatin is strongly nephrotoxic; thus it is used only topically as suspension, ointment and zinc oxide paste.

AMB is an amphoteric substance (Fig. 3.2), which is produced by the actinomycete *Streptomyces nodosus*. AMB is soluble as deoxycholate. Although it was originally empirically used to treat meningitis caused by *Coccidioides immitis*, AMB was long considered the gold standard of antifungal treatment due to its broad antifungal spectrum and its use for treatment of invasive fungal infections over 50 years in the absence of any equivalent antifungal agent. The antifungal spectrum includes *Candida* spp., *Aspergillus* spp., *Blastomyces dermatitidis*, *Coccidioides immitis*, *Cryptococcus neoformans*, *Fusarium* spp., *Sporothrix schenckii*, *Histoplasma capsulatum* and *Paracoccidioides brasiliensis*. Some activity is seen against *Mucorales* (e.g. *Rhizopus*, *Mucor*, *Rhizomucor*, *Lichtheimia*, *Cunninghamella* spp.). Amphotericin B is ineffective against *Scedosporium* sp., *Trichosporon beigelii* and in part *Candida lusitaniae*. Amphotericin B must be administered intravenously, because it is not absorbed orally. The terminal plasma half-life is 34 h, the total body distribution volume of ca 1.5 l/kg. Plasma or serum levels are of little relevance because AM B is strongly bound to lipoproteins and cell membranes.

Although AMB is nephrotoxic, a dose reduction is not feasible with rising creatinine because AMB is eliminated via the liver. A reduction of dose will result in subtherapeutic levels. The elimination of AMB occurs slowly through the biliary tract. The proper administration of AMB remains somewhat controversial. The optimal regimen, total dose or total duration of therapy is not uniformly agreed. Some authorities suggest on initial test dose of 1 mg over 1 h to

W. Graninger
Department of Medicine I, Division of Infectious Diseases and Tropical Medicine, Medical University of Vienna, Vienna, Austria

M. Diab-Elschahawi · E. Presterl (✉)
Department of Infection Control and Hospital Epidemiology, Medical University of Vienna, Vienna, Austria
e-mail: elisabeth.presterl@meduniwien.ac.at

E. Presterl (ed.), *Clinically Relevant Mycoses*, https://doi.org/10.1007/978-3-319-92300-0_3

Table 3.1 Antifungal agents—mode of action

Class	Generic name	Mode of action
Polyene	Amphotericin B Nystatin	Polyenes attach to ergosterol, a component of the fungal cell wall. The complex leads to a formation of pores and efflux of cations and damage of the fungal cell
Azoles	Fluconazole Voriconazole Ravuconazole Itraconazole Posaconazole Isavuconazole	Interaction with P450-dependent C-14 demethylation of lanosterol and thus inhibition of ergosterol formation and accumulation of aberrant and toxic sterols within the cell membrane. This leads to instability of the fungal cell wall and damage of the cell
Echinocandins	Caspofungin Micafungin Anidulafungin	Inhibition of the beta-(1, 3)-glucan synthase, thus no formation of stable glucan within the cell wall leading to instability and damage of the fungal cell walls
Allylamines	Terbinafine Naftifine	Inhibition of the ergosterol synthesis
Nucleosid-Analoga	5-Flucytosine	"False nucleic acid" to be inserted in the DNA and RNA. Thus inhibition of the protein synthesis and cell division
Others	Amorolfine	Interference with the ergosterol synthesis and formation of aberrant sterols. This leads to instability of the fungal cell wall and damage of the cell
	Ciclopirox	Binds trivalent metal ions with impact on the function of proteins and metabolism

exclude patients with idiosyncratic reactions. In the past, doses have been incremented by 5 mg/day. Today, the dose of 0.5 mg/kg will be administered as continuous infusion on day 1. The dose may be increased to 1 mg/kg/day as a continuous infusion in 5% glucose carrier medium.

AMB is available as powder (50 mg) for the intravenous infusion, as well as oral suspension (100 mg/ml), and as lozenges. The suspension is used for the treatment of superficial mucosal fungal infections (thrush). AMB is poorly soluble in water. AMB in complex with sodium deoxycholate forms a colloidal dispersion; however this dispersion is aggregated by sodium chloride of saline. Thus, AMB powder for intravenous infusion must be dissolved in 5% glucose solution. See below about the route of administration. Pharmacologically a fast saturation of the AMB plasma levels would be recommendable which is practically impossible due to its bad tolerability. There are almost always chills and fever, occasionally vomiting, during the infusion in adult persons. Neonates and infants tolerate AMB much better.

Nephrotoxicity with azotaemia, hypokalaemia and hypomagnesaemia is the leading complication of the use of AMB. This results from a combination of a reduction in glomerular filtration, renal tubular acidosis and decreased concentrating ability. Other toxic effects are normochromic anaemia, thrombocytopenia and leukopenia due to bone marrow depression. Flush syndrome, anaphylactic reactions, muscle and joint pain and cardiotoxicity with tachyarrhythmias are rare. The latter is an absolute contraindication to the administration of AMB. Efforts have been undertaken to reduce these side effects: adequate fluid intake (500–1000 ml physiological saline) and the substitution of potassium and magnesium. However, volume load results in respiratory distress by the retention of fluid in the patients with impaired renal function. For the prevention of fever and chills, premedication with acetaminophen or metamizole is helpful. Amphotericin B is better tolerated and less nephrotoxic when it is administered as a continuous infusion over 24 h [1]. The therapeutic dose is 1 mg/kg/day.

3.2.1 Lipid-Associated Formulations of AMB

To mitigate the adverse effects of AMB the so-called lipid-associated formulations of AMB were developed. These are generally less nephrotoxic than the classical formuation of AMB deoxycholate. However, moderate nephrotoxicity

Table 3.2 Antifungal agents—overview of antifungal spectrum

	Amphotericin B	Fluconazole	Itraconazole	Voriconazole	Posaconazole	Isavuconazole	Caspofungin, Micafungin, Anidulafungin	5-Flucytosin
Candida albicans	+	+	+	+	+	+	+	+
C. glabrata	+	+/–	+/–	(+)	(+)	+	+	+
C. tropicalis	+	+	+	+	+	+	+	+
C. parapsilosis	+	+	+	+	+	+	–	+
C. krusei	+	–	+	+	+	+	+	–
C. guilliermondii	–	+	+	+	+	+	+	+
Aspergillus fumigatus	+	–	+	+	+	+	+	c
A. flavus	+	–	+	+	+	+	+	c
A. niger	+	–	+	+	+		+	c
A. terreus	–	–	+	+	+		+	c
Cryptococcus neoformans	+	+	+	+	+	+	–	c
Mucorales						+		
Rhizopus spp.	+	–	–	–	+		–	
Mucor spp.	±	–	–	–	+		–	
Pseudallescheria	–	–	–	+	+	+/–	N	–
Fusarium	–	–	–	±	±	+	N	–

and infusion-related adverse reactions are fewer but can occur with higher dosages and prolonged application. There have been three lipid-associated formulations of AMB: liposomal AMB, amphotericin B lipid complex (ABLC) and amphotericin B colloidal dispersion (ABCD). The dosage for the treatment of a fungal infection is at least 3 mg/kg and for invasive mould infections at least 5 mg/kg/day.

The three formulations differ in the composition of lipid association, particle size and pharmacokinetics (Table 3.3). Liposomal AMB is now the most frequently used AMB formulation. The standard dose is 3–5 mg/kg/day. But liposomal AMB has been used in some cases to 15 mg/kg/day for rescue therapy in high-risk patients [2]. However, it is important to consider the individual clinical situation, risk factors, organ function and concomitant medication of a patient: an international multicentre randomized trial comparing two dosages of liposomal amphotericin B for treatment of invasive aspergillosis. A 1 mg/kg/day dosage is as effective as a 4 mg/(kg/day) dosage, and no advantages to the use of the higher, more expensive, dosage have been observed [3].

3.3 5-Fluorocytosine

5-Fluorocytosine (5FU) is a specific inhibitor of the thymidylate synthetase of fungi, an essential enzyme for DNA synthesis. Therefore both cell

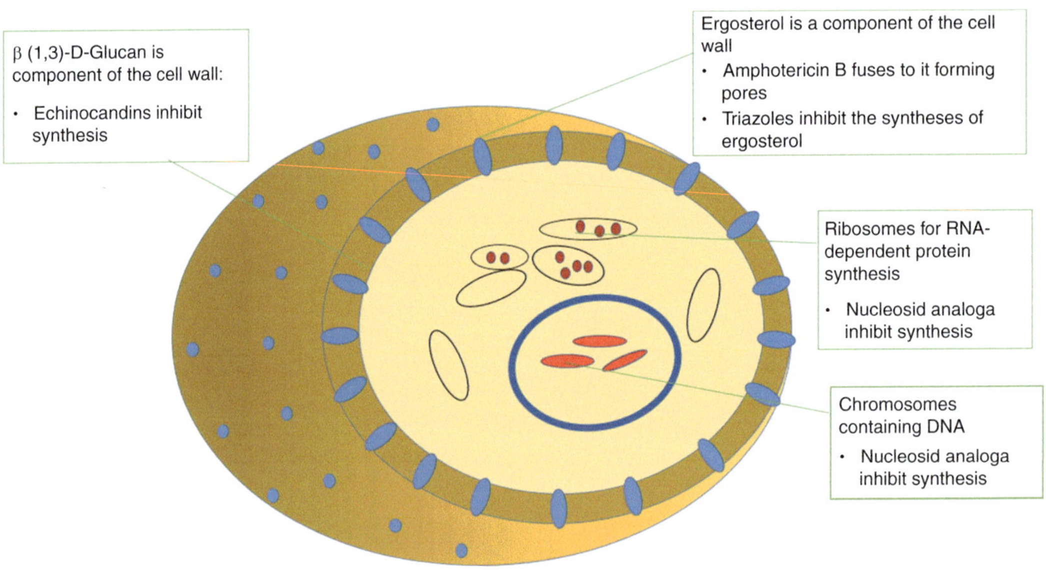

Fig. 3.1 This is a sketch of a fungal cell illustrating the mechanisms of action of antifungal agents

Fig. 3.2 Structural formular of amphotericin B

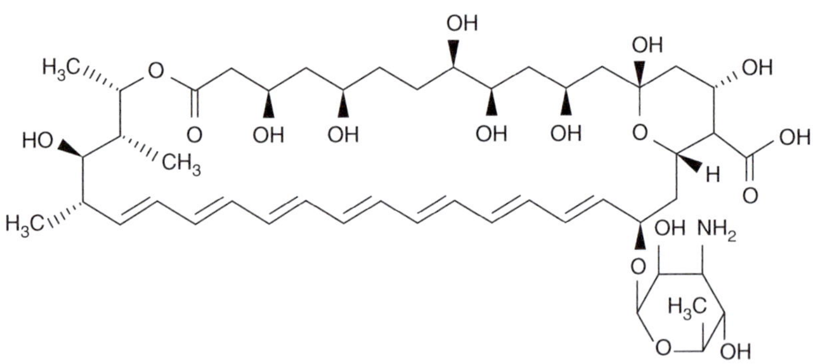

Table 3.3 Comparison of the pharmacokinetic of AMB and lipid-associated formulas

	Amphotericin B deoxycholate	Liposomal amphotericin B	Amphotericin B colloidal dispersion	Amphotericin B lipid complex
Form of the associated lipids	–	Liposomes	Discs	Ribbons
Particle size		0.06 μm	0.12 μm	1.6–11 μm
Dose investigated (mg/kg)	1	3	1.5	5
Peak serum level (μg/ml)	3.6	29	2.5	1–7
AUC (μg/ml/h)	34.2	423	56.8	9.5
Clearance (ml/h/kg)	40.2	22.2	28.4	211
Volume of distribution (litres)	111	25.9	553	2286
Elimination half-life (hours)	34	23	235	173.4

division and protein synthesis are impaired. 5FU has an excellent tissue penetration, the protein binding is low (12%), and the serum half-life is 2.5–5 h. The dose is 100–150 mg/kg/day in four divided doses (creatinine clearance >40 ml/min). 5FU is metabolized in the liver and not excreted by the kidney. With impaired renal function, it is important to adjust the dose. Overdosing may result in myelodepression. The determination of serum levels (70–80 mg/l) is recommended. In infants, the serum elimination half-life was longer; 5-fluorocytosine therefore is administered only every 12 h. Myelodepression (leukopenia, thrombocytopenia) may occur as an adverse drug effect of prolonged therapy. Today 5FU is only used for the treatment of cryptococcal meningitis. Adverse events include nausea, vomiting and skin rash. An increase of the liver enzymes may be seen in approximately 10% of patients. The antifungal spectrum is narrow and includes *Candida* spp., except *Candida krusei* and *Cryptococcus neoformans*, and also against isolates of *Cladophialophora carrionii*, *Fonsecaea* spp. and *Phialophora verrucosa*. 5FU can be considered for the treatment of urinary tract infection due to *C. glabrata* refractory to fluconazole.

3.4 Azole Antifungal Agents

Azole antifungals inhibit the enzymes for the synthesis of ergosterol. Ergosterol is a component of the fungal cell membrane, comparable to the cholesterol in the human cell membrane. Many azoles are used topically as a cream, vaginal ovules or shampoo. Miconazole was the first azole used systemically but is now obsolete due to its toxicity. Ketoconazole, another early oral azole, is also now for topical therapy only.

3.4.1 Fluconazole

Fluconazole (FLU) is a triazole (Fig. 3.3), which was developed for the treatment of *Candida* infections. The range includes *Candida albicans*, *Candida tropicalis*, *Candida parapsilosis* and dermatophytes, but not *Aspergillus* spp. or other hyphomycetes. *Candida krusei* is intrinsically resistant due to non-presence of the target enzyme. *Candida glabrata*, in some centres, the second most common type of *Candida*, occasionally has a reduced sensitivity to FLU [4]. FLU is available as *parenteral and oral* formulations. After oral administration, FLU is absorbed at more than 90%. The cerebrospinal fluid recovery rate is 60–70% of the serum concentration. The serum half-life is about 30 h. Fluconazole is excreted at approximately 80% unchanged via the kidney. In renal failure (creatinine clearance <40 ml/kg/min), the dose has to be adjusted. FLU is metabolized to a lesser extent in the liver via the cytochrome-P450 isoenzyme CYP3A4. Thus there are a few interactions with other medication. Caution is indicated when other substances are metabolized via the same mechanism, e.g. sulfonylurea derivatives, oral anticoagulants, phenytoin, cyclo-

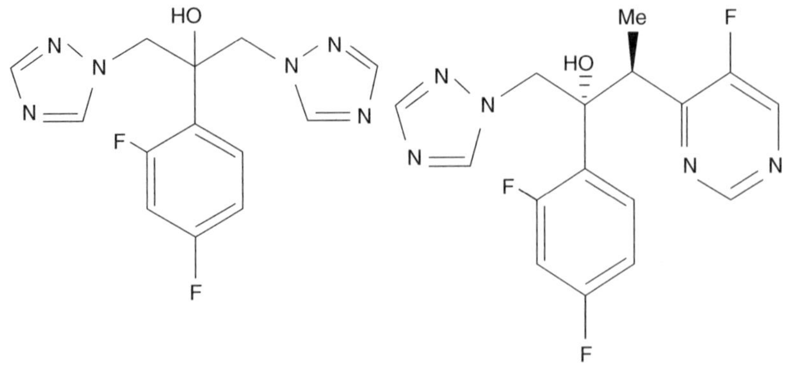

Fig. 3.3 Structural formulas of fluconazole and voriconazole

sporine, tacrolimus, zidovudine, rifabutin and theophylline, because the serum levels of these substances increase with co-administration. Co-administration of rifampicin leads to a reduction of FLU levels. FLU is usually well tolerated. Adverse effects are rare. Occasionally rashes, nausea or diarrhoea occur. At very high doses, adverse effects regarding the central nervous system, fatigue, confusion, convulsions and coma may occur. There may be increase of liver enzymes (ALT, alkaline phosphatase, bilirubin), but these are usually mild and reversible.

FLU is used for the treatment of invasive fungal infections and superficial mycoses caused mainly by *Candida* spp., particularly *C. albicans*, *C. parapsilosis* and *C. tropicalis* (see also Chap. 4—*Candida* infections).

A single dose of 150–300 mg is sufficient for the uncomplicated *Candida* vaginitis. For the treatment of dermatomycoses a dose of 150 mg/week is recommended for of 2 to 6 weeks, the infestation. In superficial *Candida* infections (oral thrush, oesophagitis), a dose of at least 400 mg is necessary because it has come mainly in patients with acquired immunodeficiency syndrome to a resistance of therapy [5, 7]. It turned out that a higher dose of at least 600–800 mg/kg effective as the original dosage of 400 mg is followed by 200 mg [6]. For invasive *Candida* infections, fluconazole has proved but more effective at a higher dose (10–20 mg/kg) [6–8]. Newborns and infants metabolize fluconazole faster; therefore the dose for this group of patients is 6–12 mg/kg/day. Fluconazole is ineffective against hyphomycete fungi, especially *Aspergillus* and *Mucoraceae*, and therefore not suitable for empirical therapy in patients with severe neutropenia and haematological diseases. In cryptococcal meningitis, amphotericin B in combination with 5-fluorocytosine is used for initial treatment. Fluconazole is used for maintenance therapy or follow-up therapy.

3.4.2 Voriconazole

Voriconazole (VOR) is a triazole and is structurally similar to the fluconazole (Fig. 3.3). In contrast to fluconazole, VOR has a broad antifungal spectrum of action against *Candida* species (including *Candida krusei* and fluconazole-resistant strains of *Candida glabrata* and *Candida albicans*), *Aspergillus* spp. and also *Aspergillus terreus*. VOR displays activity against rare pathogens, such as *Scedosporium apiospermum* and *Scedosporium prolificans*, *Fusarium* spp., *Alternaria dermatitidis* spp., *Blastomyces*, *Coccidioides immitis*, *Madurella mycetomatis*, *Paecilomyces lilacinus*, *Penicillium* spp. and also *Penicillium marneffei*, *Scopulariopsis brevicaulis* and *Trichosporon* spp. Over the past decade, the taxonomy of the genus *Trichosporon* has been subjected to extensive revision on the basis of molecular data, and the previously named *T. beigelii* (or *T. cutaneum*) corresponds, in the most recent classification, to six different species: *T. asahii*, *T. asteroides*, *T. cutaneum*, *T. inkin*, *T. mucoides*, and *T. ovoides* (Corrado Girmenia JCM April 2005). *Trichosporon beigelii*, *Acremonium* spp., *Alternaria* spp., *Histoplasma capsulatum* and many more.

The mechanism of action of VOR is based on the inhibition of the fungal cytochrome-P450-dependent sterol demethylation, an essential step in the biosynthesis of ergosterol. VOR is available as intravenous and oral formulation. The oral absorption is variable but up to 96%. The pharmacokinetics of VOR are not linear. Plasma protein binding is approximately 58%. VOR is well distributed into the cerebrospinal fluid (up to 60%). The high interindividual variability of the pharmacokinetics of VOR implies the use of drug monitoring. VOR is eliminated via the liver and less than 2% of the dose excreted unchanged in the urine. Because VOR is not soluble in water, the parenteral solution contains cyclodextrin. In patients with moderate to severe renal impairment (creatinine clearance <50 ml/min), there may be an accumulation of cyclodextrin. The clinical impact is unclear, but VOR is not recommended in renal failure (<40 ml/min). Oral VOR does not contain cyclodextrin and can be used in patients with renal failure. Because VOR is metabolized in the liver, the use in patients with impaired liver function needs dose adjustment. VOR is metabolized by the hepatic cytochrome-P450 isozymes CYP2C19, CYP2C9 and CYP3A4, resulting in interactions with other medication. The concomitant use of drugs that are also metabolized by these enzymes is contraindicated (Table 3.4). Adverse drug reactions are rare and include gastrointestinal symptoms, hepatic impairment, fever, changes in blood count and skin reactions. Reversible alteration of colour vision occurs in up to 30% of patients. Nephrotoxicity is even more rare, but most likely due the concurrent administration of cyclosporine or tacrolimus. Thus drug monitoring of these drugs has to be done to adjust the doses.

VOR has been used primarily for invasive aspergillosis (see Chap. 15—*Aspergillus* infection). The results of a randomized double-blind study in the treatment of invasive aspergillosis showed a better effectiveness compared with the treatment with AMB (response rate of 53% for VOR, response rate of 31% for AMB and other medication) [9]. VOR is used as treatment of

Table 3.4 Most frequent interference of voriconazole with the metabolism of other medications

Drug	Plasma concentration of the drug	Recommendation
Sirolimus	Markedly elevated	Not recommended
Tacrolimus	Markedly elevated	1/3 dose, serum level monitoring
Cyclosporine A	Markedly elevated	½ dose, serum level monitoring
Terfenadine, astemizole, cisapride, pimozide, chinidin	Probably elevated	Not recommended because of QT elongati on
Phenytoin	Markedly elevated	Serum level control and dose adjustment
Phencoumon	Prolonged PTT	PTT control, dose adjustment
Omeprazol	Markedly elevated	½ dose
HIV proteinase inhibitors and NNRTIs	Possibly elevated levels	
Benzodiazepines	Elevated levels	Dose adjustment
Statins	Elevated levels	Frequent side effects and toxicity monitoring
Dihydropyridine calcium channel blocker	Elevated levels	Frequent side effects and toxicity monitoring
Sulphonylurea	Possibly elevated levels	Frequent blood sugar controls and adjustment
Vinca alkaloid	Possibly elevated levels	Side effect monitoring (neurotoxicity), dose adjustment
Rifampicin Carbamazepine Barbiturate	Markedly elevated	Not recommended
Phenytoin	Decreased plasma levels	Increase of voriconazole dosage to 2 × 5 mg/kg/day
HIV proteinase inhibitors NNRTs	Possibly elevated levels	Frequent side effects and toxicity monitoring

invasive aspergillosis, chronic pulmonary aspergillosis and allergic bronchopulmonary aspergillosis. VOR is effective in the treatment of infection caused by various hyphomycetes and rare fungi (see Chap. 15), e.g. *Scedosporium* spp. and *Fusarium* spp.

The recommended dose is 6 mg/kg every 12 h during the first 24 h and then 4 mg/kg every 12 h as maintenance dose. Oral therapy starts with 2 × 400 mg on day 1 and then continues with 2 × 200 mg/day. Children receive 6 mg/kg from 2 to 12 years as a starting dose every 12 h on day 1 and then 4 mg/kg twice daily as a maintenance dose. In patients with liver cirrhosis Child-Pugh A and B, the daily dose should be reduced. Drug monitoring is strongly recommended with VOR. Because of the variable absorption and the unpredictable interactions with other complications, VOR will be replaced by posaconazole and isavuconazole.

3.4.3 Itraconazole

Itraconazole (ITR) is a lipophilic triazole (Fig. 3.4). There are oral and intravenous formulations of ITR. The absorption from the gastrointestinal tract is dependent on concurrent food intake and highest with a high-fat meal. The oral suspension is characterized both by a better absorption from the gastrointestinal tract than the capsules. ITR is bound to an extent of 99% to serum albumin. The terminal half-life is approximately 30 h. ITR has a volume distribution of 10 L. The tissue concentration is 2–3× higher than in plasma and even after discontinuation of therapy. The concentration in the skin is detectable for weeks after a treatment of a month. The concentration in cerebrospinal fluid is very low (<0.2 mg/l). The antifungal spectrum of itraconazole includes *Candida* species, dermatophytes and *Aspergillus* spp. Due to the erratic oral absorption in critically ill patients, ITR has been replaced by VOR and posaconazole for the treatment of invasive fungal infection. Due to the excellent penetration in the skin, ITR is used for the treatment of dermatomycoses.

ITR is metabolized by the isoenzymes of the cytochrome-P450 enzyme chain; thus interference with the metabolism of other drugs is common. Concurrent use of rifampicin, rifabutin, carbamazepine and phenytoin, isoniazid, phenobarbital and others decreases the levels of

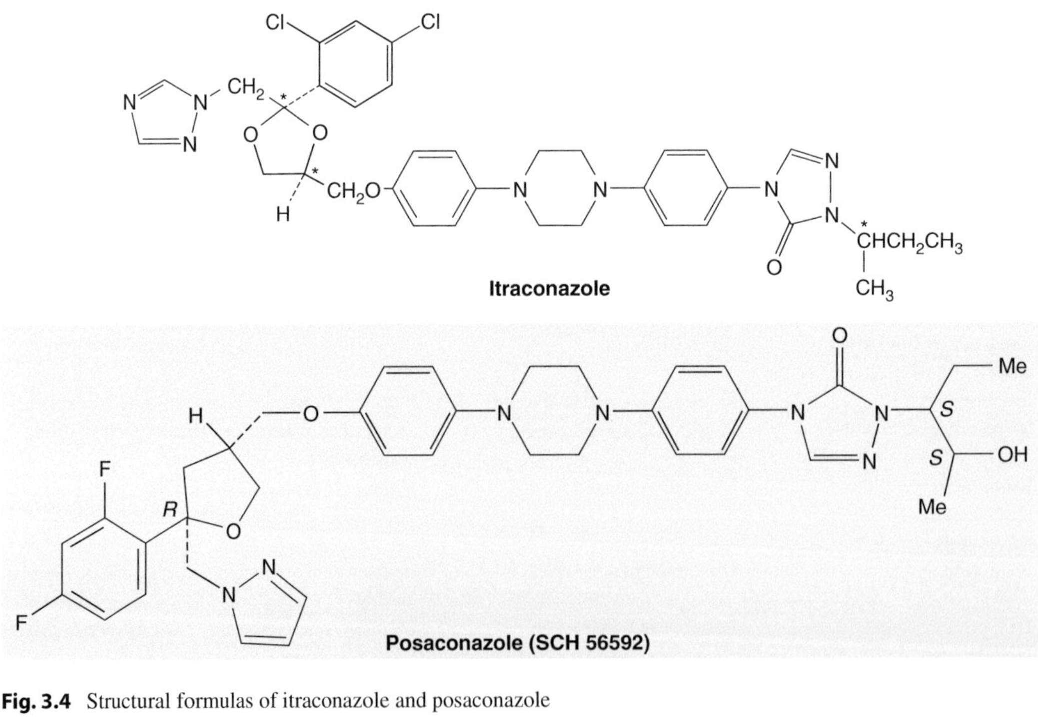

Fig. 3.4 Structural formulas of itraconazole and posaconazole

itraconazole by 60–90% and reduces the antifungal efficacy. Erythromycin, clarithromycin, ritonavir and indinavir as potent inhibitors of the isoenzyme CYP 3A4 increase itraconazole levels. Additionally, ITR may increase the concentration of other drugs through interaction and inhibition of degradation, e.g. for antihistamines, antiarrhythmics, benzodiazepines and statins. A simultaneous administration with antacids leads to a reduced absorption. Adverse drug reactions include gastrointestinal symptoms (nausea, vomiting, diarrhoea), rash or central nervous system effects (headache, dizziness, fatigue) and, rarely, polyneuropathy. Increase of the liver function tests may occur. A cross allergy with other azole antifungals can be expected.

ITR is used for the treatment of dermatomycoses. There are different treatment regimens, e.g. 2 × 200 mg/day for a week to be repeated twice every 4 weeks. For *Candida* oesophagitis, ITR oral solution is very effective because of an additional beneficial effect on the mucous membrane. The standard dose for the treatment of invasive fungal infections is 3 × 100–200 mg/day. ITR was used at a dose of 2 × 200 mg as antifungal prophylaxis in patients with long-term neutropenia due to bone marrow transplantation and leukaemia, but it has been replaced by posaconazole [10]. Drug monitoring of serum levels is recommended. The serum concentration should be about 500 μg/l.

3.4.4 Posaconazole

Posaconazole (POS) is a triazole with a broad spectrum (Fig. 3.4). In preclinical studies posaconazole demonstrated in vitro activity against *Candida albicans*, *Candida glabrata*, *Candida parapsilosis*, *Cryptococcus neoformans*, *Aspergillus* spp., *Fusarium* spp., *Scedosporium* spp. but also against *Mucorales* [11–13]. The absorption from the gastrointestinal tract is four times better when non-fasting [14]. The half-life is approximately 20 h. The volume of distribution is 346 L which is explained by a plasma protein binding of 97–98% [15] . There is penetration into the cerebrospinal fluid; however it is not predictable but illustrated by a case report of a patient with brain abscess due to *Exophiala spinifera* [16]. POS is available as an oral solution with a daily dose divided into four doses. The following regimen was used in the clinical trials: day 1 4 × 200 mg/day, followed by 2 × 400 mg daily. A new tablet formulation with a much better absorption has been developed and is now commonly used: day one 2 × 300 mg followed by 1 × 300 mg. POS is even available as an intravenous formulation. POS is a substrate of P450 cytochrome CYP3A4 isoenzymes. However, POS is but little metabolized and excreted mainly via the faeces. There are no recommendations for a dose reduction in liver or renal insufficiency. POS is the antifungal used for prophylaxis in neutropenic patients with high risk of invasive fungal infection and used for the treatment of invasive *Aspergillus* infections [17]. POS may be useful for the treatment of infections caused by *Mucorales* [18] and coccidioidomycosis [19, 20] and infection by other hyphomycetes [21].

3.4.5 Isavuconazole

Recently the new broad-spectrum azole isavuconazole with a 5-day half-life has been licenced for the treatment of invasive aspergillosis, as it had shown clinical efficacy similar to that of voriconazole in a randomized controlled double-blind trial of 516 patients with invasive aspergillosis and other mould infections [22]. Isavuconazole is cleaved from its water-soluble prodrug isavuconazonium sulphate by plasma esterases [23]. Isavuconazole is mentioned in the recent guidelines as an alternative to voriconazole [17]. Isavuconazole is available in both oral and i.v. formulations. It is given either intravenously or orally starting with a loading dose of 200 mg 3 times daily for the first 2 days followed by 200 mg once daily thereafter [22]. The toxicity profile of isavuconazole resembles that of other azoles [24]. Compared to voriconazole, isavuconazole is better tolerated by patients [22]. Regarding the cardiac effects of isavuconazole, Mellinghoff and colleagues showed in 24 out of 26 adult patients receiving isavuconazole for the treatment of invasive fungal infection a shortening of the QTc interval. This knowledge about cardiac effects should be taken into account to better manage the use of concomitant medications [25]. Significant interactions—less severe though as with voriconazole—are expected when isavuconazole is administered with drugs being metabolized by CYP. Tacrolimus and sirolimus levels augment when isavuconazole is co-administered. While the simultaneous administration of isavuconazole and methotrexate leads to increased amounts of the toxic metabolite 7-OH methotrexate, there seem to be only modest interactions with cyclosporine and glucocorticoids. Therefore according to current guidelines, clinicians should always obtain serum drug levels of azoles together with possibly interacting drugs [17]. Post-marketing surveillance of isavuconazole will be important to describe the safety profile of this new broad-spectrum azole.

3.5 Echinocandins

Echinocandins are semisynthetic lipopeptide compounds which inhibit synthesis of beta(1,3)-D-glucan, a main component of the fungal cell wall. Beta(1,3)-D-glucan does not exist in human cells. The antifungal spectrum of echinocandins includes *Candida* spp., *Aspergillus* spp., *Coccidioides*, *Histoplasma*, *Blastomyces*, *Scedosporium* spp., but also *Pneumocystis jirovecii*. Echinocandins are not active against *Cryptococcus neoformans* and *Mucorales*. Echinocandins are not absorbed from the gastrointestinal tract and must be administered parenterally.

3.5.1 Caspofungin

Caspofungin (CAS) is synthesized from a fermentation product of the fungus *Glarea lozoyensis*. Caspofungin has a broad antifungal spectrum against *Aspergillus* spp., *Candida* spp., *Histoplasma capsulatum* and *Coccidioides immitis*, though not against *Scedosporium*, *Fusarium* spp. and *Cryptococcus neoformans* [26].

The serum half-life is 9–11 h. CAS is bound to albumin at an extent of 96% and is slowly metabolized by spontaneous hydrolysis and *N*-acetylation in the liver. Excretion occurs in about 35% via the faeces and in 41% in the urine in the form of ineffective metabolites. CAS is a weak substrate for cytochrome P450 enzymes with only minimal interaction with other substances. A reduction of CAS serum levels was observed for the simultaneous use of efavirenz, nelfinavir, nevirapine, rifampin, dexamethasone, phenytoin or carbamazepine. Simultaneous use of cyclosporine increased the CAS concentration; the concentration of cyclosporine in the blood remained unchanged. In contrast, CAS reduced the tacrolimus blood concentration by 26%. Regular monitoring of blood concentrations of tacrolimus is advertised.

The recommended dose is 70 mg on the first day continued with 50 mg daily. A dose adjustment due to impaired renal function is not required. In patients with moderate hepatic insufficiency, a dose is recommended after an initial loading dose of 70 mg daily of 35 mg. For children >2 years of age, a dose of 50 mg/m^2/day is recommended. Adverse effects of CAS are rare (<3%). The most common adverse events are headache, fever, phlebitis, nausea, vomiting, flush, diarrhoea, rash and—very rare—haemolysis. CAS is used for the treatment of candidaemia and invasive *Candida* infections and empiric therapy in patients with febrile neutropenia and as second-line treatment for invasive *Aspergillus* infection [17].

3.5.2 Micafungin

Micafungin (MIC) is a modified derivative of a water-soluble lipopeptide of *Coleophoma empedri*. Its broad antifungal spectrum includes *Candida* spp. (also azole-resistant strains), *Aspergillus* spp., *Histoplasma*, *Coccidioides*, *Blastomyces* and *Paecilomyces variotii* [26–28]. MIC binds to plasma albumin by 99%. The serum half-life is approximately 14 h; the volume of distribution is 0.26 L/kg. Serum levels are 10.0 µg/ml [29] after a dose of 100 mg/day. MIC is metabolized in the liver possibly via an *O*-methyltransferase. A few data exist on potential interactions with other drugs. Micafungin is used in the treatment of serious *Candida* infections (oesophagitis), candidaemia and invasive *Candida* infections [17].

Micafungin is used as prophylaxis in patients with severe neutropenia [30].

3.5.3 Anidulafungin

Anidulafungin (ANI) is actually the longest known substance among the echinocandins. There are experimental studies in which ANI is very active against of *Pneumocystis* cysts and vegetative forms [31]. Otherwise the in vitro spectrum of activity of ANI is similar to CAS and MIC micafungin [26]. Pharmacologically, ANI differs from CAS and MIC: the half-life is 18 h, the protein binding is up to 86% and thus lower than in CAS and MIC. Interactions with other substances are inexistent because ANI is not metabolized via the cytochrome P450 enzymes [32]. With a loading dose of 150 mg, followed by 75 mg, the peak level was 3.44 mcg/ml [29]. Anidulafungin is used for the treatment of severe *Candida* infections, candidaemia and invasive *Candida* infections [32, 33]. Adverse events are rare and dose-independent.

3.6 Allylamines

Terbinafine (TER) and naftifine belong to antifungal class of the allylamines. TER is available as an oral formulation and used in dosage 2 × 125 to 250 mg/day for treatment of dermatomycoses. TER accumulates in the stratum corneum of the skin. TER has also an in vitro efficacy against *Aspergillus* spp. and *Candida* spp. Naftifine is a topically applicable allylamine. The antifungal range includes dermatophytes but also *Aspergillus* spp.

References

1. Imhof A, Walter RB, Schaffner A (2003) Continuous infusion of escalated doses of amphotericin B deoxycholate: an open-label observational study. Clin Infect Dis 36(8):943–951
2. Walsh TJ, Goodman JL, Pappas P, Bekersky I, Buell DN, Roden M et al (2001) Safety, tolerance, and pharmacokinetics of high-dose liposomal amphotericin B (AmBisome) in patients infected with Aspergillus species and other filamentous fungi: maximum tolerated dose study. Antimicrob Agents Chemother 45(12):3487–3496
3. Cornely OA, Maertens J, Bresnik M, Ebrahimi R, Ullmann AJ, Bouza E et al (2007) Liposomal amphotericin B as initial therapy for invasive mold infection: a randomized trial comparing a high-loading dose regimen with standard dosing (AmBiLoad trial). Clin Infect Dis 44(10):1289–1297
4. Rex JH, Pfaller MA, Galgiani JN, Bartlett MS, Espinel-Ingroff A, Ghannoum MA et al (1997) Development of interpretive breakpoints for antifungal susceptibility testing: conceptual framework and analysis of in vitro-in vivo correlation data for fluconazole, itraconazole, and candida infections. Subcommittee on Antifungal Susceptibility Testing of the National Committee for Clinical Laboratory Standards. Clin Infect Dis 24(2):235–247
5. Redding S, Smith J, Farinacci G, Rinaldi M, Fothergill A, Rhine-Chalberg J et al (1994) Resistance of Candida albicans to fluconazole during treatment of oropharyngeal candidiasis in a patient with AIDS: documentation by in vitro susceptibility testing and DNA subtype analysis. Clin Infect Dis 18(2):240–242
6. Voss A, de Pauw BE (1999) High-dose fluconazole therapy in patients with severe fungal infections. Eur J Clin Microbiol Infect Dis 18(3):165–174
7. Graninger W, Presteril E, Schneeweiss B, Teleky B, Georgopoulos A (1993) Treatment of Candida albicans fungaemia with fluconazole. J Infect 26(2):133–146
8. Torres HA, Kontoyiannis DP, Rolston KV (2004) High-dose fluconazole therapy for cancer patients with solid tumors and candidemia: an observational, noncomparative retrospective study. Support Care Cancer 12(7):511–516
9. Herbrecht R, Denning DW, Patterson TF, Bennett JE, Greene RE, Oestmann JW et al (2002) Voriconazole versus amphotericin B for primary therapy of invasive aspergillosis. N Engl J Med 347(6):408–415
10. Winston DJ, Busuttil RW (2002) Randomized controlled trial of oral itraconazole solution versus intravenous/oral fluconazole for prevention of fungal infections in liver transplant recipients. Transplantation 74(5):688–695
11. Gonzalez GM, Tijerina R, Najvar LK, Bocanegra R, Rinaldi MG, Loebenberg D et al (2003) Activity of posaconazole against Pseudallescheria boydii: in vitro and in vivo assays. Antimicrob Agents Chemother 47(4):1436–1438
12. Herbrecht R (2004) Posaconazole: a potent, extended-spectrum triazole anti-fungal for the treatment of serious fungal infections. Int J Clin Pract 58(6):612–624
13. Lodge BA, Ashley ED, Steele MP, Perfect JR (2004) Aspergillus fumigatus empyema, arthritis, and calcaneal osteomyelitis in a lung transplant patient successfully treated with posaconazole. J Clin Microbiol 42(3):1376–1378
14. Courtney R, Radwanski E, Lim J, Laughlin M (2004) Pharmacokinetics of posaconazole coadministered

with antacid in fasting or nonfasting healthy men. Antimicrob Agents Chemother 48(3):804–808
15. Krieter P, Flannery B, Musick T, Gohdes M, Martinho M, Courtney R (2004) Disposition of posaconazole following single-dose oral administration in healthy subjects. Antimicrob Agents Chemother 48(9):3543–3551
16. Negroni R, Helou SH, Petri N, Robles AM, Arechavala A, Bianchi MH (2004) Case study: posaconazole treatment of disseminated phaeohyphomycosis due to Exophiala spinifera. Clin Infect Dis 38(3):e15–e20
17. Patterson TF, Thompson GR, Denning DW, Fishman JA, Hadley S, Herbrecht R et al (2016) Practice guidelines for the diagnosis and management of aspergillosis: 2016 update by the infectious diseases society of America. Clin Infect Dis 63(4):e1–e60
18. Kontoyiannis DP, Lewis RE (2011) How I treat mucormycosis. Blood 118(5):1216–1224
19. Anstead GM, Corcoran G, Lewis J, Berg D, Graybill JR (2005) Refractory coccidioidomycosis treated with posaconazole. Clin Infect Dis 40(12):1770–1776
20. Gonzalez GM, Tijerina R, Najvar LK, Bocanegra R, Rinaldi M, Loebenberg D et al (2002) In vitro and in vivo activities of posaconazole against Coccidioides immitis. Antimicrob Agents Chemother 46(5):1352–1356
21. Boucher HW, Groll AH, Chiou CC, Walsh TJ (2004) Newer systemic antifungal agents : pharmacokinetics, safety and efficacy. Drugs 64(18):1997–2020
22. Maertens JA, Raad II, Marr KA, Patterson TF, Kontoyiannis DP, Cornely OA et al (2016) Isavuconazole versus voriconazole for primary treatment of invasive mould disease caused by Aspergillus and other filamentous fungi (SECURE): a phase 3, randomised-controlled, non-inferiority trial. Lancet 387(10020):760–769
23. Rybak JM, Marx KR, Nishimoto AT, Rogers PD (2015) Isavuconazole: pharmacology, pharmacodynamics, and current clinical experience with a new triazole antifungal agent. Pharmacotherapy 35(11):1037–1051
24. Falci DR, Pasqualotto AC (2013) Profile of isavuconazole and its potential in the treatment of severe invasive fungal infections. Infect Drug Resist 6:163–174
25. Mellinghoff SC, Bassetti M, Dorfel D, Hagel S, Lehners N, Plis A et al (2017) Isavuconazole shortens the QTc interval. Mycoses 61(4):256–260
26. Espinel-Ingroff A (2003) In vitro antifungal activities of anidulafungin and micafungin, licensed agents and the investigational triazole posaconazole as determined by NCCLS methods for 12,052 fungal isolates: review of the literature. Rev Iberoam Micol 20(4):121–136
27. Nakai T, Uno J, Ikeda F, Tawara S, Nishimura K, Miyaji M (2003) In vitro antifungal activity of Micafungin (FK463) against dimorphic fungi: comparison of yeast-like and mycelial forms. Antimicrob Agents Chemother 47(4):1376–1381
28. Warn PA, Morrissey G, Morrissey J, Denning DW (2003) Activity of micafungin (FK463) against an itraconazole-resistant strain of Aspergillus fumigatus and a strain of Aspergillus terreus demonstrating in vivo resistance to amphotericin B. J Antimicrob Chemother 51(4):913–919
29. Denning DW (2003) Echinocandin antifungal drugs. Lancet 362(9390):1142–1151
30. van Burik JA, Ratanatharathorn V, Stepan DE, Miller CB, Lipton JH, Vesole DH et al (2004) Micafungin versus fluconazole for prophylaxis against invasive fungal infections during neutropenia in patients undergoing hematopoietic stem cell transplantation. Clin Infect Dis 39(10):1407–1416
31. Bartlett MS, Current WL, Goheen MP, Boylan CJ, Lee CH, Shaw MM et al (1996) Semisynthetic echinocandins affect cell wall deposition of Pneumocystis carinii in vitro and in vivo. Antimicrob Agents Chemother 40(8):1811–1816
32. Dowell JA, Knebel W, Ludden T, Stogniew M, Krause D, Henkel T (2004) Population pharmacokinetic analysis of anidulafungin, an echinocandin antifungal. J Clin Pharmacol 44(6):590–598
33. Pappas PG, Kauffman CA, Andes DR, Clancy CJ, Marr KA, Ostrosky-Zeichner L et al (2016) Clinical practice guideline for the management of candidiasis: 2016 update by the infectious diseases society of America. Clin Infect Dis 62(4):e1–e50

Part II

Clinical Disease

4 Clinical Syndromes: *Candida* and Candidosis

Markus Ruhnke

4.1 Introduction

The term candidosis or candidiasis comprises several categories of infection: systemic or invasive *Candida* infections/diseases (IC), such as acute disseminated candidosis, chronic disseminated candidosis (CDC) and candidaemia as well as superficial (muco-cutaneous) *Candida* infections [1]. According to the recent consensus definition the term "fungal infection" should be replaced by "fungal disease" [2]. Candidaemia is the most frequent manifestation of systemic *Candida* infection. The serious prognosis associated with candidaemia is highlighted by a recent survey of 60 cases with candidaemia due to *C. albicans* ($n = 38$) and non-*C. albicans* ($n = 22$): 8% developed severe sepsis and 27% septic shock. The all-cause mortality was 42% [3]. Candidaemia is most often observed in non-granulocytopenic patients after abdominal surgery or catheter-related infection with secondary blood stream infection. Potential further manifestations of invasive disease are *Candida* oesophagitis (in the past often classified as muco-cutaneous candidosis), peritonitis, urinary tract infections. Less frequently, endocarditis, meningitis/meningoencephalitis or osteomyelitis are manifestations of acute disseminated candidosis. Endophthalmitis or chorioretinitis following candidaemia requires special attention, and if not diagnosed may lead to loss of vision. It may be observed in up to 15–20% of patients [4]. Superficial colonization with *Candida* spp. is a common finding in ICU patients. Candiduria is frequently found in patients with urinary catheters and does not necessarily reflect urinary tract infection [5]. Only the minority of patients have documented candidaemia following/together with candiduria. Similarly, detection of *Candida* spp. from airway samples (e.g. bronchoalveolar lavage) does not proof *Candida* pneumonia [6]. In general, most *Candida* isolates from non-sterile body sites do not represent disease [7].

4.2 Pathogens

The list of opportunistic fungi causing serious, life-threatening fungal diseases increases almost every year. In addition to *Candida*, *Aspergillus*, and *Cryptococcus* species, the opportunistic fungi include yeasts other than *Candida* species (e.g. *Geotrichum/Trichosporon* spp., *Rhodotorula* spp., *Saccharomyces* spp.), non-dematiaceous or hyaline molds, and the dematiaceous fungi [8].

Yeasts of the genus *Candida* are frequent colonizers of the skin and mucous membranes of animals and dissemination in nature is widespread. Only a few of the more than 150 described species are regularly found as infectious agents in humans. *C. albicans* is the most common isolated species (>50%) from samples taken from

M. Ruhnke
Department of Haematology and Oncology, Paracelsus-Klinik, Osnabrück, Germany

E. Presterl (ed.), *Clinically Relevant Mycoses*, https://doi.org/10.1007/978-3-319-92300-0_4

non-sterile sites (mucous membranes such as oral cavity, digestive and vaginal tract) as well as sterile sites (blood culture or tissue biopsies). Less often (<7%), other *Candida* spp. (so-called non-*Candida albicans* spp.) including *Candida tropicalis, Candida glabrata, Candida parapsilosis, Candida krusei, Candida kefyr, Candida guilliermondii, Saccharomyces cerevisiae*, rarely *Candida dubliniensis, Candida sake, Candida rugosa, Candida stellatoidea, Candida famata, Candida norvegensis, Candida inconspicua, Candida kefyr, Candida pelliculosa, Candida lipolytica, Candida pulcherrima, Candida intermedia, Candida curvata, Candida fermentati* and other "new" species such as *Candida auris* are isolated. Non-*C. albicans* species are more likely to occur in patients, who receive or have received antifungal therapy with azoles but according to recent data to echinocandins as well.

4.3 Epidemiology

4.3.1 Superficial Candidosis

Data about the "true" incidence of oral *Candida* colonization or infection in different patients groups (other than HIV-infected individuals) are rare. *C. albicans* is the most common isolated species (>70%) from samples taken from mucous membranes such as oral cavity, digestive and vaginal tract. Other species such as *Candida tropicalis, Candida parapsilosis, Candida glabrata, Candida krusei* or less often *Candida dubliniensis* are frequently cultured and/or have been found concomitantly with *C. albicans*. These non-*Candida albicans* species rarely may cause infections without simultaneous presence of *C. albicans*. These non-*Candida albicans* species may be isolated from non-sterile superficial sites in immuncompromised as well as non-immuncompromised individuals [9]. Before the introduction of protease inhibitors as part of highly active antiretroviral therapy (HAART, nowadays ART = antiretroviral therapy called) for HIV infection, the incidence of oral candidosis in HIV-infected individuals varied from 7 to 93% depending on the degree of immunosuppression of the study population [10]. The amount of asymptomatic oropharyngeal yeast carriage in persons with HIV infection is significantly correlated with HIV-Viraemia [11]. The incidence of oral candidosis is now changing in the era of HAART use. A decline in the incidence of oral candidosis is observed when HAART was administered together with a trend towards reduction in the frequency of fluconazole-resistant *C. albicans* [12].

A shift towards replacement of vaginal colonization from *C. albicans* to *C. glabrata* was observed in a study about the effect of fluconazole prophylaxis. Fluconazole had an early and persistent effect on the vaginal mycoflora, with the emergence of *C. glabrata* vaginal colonization within the first 6 months [13]. Other host factors than advanced HIV disease alone have been acclaimed to contribute to OPC: low CD4 lymphocyte count, xerostomia, age >35 years, IV drug use and certain racial populations such as black IV drug users compared to white subjects.

4.3.2 Systemic Candidosis and Candidaemia

Data are much more valid for systemic candidosis such as candidaemia. While *C. albicans* remains the most important agent among all risk groups resulting in 40–65% of all candidaemias, a shift to non-*Candida-albicans* yeasts has been reported world-wide. Candidaemia is most often caused by *C. albicans*, followed by *Candida glabrata, Candida tropicalis, Candida parapsilosis, Candida krusei, Candida lusitaniae* and *Candida guilliermondii* [8, 14–23].

Other species such as *Candida dubliniensis, Candida rugosa, Candida stellatoidea, Candida famata, Candida norvegensis, Candida inconspicua, Candida kefyr, Candida pelliculosa, Candida intermedia, Candida auris, Candida curvata, Candida fermentati* and others are only rarely recovered from blood cultures or other body fluids [24–33]. The latter less often isolated *Candida* spp. are predominantly found in blood cultures from severely immunocompromised patients (e.g. granulocytopenic patient with haematological cancer, after haematopoietic stem cell or solid organ transplantation). Most recently, *Candida auris* has been identified as a globally emerging multidrug resistant fungal pathogen causing nosocomial transmission with various forms of IC including disseminated fungal disease [34–39]. This pathogen has been misidentified as *Candida haemulonii, Candida famata, Rhodotorula* spp. and others in the past [36]. *C. auris* has been identified first in Japan in 2009, and up today has been not only found to occur sporadically world-wide but can cause outbreaks as well [28, 39]. Up to date correct identification of *Candida* spp. may require not only biochemical but molecular tests as well [40].

The aetiology of candidaemia may differ between patient groups at risk and age, different hospitals and geographic regions. Exact data on the prevalence of systemic and superficial candidosis are not available from most countries. Due to the activity of the GAFFY network (see LIFE program at www.life-worldwide.org) we become aware of systemic approach to retrieve epidemiological data about many different mycoses in many countries world-wide [41–52]. Candidaemia is the fourth most common bloodstream infection in the USA, with similar trends being reported in other countries [53, 54]. Candidaemia occurs predominantly in the ICU, but non-ICU-related candidaemia is increasingly reported [55]. Pathogens of the species *Candida* are found in 5–15% of all positive blood cultures. The rates differ among different countries, hospitals and wards [53]. In acute care hospitals in the USA, 4.8 cases of candidaemia were found per 10,000 days with central venous catheters [56]. Blumberg et al. reported a frequency of 9.8 Candida bloodstream infections per 1000 admissions in surgical ICUs in the United States [57]. Leleu et al. reported a frequency of three invasive candidosis cases per 1000 admissions in an ICU in France [58]. In the paediatric population the problem seems to be even worse. Systemic *Candida* infections represent 15.8% of all nosocomial infections and are the second most common bloodstream infection in paediatric ICUs in the USA [59]. A European point prevalence study that included all 3147 patients treated for sepsis in intensive care units documented *Candida* spp. in 17% of cases as the etiologic agent [60, 61]. In a study from Germany on device-associated nosocomial infections (NI), *C. albicans* (11.2/100NI) was the fifth most common pathogen isolated in bloodstream infections in ICUs between 1997 and 2002 [62]. In a survey conducted by the Fungal Infection Network of Switzerland between 1991 and 2000, ICUs and surgical wards accounted for about two-thirds of all episodes of candidaemia [63]. The incidence of candidaemia (on average 0.5 episodes/10,000 patient-days per year) was stable over this 10-year period and was five to 10 times higher in ICUs than in other wards [64]. Whereas the incidence and species distribution in Switzerland did not change between 1991 and 2000, an increasing incidence has been described in Scandinavian countries (from 1.7 to 2.2 cases per 100,000 inhabitants in Finland and from 6.5 to 15.6 cases in Norway) without a shift in the relative amount of different *Candida* species [63, 65–68]. A study in Denmark documented an increase in the incidence of candidaemia from 2003 to 2004 with *C. glabrata* being second after *C. albicans*. The rate of *C. glabrata* varied between 8 and 32% in reports from various hospitals within Denmark [69]. In Europe, a major epidemiological shift can be observed between North and South of Europe. In a survey from five tertiary care teaching hospitals in Italy and Spain, Candida parapsilosis complex (19.5%) was the second most frequent isolated pathogen next to *Candida albicans* (58.4%) and *Candida* glabrata less frequently detected (8.3%) [20]. The overall incidence was 1.55 cases per 1000 admissions and remained stable during the three-year study episode (2008–2010). According to a European survey in ICU patients, *C. parapsilosis* was more often isolated in neurosurgery and multiple trauma patients as well as children ≤1 years (especially in association with intravenous catheters) while *C. glabrata* was more often isolated after abdominal surgery and in elderly patients (≥60 years) [22]. According to a recent study from France (2004–2013), ICU candidaemia ranked sixth among bloodstream infections, and its average annual incidence was 0.3 per 1000 patient days. The incidence rose sharply during the study period, and ICU mortality remained high (52.4%) despite modern antifungal agents [70].

In patients with haematologic malignancies, non-*Candida-albicans* yeasts (*C. glabrata, C. tropicalis* and *C. krusei*) are more frequently found than in patients with solid tumours or in non-granulocytopenic ICU patients [22, 71, 72]. In the most recent European Organisation for Research and Treatment of Cancer (EORTC) fungaemia survey in cancer patients fungaemia including polymicrobial infection was due to: *C. albicans* in 128 (48%), and other *Candida* spp. in 145 (54%) patients [71]. Interestingly, in both surveys (1999 by Viscoli et al., and 2015 by Cornely et al.) factors associated with mortality were septic shock and lack of antifungal prophylaxis. Mortality did not change over years and remained high (30-day mortality about 39%) [71, 72].

Exposure to fluconazole, broad-spectrum antibacterial agents and severe underlying diseases are known predispositions for non-*Candida-albicans* yeasts, especially *C. glabrata* [8]. This clearly highlights the need for exact knowledge about the local epidemiology in order to start the appropriate antifungal therapy when *Candida* spp. are grown from blood cultures before the exact pathogen is identified. Echinocandin (caspofungin, micafungin) usage is associated with an increased incidence of *Candida parapsilosis* infections (e.g. breakthrough) [73–75]. Exposure to caspofungin (e.g. as prophylaxis) was observed to be associated with an increased prevalence for not only *C. parapsilosis* but *C. glabrata* and *C. krusei* as well [76].

Breakthrough Candida infections on micafungin treatment occurred predominantly in severely immunosuppressed patients with heavy prior micafungin exposure. The majority of cases were due to *C. glabrata* with an FKS mutation or wild-type *C. parapsilosis* with elevated micafungin MICs [75].

4.4 Clinical Presentation

4.4.1 Superficial Candidosis

Skin conditions contributed 1.79% to the global burden of disease measured in "disability-adjusted life year" (DALYs) from 306 diseases and injuries in 2013 [77]. Individual skin diseases varied in size with 0.38% of total burden for dermatitis (atopic, contact, and seborrheic dermatitis) as compared to 0.15% for fungal skin diseases. Fungal skin diseases are frequent and represent the leading (superficial) fungal infections in most countries world-wide. In Germany, using local data and literature estimates of the incidence and prevalence of fungal infections, about 9.6 million (12%) people suffer from a fungal infection each year [46]. These figures are dominated by fungal skin disease (FSD) with 95%. Most common FSD were Tinea pedis, Tinea corporis, and onychomycosis, respectively. The proportion of *Candida* infection of the skin (CIS) from all FSD is not known. Typical clinical features of cutaneous *Candida* infections are Candidosis intertriginosa, Candidosis genito-glutealis infantum, Candidosis interdigitalis, Folliculitis barbae candidomycetica [78]. CIS will not be discussed in detail in this book chapter and further reading in dermatological textbooks is recommended. Finally, chronic muco-cutaneous candidosis is a rare form of CIS (CMC; see below).

4.4.1.1 Oral Candidosis (OPC)

Oral candidosis or oropharyngeal candidosis (=OPC) is not only the most common fungal infection in HIV-infected individuals but is by far the most common opportunistic infection observed in this patient group, affecting nearly 90% of subjects at some stage during the course of HIV disease progression [79, 80]. However, since highly active antiretroviral therapy is commonly used in this patient cohort, a marked decline in the prevalence of OPC has been observed. In non-HIV-infected individuals the epidemiological data are not studied so intensively as in HIV-infected individuals. Predisposing factors may be either local or systemic (e.g. dentures, quantitative or qualitative saliva changes such as xerostomia, Sjögren's syndrome, radiotherapy, drug therapy, and smoking).

Patients with haematological malignancies and solid tumours often are affected by OPC. Natural physical barriers to colonization and invasion are lost during anticancer therapy. It is believed that oral candidosis is frequent (>75%) and that good oral hygiene and dental care together with antifungal agents either given prophylactically or therapeutically are important components in the care of patients receiving chemotherapy.

Various presentations of OPC have been described, from which the pseudomembranous candidosis (=oral thrush) represents the most prevalent form. The other clinical presentation includes erythematous, hyperplastic oral candidosis, and angular cheilitis ("Perlèche" or angulus infectiosus). Pseudomembranous candidosis is being characterized by removable white plaques that may be scraped away to reveal a bleeding surface. Symptoms of OPC usually include an alteration of taste ("furry" taste), inflammation in the mouth with oral pain and burning of mouth, and xerostomia. Occasionally patients complain that their breath smells like a brewery. In most cases, patients are able to maintain their oral nutritional intake, despite discomfort, and do not lose weight.

Treatment may be either locally with topical polyenes (e.g. nystatin, natamycin, or amphotericin suspension) or in more severe, in particular if oesophageal candidosis is suspected, cases with systemic active azoles such as fluconazole, itraconazole, voriconazole or posaconazole (all either as suspension or tablets/capsules).

4.4.1.2 Vulvovaginal Candidosis (VVC)

Candida species colonize the estrogenized vagina in at least 20% of all women. This statistic rises to 30% in late pregnancy and in immunosuppressed patients [81]. The predominant species is *Candida albicans*. In less than 10% of all cases, non-*Candida albicans* species, especially *C. glabrata*, but in rare cases also *Saccharomyces cerevisiae*, cause a vulvovaginitis, often with fewer clinical signs and symptoms. As in OPC, multiple factors are involved, including various *Candida* virulence factors, antibiotic usage, reproductive hormone levels, and other factors that alter the normal vaginal flora or change the avidity of epithelial cells for *Candida* species [81].

Clinical signs and symptoms are not highly specific and misdiagnosing may occur but the prominent symptoms include vulvovaginal itching and irritation. Other symptoms may be burning and dyspareunia. A diagnosis of VVC is suggested clinically by pruritus and erythema in the vulvovaginal area. However, only less than 50% of women with genital pruritus suffer from a *Candida* VCV [81]. On examination, vulvular erythema and mucosal edema may be seen together with white patches analogous to those seen in oral thrush that can be removed by gentle scraping. Diagnosis should include the microscopic investigation of the vaginal fluid by phase contrast (400×), vaginal pH-value and, in clinically and microscopically uncertain or in recurrent cases, yeast culture with species determination [81]. The success rate for treatment of acute vaginal candidosis is approximately 80%.

Vaginal preparations containing polyenes, imidazoles and ciclopiroxolamine or oral triazoles, which are not allowed during pregnancy, are all equally effective. *C. glabrata* is resistant to the usual dosages of all local antimycotics. In these situations, vaginal boric acid suppositories or vaginal flucytosine are recommended, alternatively high doses of 800 mg fluconazole/day for 2–3 weeks [81].

4.4.1.3 Oesophageal Candidosis (EC)

It is not entirely clear whether EC should be regarded as superficial or invasive/systemic candidosis. Historically, EC is regarded as invasive fungal disease, in particular when fungal mycelia are found by histopathology in deep tissue from endoscopical taken biopsies. *Candida* oesophagitis occurs in patients with chronic diseases, most of whom have been previously treated with antibiotics, steroids or omeprazole, but most frequently in those with advanced HIV infection [82]. Although a variety of both opportunistic and non-opportunistic disorders result in oesophageal disease in the HIV population, candidal oesophagitis is the most common cause of symptomatic disease. Patients with *Candida* oesophagitis may present with either dysphagia or odynophagia and develop ulcers and erosions on the oesophagus, and oral candidosis is usually present at the time of diagnosis. However, about 25% do not have OPC and as many as 40% of patients may have no symptoms and the absence of OPC does not exclude oesophageal involvement, nor do the presence of dysphagia and OPC indicate that the patient has *Candida* oesophagitis. A definite diagnosis can only be made by endoscopy/oesophagoscopy which typically reveal white removable plaque similar to oral candidosis. In immunocompromised patients (e.g. HIV) treatment is often started empirically and endoscopy only made when empirical treatment failed.

Therapy of choice would be with systemic active azoles such as fluconazole, itraconazole, voriconazole or posaconazole (all either as infusion, suspension or tablets/capsules). Alternatively, in azole-refractory case intravenous therapy with echinocandins (anidulangin, caspofungin or micafungin) or amphotericin B preparations may be used.

4.4.1.4 Chronic Muco-cutaneous Candidosis (CMC)

Chronic muco-cutaneous candidosis (CMC) refers to a heterogeneous spectrum of disorders leading to chronic or recurrent fungal infections of the skin, nails and mucosa. The chronic infections are caused by *Candida* species, usually *Candida albicans* and can be familial or sporadic, early or adult onset [83]. Apart from a selective susceptibility to *Candida* species infections, CMC is characterized by a relative limitation to the muco-cutaneous surface, mostly without a potential for systemic disease or septicaemia. According to the underlying pathomechanism CMC disorders can be divided into primary and secondary syndromes. Local or systemic immune-suppression resulting from several clinical conditions such as HIV infection, diabetes mellitus, use of immunosuppressive drugs or broad-spectrum antibiotics is the most common reason for the secondary syndromes [84]. Primary inherited syndromes present as a heterogeneous, complex group and can occur with or without associated endocrinopathies or autoimmune diseases. The autoimmune polyendocrinopathy-candidosis-ectodermal dystrophy (APECED) is a familial recessive inheritance gene defect associated with the autoimmune regulator (AIRE) found on locus 21q22.3, which is characterized by three major symptoms: Addison's disease, hypoparathyroidism and CMC. The second subgroup is a large family of CMC with hypothyroidism, which is an autosomal dominant form with a genetic defect suggested for chromosome 2p. The third group includes isolated CMC disorders. There are several other classifications based on familial or sporadic occurrence, early or adult onset, and the presence or absence of endocrinopathy. For many of CMC disorders the genetic basis or the link between the mutation and immune defect remains unknown. Inborn errors of Interleukin-17 immunity has been described in patients suffering from CMC, while inborn errors of caspase recruitment domain-containing protein 9 (CARD9) immunity underlie deep dermatophytosis and systemic candidosis [85, 86]. Recent studies identified an autosomal recessive form of susceptibility to chronic mucocutaneous candidosis which is associated with homozygous mutations in CARD9 [87].

Topical therapies are usually not effective. Systemic antifungal drugs can be effective, but the effects are often transient and development of resistance has been frequently observed. Long-term medication with azole antifungals is considered as a standard therapy. Fluconazole is still recommended as the first-line therapy, but resistance is a frequent problem. As alternative, posaconazole was reported to be effective in long-term treatment [88, 89].

4.4.2 Systemic Candidosis and Candidaemia

4.4.2.1 Terminology

Several clinical entities of systemic candidosis have been described in the literature but terminology appears to be somewhat confusing [90]. While candidaemia is defined as isolation of *Candida* spp. from the bloodstream, either catheter-related or not catheter-related, other manifestations of systemic candidosis are less clearly defined. The terms "invasive" and "systemic" candidosis are used commonly for the same disease. The term "invasive fungal infection (IFI)" is recommended in guidelines and widely used in clinical practice. However, according to the recent updated guidelines "invasive fungal disease" should be used and it would be even more correct to use the term systemic fungal disease [2, 91, 92].

Whether the term "acute invasive candidosis/candidiasis" deserves a disease by its own remains unclear. In fact, this clinical manifestation is not often described in the literature. Chronic disseminated candidosis/candidiasis (CDC) is primarily linked to hepato-splenic candidosis in patients with haematological malignancies. The general use of the term hepato-splenic candidosis (instead of CDC) would be less confusing.

Common definitions often found in the literature.

- Candidaemia (catheter-related or not catheter-related);
- Acute disseminated candidosis with/without fungaemia and disseminated organ involvement
- Invasive candidosis restricted to only one organ (e.g. endocarditis, meningoencephalitis, peritonitis)
- Chronic disseminated candidosis (CDC) or alternatively hepato-splenic candidosis in patients with haematological malignancy.

4.4.2.2 Prognostic Factors and Scores

Various risk factors have been described and specific (*Candida*) scores have been studied in prospective trials in order to identify high-risk patients before the onset of systemic disease and to lower attributable mortality (see Table 4.1 for risk factors).

In general, most *Candida* isolates from nonsterile body sites do not represent disease. However, multifocal colonization with *Candida* spp. in critically ill patients is a marker of poor prognosis. A number of studies in the ICU setting have documented that the colonization of more than one body site is associated with invasive infection [93–96]. The magnitude of colonization can be quantified by the Candida-Colonization-Index (CCI) or corrected Candida-Colonization-Index (cCCI) [93]. A prospective study from France showed that pre-emptive antifungal therapy based on the cCCI significantly reduced the rate of candidaemia [97]. For patients with severe pancreatitis, the CCI was the most accurate and discriminative test at identifying which patients with severe acute pancreatitis at risk of developing candidal infection. However, sensitivity was only 67% [98].

Table 4.1 Frequently reported risk factors of invasive candidosis in the critical care setting (adapted from Ostrosky-Zeichner [259])

Risk factors in adults	Additional risk factors for neonates
Length of stay in the ICU	Low gestational age
Broad-spectrum antibiotics	Low Apgar score
Haemodialysis, renal failure	H2 blockers
Central venous catheters	Shock
Severity of illness	Gastrointestinal disease
Total parenteral nutrition	Congenital malformations
Gastrointestinal perforation or surgery	
Pancreatitis	
Steroids and other immunosuppressants	
Mechanical ventilation	
Multiple blood transfusions	
Candida spp. colonization at multiple sites	
Diabetes mellitus	

By the addition of clinical risk factors for invasive *Candida* infections to the CCI, Leon evaluated a "*Candida* score" for the prediction of invasive infections in prospective cohort studies [99, 100]. The score includes the colonization with *Candida*, previous surgery, total parenteral nutrition, and the presence of severe sepsis. A score ≥3 was highly predictive for systemic *Candida* infections [101]. Ostrosky-Zeichner et al. developed an alternative prediction rule, including any systemic antibiotic (days 1-3) or presence of a central venous catheter (days 1-3) and at least TWO of the following—total parenteral nutrition (days 1-3), any dialysis (days 1-3), any major surgery (days -7-0), pancreatitis (days -7-0), any use of steroids (days -7-3), or use of other immunosuppressive agents (days -7-0) which was later modified (requiring artificial ventilation and CVC and broad-spectrum antibiotics together with an additional risk factor) [100, 102]. It may be concluded that the *Candida* score that combines the clinical risk factors preceding surgery, total parenteral nutrition and severe sepsis with *Candida* multi-site colonization may be considered a useful bedside scoring system [103].

Patients in the ICU are regarded as high-risk patients for developing candidaemia and poor prognosis [22, 104]. Thirty-day overall mortality rate may be as high as 50% [105]. Frequently, empiric or pre-emptive antifungal strategies are applied in these high-risk patients in particular with the availability of safe drugs such as echinocandins in order to improve prognosis [106]. However in a most recent analysis from France, independent risk factors for day-30 death in ICU were age, arterial catheter, *Candida* species, pre-exposure to caspofungin, and lack of antifungal therapy at the time of blood cultures results [105].

4.4.2.3 Candidaemia

Candidaemia is defined as the isolation of *Candida* spp. from at least one blood culture. The vast majority of systemic *Candida* cases are the result of bloodstream infection and haematogenous spreading of the fungi [107]. Typically, candidaemia may be either catheter-related infections (CRCBSI) or secondary due to dissemination from the gastrointestinal (GI) tract. Interruption of the integrity of the GI mucosa is regarded as the port of entry for *Candida* spp. in non-catheter-related candidaemias (e.g. perforation, severe mucositis, secondary or tertiary peritonitis). It is assumed that the majority of disseminated Candida infections originate from the GI tract. Gastrointestinal surgery is the major risk factor, especially when the GI tract is heavily colonized before surgery. Previous colonization of the GI tract together with colonization of other non-sterile sites are independent risk factors for candidaemia [108, 109]. There are no specific signs and symptoms which are characteristic for candidaemia or disseminated candidosis. Most patients suffer from a severe underlying disease, are seriously ill and present with persistent fever refractory to antibiotics. Fever may not be present in patients with candidaemia, especially while receiving corticosteroids. Some patients present with a sepsis-like syndrome, including fever, hypotension, and tachycardia. The sepsis syndrome cannot be distinguished from bacterial sepsis by clinical signs and symptoms.

The risk of death is very high, even fatal among patients with septic shock attributed to *Candida* infection. According to a single centre retrospective cohort study, the hospital mortality rate for patients having adequate source control and antifungal therapy administered within 24 h of the onset of shock was 52.8%, compared to a mortality rate of 97.6% in patients who did not have these goals attained [110]. The percentage of patients with septic shock from all patients with candidaemia ranges from 13 to 25%, depending on the respective study. Occasionally, patients may have only a single febrile episode and in blood cultures grow *Candida* species some days later when fever has already defervesced. This clinical scenario is always a matter of debate whether to treat a single positive blood culture or not. The same comes true for a positive culture from a catheter tip without a positive blood culture. However, even if the candidaemia may be only transient, dissemination of *Candida* has been documented [111].

Catheter-associated Candidaemia

Central venous lines should be regarded as an infectious focus and should be removed whenever possible, regardless if they are the primary portal of entry or if they are secondarily colonized [1, 112]. A rapid sterilization of the bloodstream is only achieved by the removal of infected central venous lines including implanted catheters (e.g. Port-/Hickman-/Broviac-Systems). The vast majority of the retrospective studies have demonstrated that CVC retention is a risk factor associated with a poor outcome [113]. Of note, some experts argue against current guidelines CVC removal may be not necessarily done [114]. However, this should be not the rule because catheter retention is associated with increased risk of death, independent of the severity of illness and whether patients had neutropenia. Removal should be done together with the initiation of antifungal therapy. If the central venous lines are retained, the duration of candidaemia increases (from 3 to 6 days) as does the mortality of patients [57, 112, 115, 116]. This is particularly supported by data for infections due to *C. albicans* and *C. parapsilosis*, but less for other *Candida* species. The best time for removal is controversial but should be generally done as early as possible [114]. The role of catheter removal in granulocytopenic patients is particularly controversial as the gastrointestinal mucosa, damaged by cytotoxic chemotherapy, is thought to be the main port of entry for yeasts to the bloodstream [117–119]. However, as the central venous line might be colonized, it is recommended to remove them in these patients as well as in non-granulocytopenic patients [7, 120].

4.4.2.4 Arthritis/Osteomyelitis/Spondylodiscitis

Bone infections by *Candida* spp. are rare and remain poorly studied. The usual route of infection in *Candida* arthritis, osteomyelitis and spondylodiscitis is haematogenous seeding. Among the causes of septic arthritis, fungal arthritis occurs infrequently and is most commonly caused by *Candida* species.

Most reports of *Candida arthritis* are limited to individual case descriptions and relatively small case series. According to a recent review with analysis from 112 published cases, clinical manifestations included pain (82%), oedema (71%), limited function (39%), and erythema (22%) with knees (75%) and hips (15%) most commonly infected [121].

In a systematic review of *Candida* osteomyelitis, case reports of 207 patients with *Candida osteomyelitis* from 1970 through 2011 were analysed in detail [122].

Most patients (90%) were not neutropenic. Localizing pain, tenderness, and/or edema were present in 90% of patients. Mechanisms of bone infection followed a pattern of haematogenous dissemination (67%), direct inoculation (25%), and contiguous infection (9%). Coinciding with haematogenous infection, most patients had ≥2 infected bones. The most common distribution of infected sites for adults was vertebra, rib, and sternum. In paediatric patients (≤18 years) the femur, humerus, then vertebra/ribs were the primary affected site. *Candida albicans* was the most prevalent pathogen and non-*Candida albicans* species caused 35% of cases [122].

Candida spondylodiscitis is generally associated with infection arising from catheter placement, drug abuse, provision of parenteral nutrition, and in immunocompromised patients, opportunistic infections. The thoracic and lumbar spine are affected in 95%, but spondylodiscitis of the cervical spine caused by *Candida* species is a rare disease [123]. MRI is the most sensitive method to detect spondylodiscitis but with questionable capacity to distinguish between bacterial and fungal infections [124].

4.4.2.5 Candiduria and Urinary Tract Infections

Urinary tract infections caused by *Candida* spp. make occur as pyelonephritis, cystitis, prostatitis, or epididymo-orchitis but symptoms are little different from those of the same infections produced by other pathogens. *Candida* species are commonly isolated in urine samples from hospitalized patients with urinary catheter. In general, as well-known for isolation of *Candida* from non-sterile sources, isolation of *Candida* in the urine does not necessarily mean *Candida* disease. Long-term urinary catheterization is considered to be the most significant risk factor for candiduria followed by antibiotic use and diabetes. Candiduria may be the only indicator of a more serious invasive candidosis, especially in immunocompromised patients. Consequently, mortality in patients with systemic candidosis and candiduria is high [125]. In ICU patients, although candiduria is a marker for increased mortality, it is only rarely attributable to *Candida* urinary tract infection [126]. In the ICU, candiduria can be reliably considered a surrogate marker of high density of colonization. Candiduria often coexists with *Candida* colonization of other anatomical sites [125].

In a recent study in 141 candidaemia episodes, twelve episodes of candidaemia with concomitant candiduria occurred in 11 patients (8% of all candidaemias). In six of these episodes, the strains in the blood-urine pairs belonged to different species. In two episodes, the isolates belonged to the same species but were not genetically related, and only in four (2.8% of all candidaemias), the strains were related. These findings indicate that in hospitalized patients with candidaemia, concomitant candiduria is rare and usually an independent event [127]. When *Candida* species are isolated in urine culture, repeating the urinalysis and urine culture is the first step to verify funguria [128]. Pyuria is a nonspecific finding and the morphology of the offending yeast may allow separation of *Candida glabrata* from other species. *Candida* casts in the urine are indicative of renal candidosis but are only rarely seen. The most common pathogen is *C. albicans* followed by *C. glabrata*.

In a majority of episodes in adult patients in critical care facilities candiduria represents colonization, and antifungal therapy is not required [126]. Candiduria that complicates antibiotic therapy frequently resolves shortly after antibiotics are stopped. In general, fluconazole is preferred for the treatment of *Candida* urinary tract infections (fluconazole in a loading dose of 400(-800) mg followed by 200(-400) mg daily or with appropriate adjustment for renal insufficiency). Low-dose amphotericin B (0.3–1 mg/kg single dose) may be useful for *Candida* UTIs in selected patients [128, 129]. The role of echinocandins is unclear because measurable concentrations in the urine are generally not achieved with these antifungal agents. Eradication of *Candida* bladder infections with flucytosine can be expected in about 70% of symptomatic individuals. Generally, therapy is given for only 7–10 days because resistance develops quickly when this agent is used alone for an extended period. A dose of 25 mg/kg every 6 h is recommended.

Irrigation of the bladder with antifungal agents is regarded to have limited utility. The use of amphotericin B bladder irrigation (ABBI) for treatment of asymptomatic candiduria is controversial. According to a recent meta-analysis, the evaluation of ABBI using an intermittent or continuous system of delivery showed an early candiduria clearance (24 h after therapy) of 80% and 82%, respectively [130]. The use of continuous ABBI for more than 5 days showed a better result (88% vs. 78%) than ABBI for less than 5 days. ABBI was equally efficacious in achieving overall cure, and resulted in greater clearance of candiduria compared to fluconazole [131].

4.4.2.6 Chorioretinitis and Endophthalmitis

Ocular candidosis is a major complication of candidaemia. Two distinct entities have been described, (1) *Candida* endophthalmitis with vitritis, usually presenting as fluffy balls extending into the vitreous body, and (2) *Candida* chorioretinitis, with abnormalities restricted to the chorioretinal layers. The extent of the ocular lesions may be related to the clinical setting. Endogenous endophthalmitis is characterized by haematogenous spread from the initial site of infection by candidaemia resulting in fungal invasion of retinal or choroidal vessels, vascular thrombosis and retinal necrosis.

In cases with untreated candidaemia ocular foci may not be noticed until endophthalmitis has evolved which may finally lead to blindness. Older prospective studies reported high incidences of ocular lesions in patients with candidaemia from 28% up to 37% [132, 133]. More recent data came from a prospective clinical trial that compared voriconazole with amphotericin B followed by fluconazole for the treatment of candidaemia [4]. Of 370 patients, 49 had findings consistent with the diagnosis of ocular candidosis at baseline, and an additional 11 patients developed abnormalities during treatment, totaling 60 patients with eye involvement (16%). In this study, *Candida* endophthalmitis was uncommon (1.6%). However, in a retrospective analysis of unselected patients (real world data) with candidaemia from Japan between 2011 to 2016, endogenous fungal endophthalmitis was diagnosed in 20.1% of cases (35 from 174 patients) with the majority having chorioretinitis ($n = 31$) [134].

4.4.2.7 Endocarditis

Candida infective endocarditis (IE) is uncommon but often fatal. The overall mortality is approximately 80% [135]. Some studies noted no difference in mortality with antifungal treatment versus surgical intervention, but mortality did decrease in those patients who underwent both surgical replacement and antifungal therapy.

Most epidemiologic data are derived from small case series or case reports. It is assumed that fungi comprise between 1 and 10% of organisms isolated in IE, including approximately 10% of prosthetic valve endocarditis cases [135]. In recent reviews of fungal endocarditis, 53–68% were *Candida* species and *Candida albicans* was the most common [136, 137]. Ellis et al. demonstrated that the crude survival of patients with fungal endocarditis had increased over the past 20 years, from 14% before 1970 to 41% in the period 1991–1995 [137].

The most common clinical manifestations among all patients with fungal endocarditis are fever (79.5%), new murmur (48%), haematuria (22%), pulmonary edema (22%), and evidence of a vascular embolic event (16%) [138]. According to a large series from the International Collaboration on Endocarditis—Prospective Cohort Study (ICE-PCS) where 33 cases of *Candida* endocarditis were compared to 2716 cases of non-fungal endocarditis, there was little difference in symptoms and signs at presentation between the *Candida* and non-fungal groups [138]. Symptoms may last several weeks before the diagnosis of endocarditis is made. Blood cultures are positive for *Candida* species in >80%. In the remaining cases mycological diagnosis may be made directly either by culture or histology from the infected valve. Vegetations occur predominantly on the aortic valve, followed by the mitral and tricuspid valve. Diagnostic procedure of choice is transoesophageal echocardiography for detecting vegetations.

Recent reviews reported that fluconazole-containing combination antifungal therapy, with or without concomitant valve replacement, and followed by prolonged fluconazole therapy is effective in patients with *Candida* endocarditis with survival rates over 90% [139]. Combination antifungal therapy alone appears to possibly approach the success of adjunctive surgery. The findings also suggest that in select patients in whom surgical therapy is not an alternative, combination therapy can optimize the chance for treatment success. Some studies noted no difference in mortality with antifungal treatment versus surgical intervention, but mortality did decrease in those patients who underwent both surgical replacement and antifungal therapy [135].

Thus, based on small case series the treatment of *Candida* infective endocarditis generally involves antifungal therapy infected followed by valve removal. The traditional antifungal treatment of *Candida* endocarditis is amphotericin B (6–8 weeks) or liposomal amphotericin, with or without flucytosine, often followed by fluconazole as suppression because of frequent relapse. Duration of suppression therapy is not well defined.

4.4.2.8 Hepato-splenic Candidosis (Chronic Disseminated Candidosis)

Hepato-splenic candidosis, also known as chronic disseminated candidosis (CDC) is a distinct form of disseminated *Candida* infection, with predominant involvement of the liver and to a lesser extent of the spleen. When both liver and spleen are involved, the term hepato-splenic candidosis (HSC) is used. CDC occurring in immunocompromised patients is typically associated with disseminated infection involving multiple organs. Prevalence of hepatic involvement in disseminated *Candida* infection varied depending on the publication but a mean prevalence of 14% has been suggested in earlier reports [140]. Soon, it became clear that focal hepatic *Candida* infection is a distinct clinical variant of disseminated *Candida* infection (chronic disseminated candidosis, CDC) in immunocompromised patients, mostly patients who have received intense cytotoxic chemotherapy for acute leukaemia [140–150]. CDC is a diagnosis primarily established on clinical findings with persistent fever not responsive to conventional antibiotics together with clinical findings, such as gastrointestinal symptoms with hepatomegaly, splenomegaly and laboratory signs, (e.g. elevated levels of alkaline phosphatase). Fever typically presents as recurrent fever which occurs after neutrophil recovery and CDC is diagnosed when typical lesions in liver (and sometimes spleen and/or other organs) can be seen on computed tomography, ultrasound and/or magnetic resonance imaging [142, 150–152]. Among the imaging modalities, magnetic resonance imaging (MRI) has the highest diagnostic level as a non-invasive tool for the diagnosis of hepato-splenic fungal infections [150]. Hepato-splenic candidosis may be imaged with F-18 FDG PET/CT as well [153]. This technique may not accurately allow to diagnose CDC but to monitor disease and response to antifungal therapy.

Proven CDC requires a positive histology plus cultural evidence for fungi from the liver biopsy [2]. Lesions associated with HCI were described to present as granulomas, microabscesses, centrilobular congestion, haemorrhagic necrosis, bile stasis, inflammatory parenchymal aggregates, free yeasts in sinusoids, and/or fatty changes [140, 154]. However, a liver biopsy may not always establish the definite diagnosis or some patients are ineligible for the procedure. In addition, fungal elements may not always be visible in liver tissue and mycological culture is frequently negative. This makes the evidence for proven fungal disease difficult [141, 142, 144, 147]. Fungi are usually microscopically visible in organ biopsies, but it has often been observed that yeast forms and pseudohyphae are seen only in the central area of the abscess. However, studies have reported that even when several liver biopsies were taken from white nodules negative results at histological and/or cytological examination were achieved [147]. Molecular techniques may improve diagnosis of CDC. A molecular method using a DNA microarray has been proposed to improve diagnosis of CDC, even in culture negative cases [155].

Systemic therapy is similar as for candidaemia but prolonged therapy is often required because resolution of signs and symptoms of CDC takes weeks and even many months. If the pathogen is identified which unfortunately is not often the case intravenous systemic antifungal treatment (either azoles, amphotericin B formulations or an echinocandin) may be de-escalated to oral therapy (e.g. fluconazole) once the patient condition has stabilized. It has been proposed that CDC is not necessarily a fungal disease but an immune response to the fungal infection in the liver, similar to the immune reconstitution syndrome observed in HIV positive individuals who receive antiretroviral therapy together with antifungal therapy for, e.g., cerebral cryptococcosis [156–158]. In general, rapid defervescence (median, 5 days) occurs after adjuvant corticosteroid therapy [159]. However, according to a recent report from Japan there were no significant differences in 90-day mortality between CDC patients with and without concomitant corticosteroid therapy [159].

Adjunctive treatment with corticosteroids for suppression of the immune response is currently recommended for (rapid) improvement of clinical symptoms [160, 161].

4.4.2.9 Intra-abdominal Candidosis

Candida spp. are known to colonize the gastrointestinal tract in healthy individuals since more about 50 years [162]. However, when barrier disruption occurs (e.g. in GI surgery, perforation) candidaemia and/or *Candida* peritonitis may occur as a complication of this procedure. Intra-abdominal candidosis includes peritonitis and intra-abdominal abscesses may occur in up to 40% of patients following repeated gastrointestinal (GI) surgery, GI perforation, or necrotizing pancreatitis [163]. *Candida* peritonitis is burdened by a mortality reported between 25 and 60% [164]. *Candida* was reported to be isolated in 41% of upper gastrointestinal (GI) sites, 35% of small bowel, 12% of colorectal, and less than 5% of appendicular sites [164–166]. In a recent multi-centre study, it was found that intra-abdominal candidosis mainly consisted of secondary peritonitis (41%) and abdominal abscesses (30%) [164]. Fourteen percent of cases had also candidaemia and 69% had concomitant bacterial infections. The most commonly isolated *Candida* species was *C. albicans* (64%). Diagnosis of intra-abdominal candidosis is usually made with *Candida* isolated in pure or mixed culture or peritonitis in presence of fever, abdominal pain, tenderness on palpation, ileus, and leukocytosis with isolation of *Candida* in the peritoneal fluid from laparotomy or drain effluents.

According to a multi-centre study in 271 adult intensive-care unit (ICU) patients in France (2005–2006), mortality in the ICU due to *Candida* peritonitis was high (38%) [167]. Outcome was not influenced by type of *Candida* species, fluconazole susceptibility, time to treatment, candidaemia, nosocomial acquisition, or concomitant bacterial infection. No specific factors for death were identified. Source control remains a key element in intra-abdominal candidosis, inside and outside the intensive care unit. Early antifungal treatment among ICU patients was associated with lower mortality

[168, 169]. For treatment of intra-abdominal candidosis, see Table 4.3.

4.4.2.10 Meningitis/ Meningoencephalitis

Risk factors and/or patient groups associated with *Candida* Meningitis are: (1) previous treatment with antibiotics, immunosuppressive therapy or corticosteroids, (2) carrier of intravascular catheters, (3) recent abdominal surgery, (4) premature neonate, (5) recent neurosurgery/insertion of CSF derivative systems, and (6) intravenous drug use [170]. Two major patient groups can be identified. First, patients following neurosurgery do have a potential risk for postoperative *Candida* Meningitis [171, 172]. According to a recent study, all CNS infections were associated with foreign intracranial material, with external ventricular drains (82%) in most cases [171]. The second patient group at risk is very low birth weight infants (VLBW) [173–175].

Two distinct patterns characterize candidosis of the CNS, (1) disseminated disease with acute disseminated candidosis, when patients present with a sepsis-like syndrome, persisting candidaemia, and disseminated skin or organ involvement (including CNS), and (2) localized disease with (deeply) invasive candidosis either presenting as primary or secondary meningoencephalitis, ventriculitis secondary to CSF shunt infection (e.g. after neurosurgery) or with brain abscesses [107, 171, 172, 176, 177]. Patients with *Candida* meningitis after neurosurgery do not necessarily have candidaemia as well, but previous studies reported that these patients had received antibacterial agents within four weeks prior to *Candida* meningitis, and that 50% of patients suffered from antecedent bacterial meningitis [172]. In this study overall mortality was 11% [172]. In contrast, in VLBW mortality rate was remarkably high (57%) and associated with a high incidence of deafness (50%) as well as severe retinopathy of prematurity (22%) together with frequent adverse neurologic outcomes at 2 years (60%) [178]. In an earlier report, *Candida* brain abscess in patients after bone marrow transplantation has been described [179]. *Candida* brain abscess often occurred in association with fungaemia (63% of cases) or granulocytopenia (63%). Mortality was high (97%) in these patients and treatment with conventional Amphotericin B did not have impact on survival. Most prevalent findings were fever (84%), altered mental status (42%) and cranial nerve abnormality (26%). Thirty-two percent of patients did not have any signs and symptoms suggestive for brain abscess. However, this complication occurred before antifungal prophlyaxis with triazoles was widely used. *Candida* meningitis was described to occur in otherwise healthy adults and children with inherited CARD9 deficiency which suggests a genetic disposition [177]. This genetic defect may translate in clinical therapy as demonstrated in an adult patient with relapsing *Candida* meningitis (due to *Candida albicans*) over a 11-year period who finally achieved clinical remission with adjunctive GM-CSF therapy [180].

The clinical presentation may vary depending on the host. In neonates, dyspnoea with respiratory distress syndrome together with metabolic acidosis may be seen. Adults with *Candida* meningitis do have an acute onset of symptoms, mostly fever, headache and altered mental status (decrease in the level of consciousness). Neck stiffness, as often seen in bacterial/viral meningitis may not be present [170]. These clinical presentations correspond to pathological findings in *Candida* CNS disease which compromise cerebral micro- or macroabscesses, typically showing foci of necrosis surrounded by polymorphonuclear leukocytes or noncaseating granuloma with giant cells that may contain yeasts or hyphae [170, 181, 182]. Other findings are macroabscesses and lesions of vascular origin such as cerebral infarcts by vasculitis or mycotic aneurysms, and *Candida* meningoencephalitis. *Candida* meningitis may be difficult to diagnose because the sensitivity of CSF cultures for Gram stain is low (40%) but cultures can detect *Candida* species in >75% depending on the CSF volume. CSF *Candida* mannan antigen and anti-mannan antibodies may be useful additional tests in patients with suspected *Candida* meningitis in whom cultures are negative [7, 183].

Current guidelines suggest that the first choice for treatment is a combination of intravenous amphotericin B or liposomal amphotericin B (AmBisome) and flucytosine (5-FC) [7, 183–185] (Table 4.2). Alternatives in not severely ill patients may be fluconazole or voriconazole [185]. Once the patient shows clinical improvement, therapy may be changed to fluconazole or voriconazole if the isolated species is susceptible [186]. The role of echinocandins in the therapy of *Candida* CNS disease is unclear. In a mouse model, caspofungin demonstrated dose-dependent activity and single case reports suggest activity (for caspofungin) in *Candida* meningitis [187, 188]. For treatment of *Candida* CNS disease, see Table 4.2.

4.4.2.11 Pulmonary Candidosis and Mediastinitis

Candida pneumonia has been described to occur in immunocompromised patients (e.g. haematological cancer) [189–193]. *Candida* spp. are frequently found in autopsy reports but it is often questioned whether *Candida* spp. are just colonizing the airways and/or lungs, signs of disseminated disease with pulmonal involvement (secondary to fungaemia) or a distinct organ fungal disease (pneumonia) by itself [194–199].

Clinical autopsy-controlled reports in ICU patients suggest that *Candida* pneumonia is rare when only colonization with *Candida* spp. in the tracheal secretion or BAL was found [200, 201]. Earlier reports from mechanically ventilated patients in the ICU found an incidence of definite *Candida* pneumonia of 8% [202]. In a prospec-

Table 4.2 Recommendations for adults with candidaemia modified from the ESCMID recommendations on initial targeted treatment [230]

Antifungal drug	Dosage	Evidence[a]
Monotherapy		
Polyenes		
Amphotericin B Deoxycholate (D-AMB)	0.7–1.0 mg/kg/day	D-I[e]
Liposomal Amphotericin B (L-AMB)	3 mg/kg/day	B-I
Amphotericin Lipid Complex (ABLC)	5 mg/kg/day	C-II
Amphotericin Colloidal Dispersion (ABCD)[b]	3–4 mg/kg/day	C-III
Echinocandins		
Anidulafungin	Day 1, loading 200 mg/day From day 2, 100 mg/day	A-I
Caspofungin[c]	Day 1, loading 70 mg/day From day 2, 1 × 50 mg/day	A-I
Micafungin	1 × 100 mg/day (no loading)	A-I
Azoles[d]		
Fluconazole	400–800 mg/day	C-I
Voriconazole	Day 1, 2 × 6 mg/kg/day loading From day 2, 2 × 3 mg/kg/day	B-I
Combination therapy		
Amphotericin B Deoxycholate + Fluconazole	0.7 mg/kg/day 800 mg/day	D-I[e]
Amphotericin B Deoxycholate + Flucytosine	0.7–1.0 mg/kg/day 4 × 25 mg/kg/day	D-II[e]

[a]Evidence according to ESCMID European Fungal Infection Study Group (EFISG) criteria (see [230])
[b]ABCD is not licensed in all countries
[c]Dose modification in patients with more than 80 kg and with liver failure
[d]Isavuconazole, itraconazole and posaconazole do not have a licensed indication to treat candidaemia
[e]Use of Amphotericin B deoxycholate alone or in combination is discouraged in the current ESCMID guideline because of AmB-D toxicity

tive autopsy study over 2 years in Belgium *Candida* spp. in respiratory samples were frequently isolated. However, no single case of *Candida* pneumonia was found among the patients with evidence of pneumonia on autopsy despite isolation of *Candida* spp. in respiratory secretions at lifetime [6]. Interestingly, in a different study hospital mortality for patients with *Candida* species detected in respiratory secretions was significantly increased [200].

Despite the frequent isolation of *Candida* spp. from respiratory tract samples, antifungal treatment is not recommended since pneumonia by this fungal species is exceptional in non-granulocytopenic patients [203].

Candida mediastinitis is a rare complication of open heart surgery (e.g. following sternal wound infection) with high mortality and morbidity usually associated with *C. albicans*. Other *Candida* spp. (e.g. *C. parapsilosis, C. krusei, C. famata* and others) have been reported as well in various settings. The vast majority of cases of fungal mediastinitis follow thoracic surgery after median sternotomy [204]. Descending mediastinitis may occur as a rare complication of oropharyngeal, cervical infections or as a complicating odontogenic infection (e.g. after dental extraction) and its delayed diagnosis and treatment are associated with high mortality. In cases of deep neck space candidal infections and mediastinitis, prompt, aggressive surgical intervention in combination with high doses of antifungals can be life-saving.

Treatment has been frequently given with Amphotericin B formulations in the past [204]. However, at the present time, the optimal doses and duration of antifungal treatment and the role of newer antifungals such as new broad-spectrum azoles or echinocandins need further clinical evaluation. Caspofungin, liposomal amphotericin and voriconazole were described as successful therapy in a case reports [205].

4.5 Diagnosis

Diagnostic criteria for invasive fungal disease (IFD) established by the European Organization for the Research and Treatment of Cancer (EORTC) and the Mycoses Study Group (MSG) reflect the current diagnostic standard for cancer patients [2]. However patients treated in the ICU for invasive mycoses are not formally included in the current EORTC/MSG definition criteria and criteria such as proven, probable or possible IFD may not be applicable for non-haematological patients in the ICU. An unmet medical need, with respect to candidaemia and systemic *Candida* infections, is the development of treatment strategies with echinocandins in specific ICU patient populations, in order to improve their outcome and survival.

A definite diagnosis of proven IFD requires histological and/or cultural evidence from tissue biopsies, resection material or positive cultures from normally sterile body fluids such as blood cultures [7]. Hence, biopsies should be taken whenever feasible to achieve the highest level of proof for IC. An accurate diagnosis of systemic *Candida* infections is important because an earlier diagnosis and early initiation of antifungal treatment is associated with improved patient survival [206, 207].

Blood cultures may not be the best tool to detect fungaemia with only 50% (up to 80%) sensitivity according to historical autopsy-based studies [208–210]. However, blood cultures are still the method of choice for the diagnosis of candidaemia because other standardized diagnostic methods are lacking. Two pairs of blood culture bottles (10 mL each) should be obtained for aerobic and anaerobic culture when candidaemia is suspected before the initiation of antifungal therapy [211]. Standard blood culture media detect most *Candida* species. It appears that the detection of *C. glabrata* is enhanced in anaerobic media. To increase the yield of blood cultures above 95%, up to four blood culture pairs should be obtained [212]. However, this approach is not routinely used. Assessment of sequential blood cultures (at least two pairs from peripheral veins and central lines) is the method of choice to detect fungaemia. The addition of special fungal media may further enhance the speed and recovery of yeasts from blood ("Mycosis-IC/F-Medium" or BacT/ALERT 3D) [213–215]. However, a separate blood culture bottle has to be used for this procedure. Mixed fungaemia (≥than one *Candida* spp.) may rarely occur, but prognosis for the patient is not necessarily worse as compared to fungaemia caused by a single *Candida* spp. [216]. Patients with Mixed fungaemia had more frequently experienced organ transplantation (13% vs. 0%) and surgery (60% vs. 27%) [216]. It may take over 92 h (e.g. *C. glabrata*) to have a positive blood culture (median hours to growth) for non-catheter-related candidaemia but may be as fast as 16 h (e.g. *C. tropicalis*) for catheter-related candidaemia [217]. Polymicrobial bloodstream infection (mixed infection by bacteria and fungi) may occur as well and do have a poor prognosis but no worse than fungaemia only [218].

Serologic tests may be used as adjunctive diagnostic tests. However, sensitivity (30–77%) and specificity (70–88%) varies widely between different studies. Further improvements in the sensitivity (76%) can be achieved by the combination of the *Candida* sandwich ELISA (Platelia-*Candida*, BioRad) with the detection of specific antibodies (Platelia-*Candida*) [219, 220]. The detection of circulating 1,3-beta-D-Glucan (e.g. Fungitell® Assay, Cape Cod, USA) from the cell wall of yeasts has been suggested for the diagnosis of invasive candidosis. The test cannot distinguish between infections due to different fungal pathogens such as *Candida*, *Aspergillus* and *Pneumocystis jirovecii* [221–223]. A second confirmatory test is needed to confirm *Candida* spp. as the responsible pathogens. For the early start of fungal therapy, a single-point BG assay based on a blood sample drawn at the sepsis onset, alone or in combination with CS, may guide the decision to start antifungal therapy early in patients at risk for *Candida* infection [224].

A commercial assay based on fluorescence in situ hybridisation ("peptide nucleic acid fluorescent in situ hybridization" = PNA Fish; e.g. Yeast Traffic Light™ PNA FISH™) allows for a rapid presumptive differentiation between *C. albicans, C. glabrata, C. tropicalis, C. parapsilosis* and *C. krusei*, the most commonly cultured pathogens [225]. In addition, matrix-assisted laser desorption ionization-time of flight mass spectrometry (MALDI-TOF MS) has been described for rapid routine identification of clinical yeast isolates with high diagnostic accuracy and reliability and is increasingly used for rapid identification after positive growth in blood culture bottles [226]. Most recently, a new molecular test called T2 Magnetic Resonance Assay has been licensed to diagnose candidaemia in the USA. This molecular diagnostic method can detect and speciate the five most common *Candida* spp.; namely, *Candida albicans*, *Candida glabrata*, *Candida parapsilosis*, *Candida tropicalis*, and *Candida krusei*, in approximately 5 h [227, 228]. However, this test may not identify rare *Candida* spp. and despite some promising evidence in published clinical trials, further studies are needed to determine the performance of T2MR in invasive candidosis without candidaemia.

4.6 Treatment

4.6.1 Systemic Candidosis

Despite advances in antifungal therapy over the past decades, mortality from systemic *Candida* infections (mostly candidaemia and acute invasive candidosis) remains high. Systemic *Candida* infections have a particularly strong impact among intensive care unit (ICU) patients, where these mycoses are associated with overall mortality rates of around 30–50%. Systemic *Candida* infections increased mortality and morbidity in severely ill patients. Patients with systemic *Candida* infections had longer ICU length of stays with a significantly increased relative risk for death as compared to control patients [58] (see Tables 4.2 and 4.3 for use of antifungal agents).

4.6.1.1 Prophylaxis

The prophylactic use of antifungal agents has been studied in randomized studies comparing fluconazole to placebo in the surgical intensive care unit (SICU). Fluconazole administration significantly reduced the incidence of fungal infections. However, according to a recent meta-

Table 4.3 Treatment of invasive *Candida* organ disease in adults (adapted to the recommendations of the German Speaking Mycological Society (DMykG) and the Paul-Ehrlich-Society for Chemotherapy (PEG)) [7]

Organ infection	Drug	Dosage	Comment
Meningitis/CNS	D-AMB i.v. + flucytosine L-AMB Fluconazole[a] Voriconazole[a]	0.7–1.0 mg/day 25 mg/kg/qid 3 mg/kg/day 800[b]/400 mg/day 8[b]/4 mg/kg/bid	Tissue penetration of echinocandins undefined [170]
Endophthalmitis/chorioretinitis	Fluconazole Voriconazole	800[b]/400 mg/day 8[b]/4 mg/kg/bid	Tissue penetration of echinocandins undefined [260, 261]
Endocarditis	D-AMB i.v. + flucytosine Caspofungin	0.7–1.0 mg/day 25 mg/kg/qid 70[b]/50 mg/day	[135–137, 262, 263]
Pneumonia	Anidulafungin Caspofungin Fluconazole Micafungin Voriconazole	200[b]/100 mg/day 70[b]/50 mg/day 800[b]/400 mg/day 100–200 mg/day 8[b]/4 mg/kg/qid	Diagnostic confirmation needs histologic proof
Peritonitis	Anidulafungin Caspofungin Fluconazole Micafungin Voriconazole D-AMB i.v. + flucytosine	200[b]/100 mg/day 70[b]/50 mg/day 800[b]/400 mg/day 100–200 mg/day 8[b]/4 mg/kg/bid 0.7–1.0 mg/day 25 mg/kg/qid	[264, 265]
Osteomyelitis/arthritis	Fluconazole Voriconazole	800[b]/400 mg/day 8[b]/4 mg/kg/bid	[266, 267]
Candiduria, cystitis, nephritis	Fluconazole	400[b]/200 mg/day	[268]
Chronic disseminated candidosis	Fluconazole (if isolate susceptible) Voriconazole Caspofungin L-AMB	800[b]/400 mg/day 6–12 mg/kg/day 8[b]/4 mg/kg/bid 70[b]/50 mg/day 3 mg/kg/day	Step-down therapy after 2 weeks of caspofungin/L-AMB with oral fluconazole/voriconazole/ posaconazole

[a]Good CSF penetration of azoles documented but place in primary therapy not well documented, therefore preferred for step-down therapy
[b]Loading dose on day 1 (dosage given)

analysis fluconazole prophylaxis was not associated with a survival advantage [229]. Therefore, the prophylactic use of fluconazole should be restricted to high-risk patients [230].

4.6.1.2 Empiric/Pre-emptive Antifungal Therapy

Empiric therapy with fluconazole in patients with persistent fever of unknown origin (FUO) but no definite proof of candidaemia or systemic *Candida* infection was found not to be very effective in the majority of patients and should not be routinely used [231]. In a large study from China, initial pre-emptive antifungal therapy and targeted antifungal therapy were associated with reduced hospital duration compared with patients with initial empirical antifungal therapy after confirmation of fungal infection [232]. However, time for appropriate start of antifungal therapy is critical. Inappropriate or late use of systemic antifungal therapy may inversely influence outcome and survival of patients [206, 233]. The dilemma is shown in a retrospective analysis where mortality may be as low as 15% in non-granulocytopenic patients who receive antifungal therapy (with fluconazole) starting on the day 0 when the blood culture was taken [206]. Even the administration of empiric antifungal treatment 12 h after a positive blood sample for culture is drawn is associated with greater hospital mortality [207].

4.6.1.3 Therapy for Proven Systemic IFD (Non-granulocytopenic Patient)

Important considerations when choosing the antifungal agent and the mode of application (i.v. vs. oral) in candidaemia and systemic candidosis include the localization of the infection, the severity of disease (e.g. sepsis, severe sepsis, and septic shock), impairment of organ functions (esp. liver and kidney), previous exposure to antifungals, the identified fungal strain, local resistance patterns and patient characteristics such as age. Most importantly, antifungal treatment for uncomplicated candidaemia is recommended for 14 days after the first negative blood culture and resolution of all clinical signs of infection. De-escalation strategies (switch from i.v. echinocandin therapy after initial response to oral therapy with an azole antifungal drug) are commonly used but criteria for early switch (e.g. after 3–5 days) are not clearly established and need further clinical evaluation. After improvement of clinical signs, sterilization of blood cultures and documented in vitro susceptibility of the causative yeast, step-down therapy after initial treatment with an echinocandin (anidulafungin, caspofungin and micafungin) was shown to be effective with oral fluconazole starting on day 10 of antifungal therapy, and may be recommended if oral drug intake and gastrointestinal absorption is possible [73, 234–236]. Antifungal treatment of candidaemia in granulocytopenic patients is basically similar as in non-granulocytopenic patients but echinocandins or liposomal amphotericin B are regarded as drugs of choice for initial therapy [237, 238].

Central venous lines should be regarded as an infectious focus and should be removed whenever possible, regardless if they are the primary portal of entry or if they are secondarily colonized [1, 112]. A rapid sterilization of the bloodstream is only achieved by the removal of infected central venous lines including implanted catheters (e.g. Port-/Hickman-/Broviac-Systems). Removal should be done together with the initiation of antifungal therapy. If the central venous lines are retained, the duration of candidaemia increases (from 3 to 6 days) as does the mortality of patients [57, 112, 115, 116]. This is particularly supported by data for infections due to *C. albicans* and *C. parapsilosis*, but less for other *Candida* species. The best time for removal is controversial but should generally be done as early as possible [114]. The role of catheter removal in granulocytopenic patients is particularly controversial as the gastrointestinal mucosa, damaged by cytotoxic chemotherapy, is thought to be the main port of entry for yeasts to the bloodstream [117–119]. However, as the central venous line might be colonized, it is recommended to remove them in these patients.

All antifungals have good activity against a broad range of *Candida* spp., especially *Candida albicans*. Some non-*Candida albicans* spp. are characterized by special susceptibility patterns to antifungals, e.g. *C. krusei* is resistant against fluconazole but susceptible for voriconazole. About 30% of *C. glabrata* isolates show a reduced susceptibility for fluconazole and other azoles. *C. lusitaniae* has a variable in vitro susceptibility for Amphotericin B (D-AMB) and the MICs for the echinocandins of *C. parapsilosis* and *C. C. guilliermondi* are higher than for other *Candida* species [239, 240].

The preferred antifungal therapy for candidaemia and other systemic *Candida* infections is either fluconazole (400–800 mg/day iv.; double dose as "loading dose" on day 1) or an echinocandin, such as anidulafungin (200 mg "loading dose", then 100 mg/day i.v.), caspofungin (70 mg "loading dose", then 50 mg/day iv.) or micafungin (100 mg/day iv. without "loading dose") [73, 236, 241–243]. Fluconazole is generally effective for C/IC, but is often not the optimum choice in critically ill patients. Its use may be further hampered by an increasing prevalence of infections due to *Candida* spp. with acquired or intrinsic resistance to fluconazole, such as *C. glabrata* and *C. krusei*. Recent guidelines favour the echinocandin class of antifungals as first-line therapy in haemodynamically unstable patients, in those with previous azole exposure, and in clinical settings with high local prevalence of fluconazole-resistant strains [1, 7]. Empiric therapy with fluconazole should not be used in critically ill, septic patients. Instead, an echinocandin or liposomal Amphotericin B should be used in these patients [186]. The use of D-AMB is associated with significant toxicity (infusion-related electrolyte imbalances and nephrotoxicity) and its use is therefore discouraged outside resource poor settings as a first line agent for the treatment of invasive candidosis [230] (see Table 4.2). The current recommendations reflect data from large clinical studies in adults. However, in neonates and children systemic antifungal therapy may be different (in particular the use of D-AMB is not discouraged as in adults due to better tolerability in children) and will not be discussed in detail in this review (please see current recommendations of ECIL/ESCMID [184, 244]).

The echinocandin class of antifungal agents acts by inhibition of the synthesis of 1,3-β-D-glucan in the fungal cell wall. All three available echinocandins (anidulafungin, caspofungin, and micafungin) possess fungicidal activity against most species of *Candida*, including azole-resistant species [73, 236, 243].

A direct comparison between fluconazole and anidulafungin showed a similar safety profile, a better treatment response and a trend toward better survival in patients treated with anidulafungin. This was evaluated in a randomized, double-blind, multi-centre, multinational, phase 3 study of patients with candidaemia and/or other forms of invasive *Candida* infections [236]. Global success at the end of iv therapy for anidulafungin (200 mg IV loading dose followed by 100 mg IV daily) was 75.6% compared to 60.2% for fluconazole-treated (800 mg IV loading dose followed by 400 mg IV daily) patients.

Anidulafungin was studied as monotherapy in a non-comparative trial in high-risk patients treated in the ICU [245]. The patient must have at least one of each co-factor/underlying illness to be included in this trial (post-abdominal surgery, elderly individuals >65 years, renal insufficiency/failure or dialysis, solid tumour, solid-organ (liver, kidney, lung, heart, pancreas) transplant recipients, hepatic insufficiency, or neutropenia (neutrophil count <500/mm^3) including haematology oncology patients). The most common pathogens were *Candida albicans* (55.9%), *C. glabrata* (14.7%) and *C. parapsilosis* (10.0%). Global success was 69.5% at EOT, 70.7% (at EOIVT, 60.2% at 2 weeks post-EOT, and 50.5% at 6 weeks post-EOT. Survival at day 90 was 53.8%. Anidulafungin was equally effective in all subgroups, but to a lesser extent in transplant and neutropenic patients.

A direct comparison of caspofungin and micafungin showed similar efficacy and safety. In addition, no difference in safety or efficacy was seen in patients treated with two different dosages of micafungin (100 mg/day or 150 mg/day) [235]. Further studies comparing different echinocandins are lacking. Higher dosages of caspofungin (150 mg/day vs. 70/50 mg/day) and micafungin (150 mg/day vs. 100 mg/day) showed a trend toward improved efficacy in subgroups of patients (APACHE-II score >20, granulocytopenia) and might be used in selected patients [235, 246]. Due to increased MICs and a higher rate of persistent fungaemia, the use of echinocandins in candidaemia due to *C. parapsilosis* may not be regarded as therapy of first choice. Isavuconazole was licensed in Europe and other countries in 2016 for use against invasive aspergillosis and patients with invasive mucormycosis not eligible for therapy with amphotericin B according data from large trials [247, 248]. However, a clinical trial comparing the efficacy of isavuconazole and caspofungin did not meet the primary endpoint (non-inferiority) and this broad-spectrum azole was not licensed for use in systemic *Candida* infections (unpublished data).

4.6.1.4 Catheter Management

Central venous lines should be regarded as an infectious focus and should be removed whenever possible, regardless if they are the primary portal of entry or if they are secondarily colonized [1, 112, 230]. A rapid sterilization of the bloodstream is only achieved by the removal of infected central venous lines including implanted catheters (e.g. Port-/Hickman-/Broviac-Systems). Removal should be done together with the initiation of antifungal therapy. If the central venous lines are retained, the duration of candidaemia increases (from 3 to 6 days) as does the mortality of patients [57, 112, 115, 116]. This is particularly supported by data for infections due to *C. albicans* and *C. parapsilosis*, but less for other *Candida* species. The best time for removal is controversial but should generally be done as early as possible [114]. The role of catheter removal in granulocytopenic patients is particularly controversial as the gastrointestinal mucosa, damaged by cytotoxic chemotherapy, is thought to be the main port of entry for yeasts to the bloodstream [117–119]. However, as the central venous line might be colonized, it is recommended to remove them in these patients as well when no rapid improvement occurs during antifungal therapy.

4.7 Infection Control

The Centers for Disease Control (CDC, USA) released a comprehensive report on "Antibiotic Resistance Threats in 2013" in order to raise public awareness for the prevention of multi-drug resistant pathogens (MDRP). It underscores the importance of enforcing public health strategies such as infection control, protection of the food supply, antibiotic stewardship, and reduction of person-to-person spread through screening, treatment and education of health care workers (HCW) and patients [249]. According to the ESCMID guidelines for the management of the infection control measures to reduce transmission of multidrug-resistant Gram-negative bacteria (MDR-GNB) in hospitalized patients, the various types of IPC interventions used to prevent and control the spread of MDR-GNB are recommended, such as (a) hand hygiene measures, (b) active screening cultures, (c) contact precautions, (d) environmental cleaning, and (e) antimicrobial stewardship [250]. Basically, these measures apply not only to bacterial but fungal pathogens such as *Candida* spp. as well. In particular, strict hand hygiene measures are the most important component of infection control in the hospital [8, 251, 252]. Yeast carriage on hands and transmission of *Candida* spp. (e.g. *Candida parapsilosis*) from healthcare workers to patients were repeatedly reported in the literature [8, 253, 254].

Daily antiseptic whole-body washing in ICU and HSCT patients has been shown to be a highly effective therapeutic intervention to reduce severe nosocomial infections. A randomized multicentre trial in eight ICU units and one HSCT unit in the USA demonstrated that daily bathing with chlorhexidine-impregnated washcloths reduced the acquisition of fungal (and multidrug-resistant pathogens and hospital-acquired bacterial) bloodstream infections [255].

4.8 Antifungal Stewardship

The concept of anti-infective or antifungal stewardship (AFS) may be defined as an ongoing effort by a healthcare institution to optimize antimicrobial use in order to improve patient outcomes, ensure cost-effective therapy, and reduce adverse sequelae [256]. This includes the appropriate use of antimicrobials by selecting the proper drug, dosage, duration, and route of administration. Antimicrobial resistance—a consequence of the use and misuse of antimicrobial medicines—occurs when a microorganism becomes resistant to an antimicrobial drug to which it was previously sensitive [257]. Concepts may not only include the appropriate use of antimicrobials by selecting the proper drug, dosage, duration, route of administration, but and finally costs as well. An understanding of the pharmacokinetics and pharmacodynamics (PK/PD) of these drugs has been demonstrated to be important to optimize drug choice and dosing regimen. Optimizing the use of currently available antifungal agents is not only influenced by antifungal drug properties (spectrum of activity, PK/PD, mode of action, route of application) but by their high cost and drug-related toxicities as well. AFS programs should be organized by an interdisciplinary team of clinicians, pharmacists, microbiologists and infection control experts with the lead of an infectious disease specialist preferably in each large hospital/institution dealing with high-risk patients for invasive fungal infections. These programs should consider various aspects of IC/C including: (1) the local fungal epidemiology, (2) information on antifungal resistance rates, (3) establishing and application of therapeutic guidelines, (4) implementation of treatment strategies for empirical, pre-emptive therapy including PK/PD data for antifungal drugs, deescalation and "switch strategies" (from intravenous to oral medication) in defined patient populations, (5) catheter management and application of routine diagnostic procedures such as ophthalmological and cardiac evaluations, as well as (6) the best available diagnostic tests for diagnosing IC and candidaemia. The role of automatic ID consultation for inpatients with fungaemia has been shown not to affect the time to administration of appropriate therapy, but improvement was observed for several process indicators, including rates of appropriate antifungal therapy selection, time to removal of CVCs, and performance of ophthalmologic examinations [258].

References

1. Pappas PG, Kauffman CA, Andes D, Benjamin DK Jr, Calandra TF, Edwards JE Jr et al (2009) Clinical practice guidelines for the management of candidiasis: 2009 update by the Infectious Diseases Society of America. Clin Infect Dis 48(5):503–535
2. dePauw B, Walsh TJ, Donnelly JP, Stevens DA, Edwards JE, Calandra T et al (2008) Revised definitions of invasive fungal disease from the European Organization for Research and Treatment of Cancer/Invasive Fungal Infections Cooperative Group and the National Institute of Allergy and Infectious Diseases Mycoses Study Group (EORTC/MSG) Consensus Group. Clin Infect Dis 46(12):1813–1821
3. Wisplinghoff H, Seifert H, Coimbra M, Wenzel RP, Edmond MB (2001) Systemic inflammatory response syndrome in adult patients with nosocomial bloodstream infection due to Staphylococcus aureus. Clin Infect Dis 33(5):733–736
4. Oude Lashof AM, Rothova A, Sobel JD, Ruhnke M, Pappas PG, Viscoli C et al (2011) Ocular manifestations of candidemia. Clin Infect Dis 53(3):262–268
5. Kauffman CA, Vazquez JA, Sobel JD, Gallis HA, McKinsey DS, Karchmer AW et al (2000) Prospective multicenter surveillance study of funguria in hospitalized patients. The National Institute for Allergy and Infectious Diseases (NIAID) Mycoses Study Group. Clin Infect Dis 30(1):14–18
6. Meersseman W, Lagrou K, Spriet I, Maertens J, Verbeken E, Peetermans WE et al (2009) Significance of the isolation of Candida species from airway samples in critically ill patients: a prospective, autopsy study. Intensive Care Med 35(9):1526–1531
7. Ruhnke M, Rickerts V, Cornely OA, Buchheidt D, Glockner A, Heinz W et al (2011) Diagnosis and therapy of Candida infections: joint recommendations of the German Speaking Mycological Society and the Paul-Ehrlich-Society for Chemotherapy. Mycoses 54(4):279–310
8. Pfaller MA, Diekema DJ (2007) Epidemiology of invasive candidiasis: a persistent public health problem. Clin Microbiol Rev 20(1):133–163
9. Ruhnke M (2006) Epidemiology of Candida albicans infections and role of non-Candida-albicans yeasts. Curr Drug Targets 7(4):495–504
10. Greenspan D, Greenspan JS (1996) HIV-related oral disease. Lancet 348(9029):729–733
11. Gottfredsson M, Cox GM, Indridason OS, de Almeida GM, Heald AE, Perfect JR (1999) Association of plasma levels of human immunodeficiency virus type 1 RNA and oropharyngeal Candida colonization. J Infect Dis 180(2):534–537
12. Martins MD, Lozano-Chiu M, Rex JH (1998) Declining rates of oropharyngeal candidiasis and carriage of Candida albicans associated with trends toward reduced rates of carriage of fluconazole-resistant C. albicans in human immunodeficiency virus-infected patients. Clin Infect Dis 27(5):1291–1294
13. Vazquez JA, Sobel JD, Peng G, Steele-Moore L, Schuman P, Holloway W et al (1999) Evolution of vaginal Candida species recovered from human immunodeficiency virus-infected women receiving fluconazole prophylaxis: the emergence of Candida glabrata? Terry Beirn Community Programs for Clinical Research in AIDS (CPCRA). Clin Infect Dis 28(5):1025–1031
14. Pfaller MA, Diekema DJ, Mendez M, Kibbler C, Erzsebet P, Chang SC et al (2006) Candida guilliermondii, an opportunistic fungal pathogen with decreased susceptibility to fluconazole: geographic and temporal trends from the ARTEMIS DISK antifungal surveillance program. J Clin Microbiol 44(10):3551–3556
15. Pfaller MA, Diekema DJ, Gibbs DL, Newell VA, Nagy E, Dobiasova S et al (2008) Candida krusei, a multidrug-resistant opportunistic fungal pathogen: geographic and temporal trends from the ARTEMIS DISK Antifungal Surveillance Program, 2001 to 2005. J Clin Microbiol 46(2):515–521
16. Pfaller MA, Diekema DJ, Colombo AL, Kibbler C, Ng KP, Gibbs DL et al (2006) Candida rugosa, an

emerging fungal pathogen with resistance to azoles: geographic and temporal trends from the ARTEMIS DISK antifungal surveillance program. J Clin Microbiol 44(10):3578–3582
17. Pfaller MA, Castanheira M, Messer SA, Moet GJ, Jones RN (2010) Variation in Candida spp. distribution and antifungal resistance rates among bloodstream infection isolates by patient age: report from the SENTRY Antimicrobial Surveillance Program (2008-2009). Diagn Microbiol Infect Dis 68(3):278–283
18. Almirante B, Rodriguez D, Park BJ, Cuenca-Estrella M, Planes AM, Almela M et al (2005) Epidemiology and predictors of mortality in cases of Candida bloodstream infection: results from population-based surveillance, Barcelona, Spain, from 2002 to 2003. J Clin Microbiol 43(4):1829–1835
19. Arendrup MC, Dzajic E, Jensen RH, Johansen HK, Kjaeldgaard P, Knudsen JD et al (2013) Epidemiological changes with potential implication for antifungal prescription recommendations for fungaemia: data from a nationwide fungaemia surveillance programme. Clin Microbiol Infect 19(8):E343–E353
20. Bassetti M, Merelli M, Righi E, Az-Martin A, Rosello EM, Luzzati R et al (2013) Epidemiology, species distribution, antifungal susceptibility, and outcome of candidemia across five sites in Italy and Spain. J Clin Microbiol 6(9):e24198
21. Borg-von-Zepelin M, Kunz L, Ruchel R, Reichard U, Weig M, Gross U (2007) Epidemiology and antifungal susceptibilities of Candida spp. to six antifungal agents: results from a surveillance study on fungaemia in Germany from July 2004 to August 2005. J Antimicrob Chemother 60(2):424–428
22. Klingspor L, Tortorano AM, Peman J, Willinger B, Hamal P, Sendid B et al (2015) Invasive Candida infections in surgical patients in intensive care units: a prospective, multicentre survey initiated by the European Confederation of Medical Mycology (ECMM) (2006-2008). Clin Microbiol Infect 21(1):87
23. Presterl E, Daxbock F, Graninger W, Willinger B (2007) Changing pattern of candidaemia 2001-2006 and use of antifungal therapy at the University Hospital of Vienna, Austria. Clin Microbiol Infect 13(11):1072–1076
24. Colombo AL, Melo AS, Crespo Rosas RF, Salomao R, Briones M, Hollis RJ et al (2003) Outbreak of Candida rugosa candidemia: an emerging pathogen that may be refractory to amphotericin B therapy. Diagn Microbiol Infect Dis 46(4):253–257
25. Horn DL, Neofytos D, Anaissie EJ, Fishman JA, Steinbach WJ, Olyaei AJ et al (2009) Epidemiology and outcomes of candidemia in 2019 patients: data from the prospective antifungal therapy alliance registry. Clin Infect Dis 48(12):1695–1703
26. Pfaller MA, Moet GJ, Messer SA, Jones RN, Castanheira M (2011) Candida bloodstream infections: comparison of species distributions and antifungal resistance patterns in community-onset and nosocomial isolates in the SENTRY Antimicrobial Surveillance Program, 2008-2009. Antimicrob Agents Chemother 55(2):561–566
27. Pfaller MA, Diekema DJ, Jones RN, Sader HS, Fluit AC, Hollis RJ et al (2001) International surveillance of bloodstream infections due to Candida species: frequency of occurrence and in vitro susceptibilities to fluconazole, ravuconazole, and voriconazole of isolates collected from 1997 through 1999 in the SENTRY antimicrobial surveillance program. J Clin Microbiol 39(9):3254–3259
28. Lockhart SR, Etienne KA, Vallabhaneni S, Farooqi J, Chowdhary A, Govender NP et al (2017) Simultaneous emergence of multidrug-resistant Candida auris on 3 continents confirmed by whole-genome sequencing and epidemiological analyses. Clin Infect Dis 64(2):134–140
29. Beyda ND, Chuang SH, Alam MJ, Shah DN, Ng TM, McCaskey L et al (2013) Treatment of Candida famata bloodstream infections: case series and review of the literature. J Antimicrob Chemother 68(2):438–443
30. Guitard J, Angoulvant A, Letscher-Bru V, L'ollivier C, Cornet M, Dalle F et al (2013) Invasive infections due to Candida norvegensis and Candida inconspicua: report of 12 cases and review of the literature. Med Mycol 51(8):795–799
31. Meis JF, Ruhnke M, de Pauw BE, Odds FC, Siegert W, Verweij PE (1999) Candida dubliniensis candidemia in patients with chemotherapy-induced neutropenia and bone marrow transplantation. Emerg Infect Dis 5(1):150–153
32. Hirayama T, Miyazaki T, Yamagishi Y, Mikamo H, Ueda T, Nakajima K et al (2018) Clinical and microbiological characteristics of Candida guilliermondii and Candida fermentati. Antimicrob Agents Chemother 62(6):e02528
33. Liu WL, Lai CC, Li MC, Wu CJ, Ko WC, Hung YL et al (2017) Clinical manifestations of candidemia caused by uncommon Candida species and antifungal susceptibility of the isolates in a regional hospital in Taiwan, 2007–2014. J Microbiol Immunol Infect. https://doi.org/10.1016/j.jmii.2017.08.007
34. Vallabhaneni S, Kallen A, Tsay S, Chow N, Welsh R, Kerins J et al (2016) Investigation of the first seven reported cases of Candida auris, a globally emerging invasive, multidrug-resistant fungus - United States, May 2013-August 2016. Morb Mortal Wkly Rep 65(44):1234–1237
35. Calvo B, Melo AS, Perozo-Mena A, Hernandez M, Francisco EC, Hagen F et al (2016) First report of Candida auris in America: clinical and microbiological aspects of 18 episodes of candidemia. J Infect 73(4):369–374
36. Chowdhary A, Voss A, Meis JF (2016) Multidrug-resistant Candida auris: 'new kid on the block' in hospital-associated infections? J Hosp Infect 94(3):209–212
37. McCarthy M (2016) Hospital transmitted Candida auris infections confirmed in the US. BMJ 355:i5978

38. Morales-Lopez SE, Parra-Giraldo CM, Ceballos-Garzon A, Martinez HP, Rodriguez GJ, Varez-Moreno CA et al (2017) Invasive Infections with Multidrug-Resistant Yeast Candida auris, Colombia. Emerg Infect Dis 23(1):162–164
39. Schelenz S, Hagen F, Rhodes JL, Abdolrasouli A, Chowdhary A, Hall A et al (2016) First hospital outbreak of the globally emerging Candida auris in a European hospital. Antimicrob Resist Infect Control 5:35
40. Zhang L, Xiao M, Wang H, Gao R, Fan X, Brown M et al (2014) Yeast identification algorithm based on use of the Vitek MS system selectively supplemented with ribosomal DNA sequencing: proposal of a reference assay for invasive fungal surveillance programs in China. J Clin Microbiol 52(2):572–577
41. Dorgan E, Denning DW, McMullan R (2015) Burden of fungal disease in Ireland. J Med Microbiol 64(Pt 4):423–426
42. Gugnani HC, Denning DW (2015) Burden of serious fungal infections in the Dominican Republic. J Infect Public Health 9(1):7–12
43. Mortensen KL, Denning DW, Arendrup MC (2015) The burden of fungal disease in Denmark. Mycoses 58(Suppl 5):15–21
44. Oladele RO, Denning DW (2014) Burden of serious fungal infection in Nigeria. West Afr J Med 33(2):107–114
45. Rodriguez-Tudela JL, Astruey-Izquierdo A, Gago S, Cuenca-Estrella M, Leon C, Miro JM et al (2015) Burden of serious fungal infections in Spain. Clin Microbiol Infect 21(2):183–189
46. Ruhnke M, Groll AH, Mayser P, Ullmann AJ, Mendling W, Hof H et al (2015) Estimated burden of fungal infections in Germany. Mycoses 58(Suppl 5):22–28
47. Ben R, Denning DW (2015) Estimating the burden of fungal diseases in Israel. Isr Med Assoc J 17(6):374–379
48. Chrdle A, Mallatova N, Vasakova M, Haber J, Denning DW (2015) Burden of serious fungal infections in the Czech Republic. Mycoses 58(Suppl 5):6–14
49. Corzo-Leon DE, Rmstrong-James D, Denning DW (2015) Burden of serious fungal infections in Mexico. Mycoses 58(Suppl 5):34–44
50. Klimko N, Kozlova Y, Khostelidi S, Shadrivova O, Borzova Y, Burygina E et al (2015) The burden of serious fungal diseases in Russia. Mycoses 58(Suppl 5):58–62
51. Lagrou K, Maertens J, Van EE, Denning DW (2015) Burden of serious fungal infections in Belgium. Mycoses 58(Suppl 5):1–5
52. Pegorie M, Denning DW, Welfare W (2016) Estimating the burden of invasive and serious fungal disease in the United Kingdom. J Infect 74(1):60–71
53. Wisplinghoff H, Bischoff T, Tallent SM, Seifert H, Wenzel RP, Edmond MB (2004) Nosocomial bloodstream infections in US hospitals: analysis of 24,179 cases from a prospective nationwide surveillance study. Clin Infect Dis 39(3):309–317
54. Wisplinghoff H, Ebbers J, Geurtz L, Stefanik D, Major Y, Edmond MB et al (2014) Nosocomial bloodstream infections due to Candida spp. in the USA: species distribution, clinical features and antifungal susceptibilities. Int J Antimicrob Agents 43(1):78–81
55. Ylipalosaari P, La-Kokko TI, Karhu J, Koskela M, Laurila J, Ohtonen P et al (2012) Comparison of the epidemiology, risk factors, outcome and degree of organ failures of patients with candidemia acquired before or during ICU treatment. Crit Care 16(2):R62
56. Trick WE, Fridkin SK, Edwards JR, Hajjeh RA, Gaynes RP (2002) Secular trend of hospital-acquired candidemia among intensive care unit patients in the United States during 1989-1999. Clin Infect Dis 35(5):627–630
57. Blumberg HM, Jarvis WR, Soucie JM, Edwards JE, Patterson JE, Pfaller MA et al (2001) Risk factors for candidal bloodstream infections in surgical intensive care unit patients: the NEMIS prospective multicenter study. The National Epidemiology of Mycosis Survey. Clin Infect Dis 33(2):177–186
58. Leleu G, Aegerter P, Guidet B (2002) Systemic candidiasis in intensive care units: a multicenter, matched-cohort study. J Crit Care 17(3):168–175
59. Grohskopf LA, Sinkowitz-Cochran RL, Garrett DO, Sohn AH, Levine GL, Siegel JD et al (2002) A national point-prevalence survey of pediatric intensive care unit-acquired infections in the United States. J Pediatr 140(4):432–438
60. Vincent JL, Sakr Y, Sprung CL, Ranieri VM, Reinhart K, Gerlach H et al (2006) Sepsis in European intensive care units: results of the SOAP study. Crit Care Med 34(2):344–353
61. Vincent JL, Bihari DJ, Suter PM, Bruining HA, White J, Nicolas-Chanoin MH et al (1995) The prevalence of nosocomial infection in intensive care units in Europe. Results of the European Prevalence of Infection in Intensive Care (EPIC) Study. EPIC International Advisory Committee. JAMA 274(8):639–644
62. Geffers C, Zuschneid I, Sohr D, Ruden H, Gastmeier P (2004) Microbiological isolates associated with nosocomial infections in intensive care units: data of 274 intensive care units participating in the German Nosocomial Infections Surveillance System (KISS). Anasthesiol Intensivmed Notfallmed Schmerzther 39(1):15–19
63. Marchetti O, Bille J, Fluckiger U, Eggimann P, Ruef C, Garbino J et al (2004) Epidemiology of candidemia in Swiss tertiary care hospitals: secular trends, 1991-2000. Clin Infect Dis 38(3):311–320
64. Mean M, Marchetti O, Calandra T (2008) Bench-to-bedside review: Candida infections in the intensive care unit. Crit Care 12(1):204
65. Arendrup MC, Fuursted K, Gahrn-Hansen B, Schonheyder HC, Knudsen JD, Jensen IM et al (2008) Semi-national surveillance of fungaemia in Denmark 2004-2006: increasing incidence of fun-

gaemia and numbers of isolates with reduced azole susceptibility. Clin Microbiol Infect 14(5):487–494
66. Klingspor L, Tornqvist E, Johansson A, Petrini B, Forsum U, Hedin G (2004) A prospective epidemiological survey of candidaemia in Sweden. Scand J Infect Dis 36(1):52–55
67. Poikonen E, Lyytikainen O, Anttila VJ, Ruutu P (2003) Candidemia in Finland, 1995-1999. Emerg Infect Dis 9(8):985–990
68. Sandven P, Bevanger L, Digranes A, Haukland HH, Mannsaker T, Gaustad P (2006) Candidemia in Norway (1991 to 2003): results from a nationwide study. J Clin Microbiol 44(6):1977–1981
69. Arendrup MC, Fuursted K, Gahrn-Hansen B, Jensen IM, Knudsen JD, Lundgren B et al (2005) Seminational surveillance of fungemia in Denmark: notably high rates of fungemia and numbers of isolates with reduced azole susceptibility. J Clin Microbiol 43(9):4434–4440
70. Baldesi O, Bailly S, Ruckly S, Lepape A, L'Heriteau F, Aupee M et al (2017) ICU-acquired candidaemia in France: epidemiology and temporal trends, 2004-2013 - a study from the REA-RAISIN network. J Infect 75(1):59–67
71. Cornely OA, Gachot B, Akan H, Bassetti M, Uzun O, Kibbler C et al (2015) Epidemiology and outcome of fungemia in a cancer Cohort of the Infectious Diseases Group (IDG) of the European Organization for Research and Treatment of Cancer (EORTC 65031). Clin Infect Dis 61(3):324–331
72. Viscoli C, Girmenia C, Marinus A, Collette L, Martino P, Vandercam B et al (1999) Candidemia in cancer patients: a prospective, multicenter surveillance study by the Invasive Fungal Infection Group (IFIG) of the European Organization for Research and Treatment of Cancer (EORTC). Clin Infect Dis 28(5):1071–1079
73. Mora-Duarte J, Betts R, Rotstein C, Colombo AL, Thompson-Moya L, Smietana J et al (2002) Comparison of caspofungin and amphotericin B for invasive candidiasis. N Engl J Med 347(25):2020–2029
74. Forrest GN, Weekes E, Johnson JK (2008) Increasing incidence of Candida parapsilosis candidemia with caspofungin usage. J Infect 56(2):126–129
75. Pfeiffer CD, Garcia-Effron G, Zaas AK, Perfect JR, Perlin DS, Alexander BD (2010) Breakthrough invasive candidiasis in patients on micafungin. J Clin Microbiol 48(7):2373–2380
76. Lortholary O, Desnos-Ollivier M, Sitbon K, Fontanet A, Bretagne S, Dromer F (2011) Recent exposure to caspofungin or fluconazole influences the epidemiology of candidemia: a prospective multicenter study involving 2,441 patients. Antimicrob Agents Chemother 55(2):532–538
77. Karimkhani C, Dellavalle RP, Coffeng LE, Flohr C, Hay RJ, Langan SM et al (2017) Global skin disease morbidity and mortality: an update from the global burden of disease study 2013. JAMA Dermatol 153(5):406–412
78. Seebacher C, Abeck D, Brasch J, Effendy I, Ginter-Hanselmayer G, Haake N et al (2006) Candidiasis of the skin. J Dtsch Dermatol Ges 4(7):591–596
79. Ledergerber B, Egger M, Erard V, Weber R, Hirschel B, Furrer H et al (1999) AIDS-related opportunistic illnesses occurring after initiation of potent antiretroviral therapy: the Swiss HIV Cohort Study. JAMA 282(23):2220–2226
80. Thoden J, Potthoff A, Bogner JR, Brockmeyer NH, Esser S, Grabmeier-Pfistershammer K et al (2013) Therapy and prophylaxis of opportunistic infections in HIV-infected patients: a guideline by the German and Austrian AIDS societies (DAIG/OAG) (AWMF 055/066). Infection 41(Suppl 2):S91–S115
81. Mendling W, Brasch J, Cornely OA, Effendy I, Friese K, Ginter-Hanselmayer G et al (2015) Guideline: vulvovaginal candidosis (AWMF 015/072), S2k (excluding chronic mucocutaneous candidosis). Mycoses 58(Suppl 1):1–15
82. Chocarro Martinez A, Galindo Tobal F, Ruiz-Irastorza G, Gonzalez Lopez A, Alvarez Navia F, Ochoa Sangrador C et al (2000) Risk factors for esophageal candidiasis. Eur J Clin Microbiol Infect Dis 19(2):96–100
83. Kirkpatrick CH (2001) Chronic mucocutaneous candidiasis. Pediatr Infect Dis J 20(2):197–206
84. Glocker E, Grimbacher B (2010) Chronic mucocutaneous candidiasis and congenital susceptibility to Candida. Curr Opin Allergy Clin Immunol 10(6):542–550
85. Lanternier F, Cypowyj S, Picard C, Bustamante J, Lortholary O, Casanova JL et al (2013) Primary immunodeficiencies underlying fungal infections. Curr Opin Pediatr 25(6):736–747
86. Puel A, Cypowyj S, Bustamante J, Wright JF, Liu L, Lim HK et al (2011) Chronic mucocutaneous candidiasis in humans with inborn errors of interleukin-17 immunity. Science 332(6025):65–68
87. Glocker EO, Hennigs A, Nabavi M, Schaffer AA, Woellner C, Salzer U et al (2009) A homozygous CARD9 mutation in a family with susceptibility to fungal infections. N Engl J Med 361(18):1727–1735
88. Skiest DJ, Vazquez JA, Anstead GM, Graybill JR, Reynes J, Ward D et al (2007) Posaconazole for the treatment of azole-refractory oropharyngeal and esophageal candidiasis in subjects with HIV infection. Clin Infect Dis 44(4):607–614
89. Firinu D, Massidda O, Lorrai MM, Serusi L, Peralta M, Barca MP et al (2011) Successful treatment of chronic mucocutaneous candidiasis caused by azole-resistant Candida albicans with posaconazole. Clin Dev Immunol 2011:283239
90. Bodey GP, Anaissie EJ, Edwards JE Jr (1993) Definitions of Candida infections. In: Bodey GP (ed) Candidiasis. Raven Press, Ltd., New York, pp 407–408
91. Hof H (2010) IFI = invasive fungal infections. What is that? A misnomer, because a non-invasive

fungal infection does not exist! Int J Infect Dis 14(6):e458–e459

92. Ascioglu S, Rex JH, De Pauw B, Bennett JE, Bille J, Crokaert F et al (2002) Defining opportunistic invasive fungal infections in immunocompromised patients with cancer and hematopoietic stem cell transplants: an international consensus. Clin Infect Dis 34(1):7–14
93. Pittet D, Monod M, Suter PM, Frenk E, Auckenthaler R (1994) Candida colonization and subsequent infections in critically ill surgical patients. Ann Surg 220(6):751–758
94. Solomkin JS (1996) Timing of treatment for nonneutropenic patients colonized with Candida. Am J Surg 172(6A):44S–48S
95. Eggimann P, Garbino J, Pittet D (2003) Management of Candida species infections in critically ill patients. Lancet Infect Dis 3(12):772–785
96. Playford EG, Lipman J, Kabir M, McBryde ES, Nimmo GR, Lau A et al (2009) Assessment of clinical risk predictive rules for invasive candidiasis in a prospective multicentre cohort of ICU patients. Intensive Care Med 35(12):2141–2145
97. Piarroux R, Grenouillet F, Balvay P, Tran V, Blasco G, Millon L et al (2004) Assessment of preemptive treatment to prevent severe candidiasis in critically ill surgical patients. Crit Care Med 32(12):2443–2449
98. Hall AM, Poole LA, Renton B, Wozniak A, Fisher M, Neal T et al (2013) Prediction of invasive candidal infection in critically ill patients with severe acute pancreatitis. Crit Care 17(2):R49
99. Leon C, Ruiz-Santana S, Saavedra P, Almirante B, Nolla-Salas J, Varez-Lerma F et al (2006) A bedside scoring system ("Candida score") for early antifungal treatment in nonneutropenic critically ill patients with Candida colonization. Crit Care Med 34(3):730–737
100. Ostrosky-Zeichner L, Sable C, Sobel J, Alexander BD, Donowitz G, Kan V et al (2007) Multicenter retrospective development and validation of a clinical prediction rule for nosocomial invasive candidiasis in the intensive care setting. Eur J Clin Microbiol Infect Dis 26(4):271–276
101. Leon C, Ruiz-Santana S, Saavedra P, Galvan B, Blanco A, Castro C et al (2009) Usefulness of the "Candida score" for discriminating between Candida colonization and invasive candidiasis in non-neutropenic critically ill patients: a prospective multicenter study. Crit Care Med 37(5):1624–1633
102. Ostrosky-Zeichner L, Pappas PG, Shoham S, Reboli A, Barron MA, Sims C et al (2009) Improvement of a clinical prediction rule for clinical trials on prophylaxis for invasive candidiasis in the intensive care unit. Mycoses 54(1):46–51
103. Kratzer C, Graninger W, Lassnigg A, Presterl E (2011) Design and use of Candida scores at the intensive care unit. Mycoses 54(6):467–474
104. Leroy O, Gangneux JP, Montravers P, Mira JP, Gouin F, Sollet JP et al (2009) Epidemiology, management, and risk factors for death of invasive Candida infections in critical care: a multicenter, prospective, observational study in France (2005-2006). Crit Care Med 37(5):1612–1618
105. Lortholary O, Renaudat C, Sitbon K, Madec Y, Oeud-Ndam L, Wolff M et al (2014) Worrisome trends in incidence and mortality of candidemia in intensive care units (Paris area, 2002-2010). Intensive Care Med 40(9):1303–1312
106. Eggimann P, Ostrosky-Zeichner L (2010) Early antifungal intervention strategies in ICU patients. Curr Opin Crit Care 16(5):465–469
107. Kullberg BJ, Arendrup MC (2015) Invasive candidiasis. N Engl J Med 373(15):1445–1456
108. Eggimann P, Pittet D (2014) Candida colonization index and subsequent infection in critically ill surgical patients: 20 years later. Intensive Care Med 40(10):1429–1448
109. Eggimann P, Garbino J, Pittet D (2003) Epidemiology of Candida species infections in critically ill non-immunosuppressed patients. Lancet Infect Dis 3(11):685–702
110. Kollef M, Micek S, Hampton N, Doherty JA, Kumar A (2012) Septic shock attributed to Candida infection: importance of empiric therapy and source control. Clin Infect Dis 54(12):1739–1746
111. Lecciones JA, Lee JW, Navarro EE, Witebsky FG, Marshall D, Steinberg SM et al (1992) Vascular catheter-associated fungemia in patients with cancer: analysis of 155 episodes. Clin Infect Dis 14(4): 875–883
112. Rex JH, Bennett JE, Sugar AM, Pappas PG, Serody J, Edwards JE et al (1995) Intravascular catheter exchange and duration of candidemia. NIAID Mycoses Study Group and the Candidemia Study Group. Clin Infect Dis 21(4):994–996
113. Raad I, Hanna H, Boktour M, Girgawy E, Danawi H, Mardani M et al (2004) Management of central venous catheters in patients with cancer and candidemia. Clin Infect Dis 38(8):1119–1127
114. Nucci M, Anaissie E, Betts RF, Dupont BF, Wu C, Buell DN et al (2010) Early removal of central venous catheter in patients with candidemia does not improve outcome: analysis of 842 patients from 2 randomized clinical trials. Clin Infect Dis 51(3):295–303
115. Wenzel RP, Gennings C (2005) Bloodstream infections due to Candida species in the intensive care unit: identifying especially high-risk patients to determine prevention strategies. Clin Infect Dis 41(Suppl 6):S389–S393
116. Labelle AJ, Micek ST, Roubinian N, Kollef MH (2008) Treatment-related risk factors for hospital mortality in Candida bloodstream infections. Crit Care Med 36(11):2967–2972
117. Anaissie EJ, Rex JH, Uzun O, Vartivarian S (1998) Predictors of adverse outcome in cancer patients with candidemia. Am J Med 104(3):238–245
118. Raad I, Hanna H, Maki D (2007) Intravascular catheter-related infections: advances in diagnosis,

prevention, and management. Lancet Infect Dis 7(10):645–657
119. Wolf HH, Leithauser M, Maschmeyer G, Salwender H, Klein U, Chaberny I et al (2008) Central venous catheter-related infections in hematology and oncology: guidelines of the Infectious Diseases Working Party (AGIHO) of the German Society of Hematology and Oncology (DGHO). Ann Hematol 87(11):863–876
120. Pappas PG, Kauffman CA, Andes DR, Clancy CJ, Marr KA, Ostrosky-Zeichner L et al (2016) Executive summary: clinical practice guideline for the management of candidiasis: 2016 update by the Infectious Diseases Society of America. Clin Infect Dis 62(4):409–417
121. Gamaletsou MN, Rammaert B, Bueno MA, Sipsas NV, Moriyama B, Kontoyiannis DP et al (2016) Candida arthritis: analysis of 112 pediatric and adult cases. Open Forum Infect Dis 3(1):ofv207
122. Gamaletsou MN, Kontoyiannis DP, Sipsas NV, Moriyama B, Alexander E, Roilides E et al (2012) Candida osteomyelitis: analysis of 207 pediatric and adult cases (1970-2011). Clin Infect Dis 55(10):1338–1351
123. Richaud C, De Lastours V, Panhard X, Petrover D, Bruno F, Lefort A (2017) Candida vertebral osteomyelitis (CVO) 28 cases from a 10-year retrospective study in France. Medicine 96(31):e7525
124. Stolberg-Stolberg J, Horn D, Rosslenbroich S, Riesenbeck O, Kampmeier S, Mohr M et al (2017) Management of destructive Candida albicans spondylodiscitis of the cervical spine: a systematic analysis of literature illustrated by an unusual case. Eur Spine J 26(4):1009–1018
125. Viale P (2009) Candida colonization and candiduria in critically ill patients in the intensive care unit. Drugs 69(Suppl 1):51–57
126. Sobel JD, Fisher JF, Kauffman CA, Newman CA (2011) Candida urinary tract infections--epidemiology. Clin Infect Dis 52(Suppl 6):S433–S436
127. Drogari-Apiranthitou M, Anyfantis I, Galani I, Kanioura L, Daikos GL, Petrikkos G (2017) Association between candiduria and candidemia: a clinical and molecular analysis of cases. Mycopathologia 182(11-12):1045–1052
128. Kauffman CA, Fisher JF, Sobel JD, Newman CA (2011) Candida urinary tract infections--diagnosis. Clin Infect Dis 52(Suppl 6):S452–S456
129. Fisher JF, Sobel JD, Kauffman CA, Newman CA (2011) Candida urinary tract infections--treatment. Clin Infect Dis 52(Suppl 6):S457–S466
130. Tuon FF, Amato VS, Penteado F Sr (2009) Bladder irrigation with amphotericin B and fungal urinary tract infection--systematic review with meta-analysis. Int J Infect Dis 13(6):701–706
131. Sullivan KA, Caylor MM, Lin FC, Campbell-Bright S (2017) Comparison of amphotericin B bladder irrigations versus fluconazole for the treatment of candiduria in intensive care unit patients. J Pharm Pract 30(3):347–352
132. Brooks RG (1989) Prospective study of Candida endophthalmitis in hospitalized patients with candidemia. Arch Intern Med 149(10):2226–2228
133. Parke DW, Jones DB, Gentry LO (1982) Endogenous endophthalmitis among patients with candidemia. Ophthalmology 89(7):789–796
134. Kato H, Yoshimura Y, Suido Y, Ide K, Sugiyama Y, Matsuno K et al (2018) Prevalence of, and risk factors for, hematogenous fungal endophthalmitis in patients with Candida bloodstream infection. Infection. https://doi.org/10.1007/s15010-018-1163-z
135. Steinbach WJ, Perfect JR, Cabell CH, Fowler VG, Corey GR, Li JS et al (2005) A meta-analysis of medical versus surgical therapy for Candida endocarditis. J Infect 51(3):230–247
136. Pierrotti LC, Baddour LM (2002) Fungal endocarditis, 1995-2000. Chest 122(1):302–310
137. Ellis ME, Al-Abdely H, Sandridge A, Greer W, Ventura W (2001) Fungal endocarditis: evidence in the world literature, 1965-1995. Clin Infect Dis 32(1):50–62
138. Baddley JW, Benjamin DK Jr, Patel M, Miro J, Athan E, Barsic B et al (2008) Candida infective endocarditis. Eur J Clin Microbiol Infect Dis 27(7): 519–529
139. Smego RA Jr, Ahmad H (2011) The role of fluconazole in the treatment of Candida endocarditis: a meta-analysis. Medicine 90(4):237–249
140. Lewis JH, Patel HR, Zimmerman HJ (1982) The spectrum of hepatic candidiasis. Hepatology 2(4):479–487
141. Jones JM (1981) Granulomatous hepatitis due to Candida albicans in patients with acute leukemia. Ann Intern Med 94(4 pt 1):475–477
142. Tashjian LS, Abramson JS, Peacock JE Jr (1984) Focal hepatic candidiasis: a distinct clinical variant of candidiasis in immunocompromised patients. Rev Infect Dis 6(5):689–703
143. Haron E, Feld R, Tuffnell P, Patterson B, Hasselback R, Matlow A (1987) Hepatic candidiasis: an increasing problem in immunocompromised patients. Am J Med 83(1):17–26
144. Thaler M, Pastakia B, Shawker TH, O'Leary T, Pizzo PA (1988) Hepatic candidiasis in cancer patients: the evolving picture of the syndrome. Ann Intern Med 108(1):88–100
145. Blade J, Lopez-Guillermo A, Rozman C, Granena A, Bruguera M, Bordas J et al (1992) Chronic systemic candidiasis in acute leukemia. Ann Hematol 64(5):240–244
146. Woolley I, Curtis D, Szer J, Fairley C, Vujovic O, Ugoni A et al (1997) High dose cytosine arabinoside is a major risk factor for the development of hepatosplenic candidiasis in patients with leukemia. Leuk Lymphoma 27(5-6):469–474
147. Anttila VJ, Elonen E, Nordling S, Sivonen A, Ruutu T, Ruutu P (1997) Hepatosplenic candidiasis in patients with acute leukemia: incidence and prognostic implications. Clin Infect Dis 24(3):375–380

148. Kontoyiannis DP, Luna MA, Samuels BI, Bodey GP (2000) Hepatosplenic candidiasis. A manifestation of chronic disseminated candidiasis. Infect Dis Clin N Am 14(3):721–739
149. Chen CY, Chen YC, Tang JL, Yao M, Huang SY, Tsai W et al (2003) Hepatosplenic fungal infection in patients with acute leukemia in Taiwan: incidence, treatment, and prognosis. Ann Hematol 82(2):93–97
150. Masood A, Sallah S (2005) Chronic disseminated candidiasis in patients with acute leukemia: emphasis on diagnostic definition and treatment. Leuk Res 29(5):493–501
151. Shirkhoda A, Lopez-Berestein G, Holbert JM, Luna MA (1986) Hepatosplenic fungal infection: CT and pathologic evaluation after treatment with liposomal amphotericin B. Radiology 159(2):349–353
152. Semelka RC, Shoenut JP, Greenberg HM, Bow EJ (1992) Detection of acute and treated lesions of hepatosplenic candidiasis: comparison of dynamic contrast-enhanced CT and MR imaging. J Magn Reson Imaging 2(3):341–345
153. Teyton P, Baillet G, Hindie E, Filmont JE, Sarandi F, Toubert ME et al (2009) Hepatosplenic candidiasis imaged with F-18 FDG PET/CT. Clin Nucl Med 34(7):439–440
154. Johnson TL, Barnett JL, Appelman HD, Nostrant T (1988) Candida hepatitis. Histopathologic diagnosis. Am J Surg Pathol 12(9):716–720
155. Fleischhacker M, Schulz S, Johrens K, von Lilienfeld-Toal M, Held T, Fietze E et al (2011) Diagnosis of chronic disseminated candidosis from liver biopsies by a novel PCR in patients with haematological malignancies. Clin Microbiol Infect 18(10):1010–1016
156. Gupta AO, Singh N (2011) Immune reconstitution syndrome and fungal infections. Curr Opin Infect Dis 24(6):527–533
157. Hu Z, Wei H, Meng F, Xu C, Cheng C, Yang Y (2013) Recurrent cryptococcal immune reconstitution inflammatory syndrome in an HIV-infected patient after anti-retroviral therapy: a case report. Ann Clin Microbiol Antimicrob 12:40
158. Lortholary O, Fontanet A, Memain N, Martin A, Sitbon K, Dromer F (2005) Incidence and risk factors of immune reconstitution inflammatory syndrome complicating HIV-associated cryptococcosis in France. AIDS 19(10):1043–1049
159. Jang YR, Kim MC, Kim T, Chong YP, Lee SO, Choi SH et al (2018) Clinical characteristics and outcomes of patients with chronic disseminated candidiasis who need adjuvant corticosteroid therapy. Med Mycol 56(6):782–786
160. Legrand F, Lecuit M, Dupont B, Bellaton E, Huerre M, Rohrlich PS et al (2008) Adjuvant corticosteroid therapy for chronic disseminated candidiasis. Clin Infect Dis 46(5):696–702
161. Lortholary O, Petrikkos G, Akova M, Arendrup MC, Rikan-Akdagli S, Bassetti M et al (2012) ESCMID* guideline for the diagnosis and management of Candida diseases 2012: patients with HIV infection or AIDS. Clin Microbiol Infect 18(Suppl 7):68–77
162. Cohen R, Roth FJ, Delgado E, Ahearn DG, Kalser MH (1969) Fungal flora of the normal human small and large intestine. N Engl J Med 280(12):638–641
163. Bassetti M, Marchetti M, Chakrabarti A, Colizza S, Garnacho-Montero J, Kett DH et al (2013) A research agenda on the management of intra-abdominal candidiasis: results from a consensus of multinational experts. Intensive Care Med 39(12):2092–2106
164. Bassetti M, Righi E, Ansaldi F, Merelli M, Scarparo C, Antonelli M et al (2015) A multicenter multinational study of abdominal candidiasis: epidemiology, outcomes and predictors of mortality. Intensive Care Med 41(9):1601–1610
165. Sandven P, Qvist H, Skovlund E, Giercksky KE (2002) Significance of Candida recovered from intraoperative specimens in patients with intra-abdominal perforations. Crit Care Med 30(3):541–547
166. de Ruiter J, Weel J, Manusama E, Kingma WP, van der Voort PH (2009) The epidemiology of intra-abdominal flora in critically ill patients with secondary and tertiary abdominal sepsis. Infection 37(6):522–527
167. Montravers P, Mira JP, Gangneux JP, Leroy O, Lortholary O (2011) A multicentre study of antifungal strategies and outcome of Candida spp. peritonitis in intensive-care units. Clin Microbiol Infect 17(7):1061–1067
168. Lagunes L, Rey-Perez A, Martin-Gomez MT, Vena A, de Egea V, Munoz P et al (2017) Association between source control and mortality in 258 patients with intra-abdominal candidiasis: a retrospective multi-centric analysis comparing intensive care versus surgical wards in Spain. Eur J Clin Microbiol Infect Dis 36(1):95–104
169. Montravers P, Perrigault PF, Timsit JF, Mira JP, Lortholary O, Leroy O et al (2017) Antifungal therapy for patients with proven or suspected Candida peritonitis: Amarcand2, a prospective cohort study in French intensive care units. Clin Microbiol Infect 23(2):117
170. Sanchez-Portocarrero J, Perez-Cecilia E, Corral O, Romero-Vivas J, Picazo JJ (2000) The central nervous system and infection by Candida species. Diagn Microbiol Infect Dis 37(3):169–179
171. O'Brien D, Stevens NT, Lim CH, O'Brien DF, Smyth E, Fitzpatrick F et al (2011) Candida infection of the central nervous system following neurosurgery: a 12-year review. Acta Neurochir 153(6):1347–1350
172. Nguyen MH, Yu VL (1995) Meningitis caused by Candida species: an emerging problem in neurosurgical patients. Clin Infect Dis 21(2):323–327
173. Fernandez M, Moylett EH, Noyola DE, Baker CJ (2000) Candidal meningitis in neonates: a 10-year review. Clin Infect Dis 31(2):458–463
174. Faix RG (1984) Systemic Candida infections in infants in intensive care nurseries: high incidence of central nervous system involvement. J Pediatr 105(4):616–622

175. Barton M, O'Brien K, Robinson JL, Davies DH, Simpson K, Asztalos E et al (2014) Invasive candidiasis in low birth weight preterm infants: risk factors, clinical course and outcome in a prospective multicenter study of cases and their matched controls. BMC Infect Dis 14:327
176. Montero A, Romero J, Vargas JA, Regueiro CA, Sanchez-Aloz G, De PF et al (2000) Candida infection of cerebrospinal fluid shunt devices: report of two cases and review of the literature. Acta Neurochir 142(1):67–74
177. Lanternier F, Mahdaviani SA, Barbati E, Chaussade H, Koumar Y, Levy R et al (2015) Inherited CARD9 deficiency in otherwise healthy children and adults with Candida species-induced meningoencephalitis, colitis, or both. J Allergy Clin Immunol 135(6):1558–1568
178. Friedman S, Richardson SE, Jacobs SE, O'Brien K (2000) Systemic Candida infection in extremely low birth weight infants: short term morbidity and long term neurodevelopmental outcome. Pediatr Infect Dis J 19(6):499–504
179. Hagensee ME, Bauwens JE, Kjos B, Bowden RA (1994) Brain abscess following marrow transplantation: experience at the Fred Hutchinson Cancer Research Center, 1984-1992. Clin Infect Dis 19(3):402–408
180. Gavino C, Cotter A, Lichtenstein D, Lejtenyi D, Fortin C, Legault C et al (2014) CARD9 deficiency and spontaneous central nervous system candidiasis: complete clinical remission with GM-CSF therapy. Clin Infect Dis 59(1):81–84
181. Sundaram C, Umabala P, Laxmi V, Purohit AK, Prasad VS, Panigrahi M et al (2006) Pathology of fungal infections of the central nervous system: 17 years' experience from Southern India. Histopathology 49(4):396–405
182. Pendlebury WW, Perl DP, Munoz DG (1989) Multiple microabscesses in the central nervous system: a clinicopathologic study. J Neuropathol Exp Neurol 48(3):290–300
183. Tunkel AR, Hasbun R, Bhimraj A, Byers K, Kaplan SL, Michael SW et al (2017) 2017 Infectious Diseases Society of America's clinical practice guidelines for healthcare-associated ventriculitis and meningitis. Clin Infect Dis. https://doi.org/10.1093/cid/ciw861
184. Hope WW, Castagnola E, Groll AH, Roilides E, Akova M, Arendrup MC et al (2012) ESCMID* guideline for the diagnosis and management of Candida diseases 2012: prevention and management of invasive infections in neonates and children caused by Candida spp. Clin Microbiol Infect 18(Suppl 7):38–52
185. Schmidt-Hieber M, Silling G, Schalk E, Heinz W, Panse J, Penack O et al (2016) CNS infections in patients with hematological disorders (including allogeneic stem-cell transplantation)-Guidelines of the Infectious Diseases Working Party (AGIHO) of the German Society of Hematology and Medical Oncology (DGHO). Ann Oncol 27(7):1207–1225
186. Pappas PG, Kauffman CA, Andes DR, Clancy CJ, Marr KA, Ostrosky-Zeichner L et al (2016) Clinical practice guideline for the management of candidiasis: 2016 update by the Infectious Diseases Society of America. Clin Infect Dis 62(4):e1–e50
187. Liu KH, Wu CJ, Chou CH, Lee HC, Lee NY, Hung ST et al (2004) Refractory candidal meningitis in an immunocompromised patient cured by caspofungin. J Clin Microbiol 42(12):5950–5953
188. Flattery AM, Hickey E, Gill CJ, Powles MA, Misura AS, Galgoci AM et al (2011) Efficacy of caspofungin in a juvenile mouse model of central nervous system candidiasis. Antimicrob Agents Chemother 55(7):3491–3497
189. Kume H, Yamazaki T, Abe M, Tanuma H, Okudaira M, Okayasu I (2006) Epidemiology of visceral mycoses in patients with leukemia and MDS - analysis of the data in annual of pathological autopsy cases in Japan in 1989, 1993, 1997 and 2001. Nippon Ishinkin Gakkai Zasshi 47(1):15–24
190. von EM, Zuhlsdorf M, Roos N, Hesse M, Schulten R, van de Loo J (1995) Pulmonary fungal infections in patients with hematological malignancies--diagnostic approaches. Ann Hematol 70(3):135–141
191. Blaschke S, Don M, Schillinger W, Ruchel R (2002) Candida pneumonia in patients without definitive immunodeficiency. Mycoses 45(Suppl 3):22–26
192. Chen KY, Ko SC, Hsueh PR, Luh KT, Yang PC (2001) Pulmonary fungal infection: emphasis on microbiological spectra, patient outcome, and prognostic factors. Chest 120(1):177–184
193. Dermawan JKT, Ghosh S, Keating MK, Gopalakrishna KV, Mukhopadhyay S (2018) Candida pneumonia with severe clinical course, recovery with antifungal therapy and unusual pathologic findings: a case report. Medicine 97(2):e9650
194. Yamazaki T, Kume H, Murase S, Yamashita E, Arisawa M (1999) Epidemiology of visceral mycoses: analysis of data in annual of the pathological autopsy cases in Japan. J Clin Microbiol 37(6):1732–1738
195. Kume H, Yamazaki T, Abe M, Tanuma H, Okudaira M, Okayasu I (2003) Increase in aspergillosis and severe mycotic infection in patients with leukemia and MDS: comparison of the data from the Annual of the Pathological Autopsy Cases in Japan in 1989, 1993 and 1997. Pathol Int 53(11):744–750
196. Chamilos G, Luna M, Lewis RE, Bodey GP, Chemaly R, Tarrand JJ et al (2006) Invasive fungal infections in patients with hematologic malignancies in a tertiary care cancer center: an autopsy study over a 15-year period (1989-2003). Haematologica 91(7):986–989
197. Donhuijsen K, Petersen P, Schmid WK (2008) Trend reversal in the frequency of mycoses in hematological neoplasias: autopsy results from 1976 to 2005. Dtsch Arztebl Int 105(28-29):501–506
198. Lehrnbecher T, Frank C, Engels K, Kriener S, Groll AH, Schwabe D (2010) Trends in the postmortem

epidemiology of invasive fungal infections at a university hospital. J Infect 61(3):259–265
199. Suzuki Y, Kume H, Togano T, Kanoh Y, Ohto H (2013) Epidemiology of visceral mycoses in autopsy cases in Japan: the data from 1989 to 2009 in the annual of pathological autopsy cases in Japan. Med Mycol 51(5):522–526
200. Delisle MS, Williamson DR, Albert M, Perreault MM, Jiang X, Day AG et al (2011) Impact of Candida species on clinical outcomes in patients with suspected ventilator-associated pneumonia. Can Respir J 18(3):131–136
201. Delisle MS, Williamson DR, Perreault MM, Albert M, Jiang X, Heyland DK (2008) The clinical significance of Candida colonization of respiratory tract secretions in critically ill patients. J Crit Care 23(1):11–17
202. el-Ebiary M, Torres A, Fabregas N, de la Bellacasa JP, Gonzalez J, Ramirez J et al (1997) Significance of the isolation of Candida species from respiratory samples in critically ill, non-neutropenic patients. An immediate postmortem histologic study. Am J Respir Crit Care Med 156(2 Pt 1):583–590
203. Garnacho-Montero J, Olaechea P, varez-Lerma F, varez-Rocha L, Blanquer J, Galvan B et al (2013) Epidemiology, diagnosis and treatment of fungal respiratory infections in the critically ill patient. Rev Esp Quimioter 26(2):173–188
204. Clancy CJ, Nguyen MH, Morris AJ (1997) Candidal mediastinitis: an emerging clinical entity. Clin Infect Dis 25(3):608–613
205. Kofteridis DP, Mantadakis E, Karatzanis AD, Bourolias CA, Papazoglou G, Velegrakis GA et al (2008) Non-Candida albicans Candida mediastinitis of odontogenic origin in a diabetic patient. Med Mycol 46(4):345–348
206. Garey KW, Rege M, Pai MP, Mingo DE, Suda KJ, Turpin RS et al (2006) Time to initiation of fluconazole therapy impacts mortality in patients with candidemia: a multi-institutional study. Clin Infect Dis 43(1):25–31
207. Morrell M, Fraser VJ, Kollef MH (2005) Delaying the empiric treatment of candida bloodstream infection until positive blood culture results are obtained: a potential risk factor for hospital mortality. Antimicrob Agents Chemother 49(9):3640–3645
208. Bodey G, Bueltmann B, Duguid W, Gibbs D, Hanak H, Hotchi M et al (1992) Fungal infections in cancer patients: an international autopsy survey. Eur J Clin Microbiol Infect Dis 11(2):99–109
209. Jones JM (1990) Laboratory diagnosis of invasive candidiasis. Clin Microbiol Rev 3(1):32–45
210. Ness MJ, Vaughan WP, Woods GL (1989) Candida antigen latex test for detection of invasive candidiasis in immunocompromised patients. J Infect Dis 159(3):495–502
211. Ruhnke M, Böhme A, Buchheidt D, Donhuijsen K, Einsele H, Enzensberger R et al (2003) Diagnosis of invasive fungal infections in hematology and oncology--guidelines of the Infectious Diseases Working Party (AGIHO) of the German Society of Hematology and Oncology (DGHO). Ann Hematol 82(Suppl 2):S141–S148
212. Lee A, Mirrett S, Reller LB, Weinstein MP (2007) Detection of bloodstream infections in adults: how many blood cultures are needed? J Clin Microbiol 45(11):3546–3548
213. Horvath LL, George BJ, Hospenthal DR (2007) Detection of fifteen species of Candida in an automated blood culture system. J Clin Microbiol 45(9):3062–3064
214. Horvath LL, George BJ, Murray CK, Harrison LS, Hospenthal DR (2004) Direct comparison of the BACTEC 9240 and BacT/ALERT 3D automated blood culture systems for candida growth detection. J Clin Microbiol 42(1):115–118
215. Fricker-Hidalgo H, Lebeau B, Pelloux H, Grillot R (2004) Use of the BACTEC 9240 system with mycosis-IC/F blood culture bottles for detection of fungemia. J Clin Microbiol 42(4):1855–1856
216. Jensen J, Munoz P, Guinea J, Rodriguez-Creixems M, Pelaez T, Bouza E (2007) Mixed fungemia: incidence, risk factors, and mortality in a general hospital. Clin Infect Dis 44(12):e109–e114
217. Bouza E, Alcala L, Munoz P, Martin-Rabadan P, Guembe M, Rodriguez-Creixems M (2013) Can microbiologists help to assess catheter involvement in candidaemic patients before removal? Clin Microbiol Infect 19(2):E129–E135
218. Bouza E, Burillo A, Munoz P, Guinea J, Marin M, Rodriguez-Creixems M (2013) Mixed bloodstream infections involving bacteria and Candida spp. J Antimicrob Chemother 68(8):1881–1888
219. Sendid B, Poirot JL, Tabouret M, Bonnin A, Caillot D, Camus D et al (2002) Combined detection of mannanaemia and antimannan antibodies as a strategy for the diagnosis of systemic infection caused by pathogenic Candida species. J Med Microbiol 51(5):433–442
220. Sendid B, Caillot D, Baccouch-Humbert B, Klingspor L, Grandjean M, Bonnin A et al (2003) Contribution of the Platelia Candida-specific antibody and antigen tests to early diagnosis of systemic Candida tropicalis infection in neutropenic adults. J Clin Microbiol 41(10):4551–4558
221. Odabasi Z, Mattiuzzi G, Estey E, Kantarjian H, Saeki F, Ridge RJ et al (2004) Beta-D-glucan as a diagnostic adjunct for invasive fungal infections: validation, cutoff development, and performance in patients with acute myelogenous leukemia and myelodysplastic syndrome. Clin Infect Dis 39(2):199–205
222. Ostrosky-Zeichner L, Alexander BD, Kett DH, Vazquez J, Pappas PG, Saeki F et al (2005) Multicenter clinical evaluation of the (1-->3) beta-D-glucan assay as an aid to diagnosis of fungal infections in humans. Clin Infect Dis 41(5):654–659
223. Presterl E, Parschalk B, Bauer E, Lassnigg A, Hajdu S, Graninger W (2009) Invasive fungal infections and (1,3)-beta-D-glucan serum concentrations in

long-term intensive care patients. Int J Infect Dis 13(6):707–712

224. Posteraro B, De PG, Tumbarello M, Torelli R, Pennisi MA, Bello G et al (2011) Early diagnosis of candidemia in intensive care unit patients with sepsis: a prospective comparison of (1-->3)-beta-D-glucan assay, Candida score, and colonization index. Crit Care 15(5):R249
225. Shepard JR, Addison RM, Alexander BD, la-Latta P, Gherna M, Haase G et al (2008) Multicenter evaluation of the Candida albicans/Candida glabrata peptide nucleic acid fluorescent in situ hybridization method for simultaneous dual-color identification of C. albicans and C. glabrata directly from blood culture bottles. J Clin Microbiol 46(1):50–55
226. Marklein G, Josten M, Klanke U, Muller E, Horre R, Maier T et al (2009) Matrix-assisted laser desorption ionization-time of flight mass spectrometry for fast and reliable identification of clinical yeast isolates. J Clin Microbiol 47(9):2912–2917
227. Mylonakis E, Clancy CJ, Ostrosky-Zeichner L, Garey KW, Alangaden GJ, Vazquez JA et al (2015) T2 magnetic resonance assay for the rapid diagnosis of candidemia in whole blood: a clinical trial. Clin Infect Dis 60(6):892–899
228. Zacharioudakis IM, Zervou FN, Mylonakis E (2018) T2 magnetic resonance assay: overview of available data and clinical implications. J Fungi 4(2):E45
229. Shorr AF, Chung K, Jackson WL, Waterman PE, Kollef MH (2005) Fluconazole prophylaxis in critically ill surgical patients: a meta-analysis. Crit Care Med 33(9):1928–1935
230. Cornely OA, Bassetti M, Calandra T, Garbino J, Kullberg BJ, Lortholary O et al (2012) ESCMID* guideline for the diagnosis and management of Candida diseases 2012: non-neutropenic adult patients. Clin Microbiol Infect 18(Suppl 7):19–37
231. Schuster MG, Edwards JE Jr, Sobel JD, Darouiche RO, Karchmer AW, Hadley S et al (2008) Empirical fluconazole versus placebo for intensive care unit patients: a randomized trial. Ann Intern Med 149(2):83–90
232. Cui N, Wang H, Su L, Qiu H, Li R, Liu D (2017) Initial therapeutic strategy of invasive candidiasis for intensive care unit patients: a retrospective analysis from the China-SCAN study. BMC Infect Dis 17(1):93
233. Zilberberg MD, Kollef MH, Arnold H, Labelle A, Micek ST, Kothari S et al (2010) Inappropriate empiric antifungal therapy for candidemia in the ICU and hospital resource utilization: a retrospective cohort study. BMC Infect Dis 10:150
234. Kullberg BJ, Sobel JD, Ruhnke M, Pappas PG, Viscoli C, Rex JH et al (2005) Voriconazole versus a regimen of amphotericin B followed by fluconazole for candidaemia in non-neutropenic patients: a randomised non-inferiority trial. Lancet 366(9495):1435–1442
235. Pappas PG, Rotstein CM, Betts RF, Nucci M, Talwar D, De Waele JJ et al (2007) Micafungin versus caspofungin for treatment of candidemia and other forms of invasive candidiasis. Clin Infect Dis 45(7):883–893
236. Reboli AC, Rotstein C, Pappas PG, Chapman SW, Kett DH, Kumar D et al (2007) Anidulafungin versus fluconazole for invasive candidiasis. N Engl J Med 356(24):2472–2482
237. Mousset S, Buchheidt D, Heinz W, Ruhnke M, Cornely OA, Egerer G et al (2013) Treatment of invasive fungal infections in cancer patients-updated recommendations of the Infectious Diseases Working Party (AGIHO) of the German Society of Hematology and Oncology (DGHO). Ann Hematol 93(1):13–32
238. Tissot F, Agrawal S, Pagano L, Petrikkos G, Groll AH, Skiada A et al (2017) ECIL-6 guidelines for the treatment of invasive candidiasis, aspergillosis and mucormycosis in leukemia and hematopoietic stem cell transplant patients. Haematologica 102(3):433–444
239. Ostrosky-Zeichner L, Rex JH, Pappas PG, Hamill RJ, Larsen RA, Horowitz HW et al (2003) Antifungal susceptibility survey of 2,000 bloodstream Candida isolates in the United States. Antimicrob Agents Chemother 47(10):3149–3154
240. Pfaller MA, Boyken L, Hollis RJ, Messer SA, Tendolkar S, Diekema DJ (2005) In vitro activities of anidulafungin against more than 2,500 clinical isolates of Candida spp., including 315 isolates resistant to fluconazole. J Clin Microbiol 43(11):5425–5427
241. Rex JH, Bennett JE, Sugar AM, Pappas PG, van der Horst CM, Edwards JE et al (1994) A randomized trial comparing fluconazole with amphotericin B for the treatment of candidemia in patients without neutropenia. Candidemia Study Group and the National Institute. N Engl J Med 331(20):1325–1330
242. Rex JH, Pappas PG, Karchmer AW, Sobel J, Edwards JE, Hadley S et al (2003) A randomized and blinded multicenter trial of high-dose fluconazole plus placebo versus fluconazole plus amphotericin B as therapy for candidemia and its consequences in nonneutropenic subjects. Clin Infect Dis 36(10):1221–1228
243. Kuse ER, Chetchotisakd P, da Cunha CA, Ruhnke M, Barrios C, Raghunadharao D et al (2007) Micafungin versus liposomal amphotericin B for candidaemia and invasive candidosis: a phase III randomised double-blind trial. Lancet 369(9572):1519–1527
244. Groll AH, Castagnola E, Cesaro S, Dalle JH, Engelhard D, Hope W et al (2014) Fourth European Conference on Infections in Leukaemia (ECIL-4): guidelines for diagnosis, prevention, and treatment of invasive fungal diseases in paediatric patients with cancer or allogeneic haemopoietic stem-cell transplantation. Lancet Oncol 15(8):e327–e340
245. Ruhnke M, Paiva JA, Meersseman W, Pachl J, Grigoras I, Sganga G et al (2012) Anidulafungin for the treatment of candidaemia/invasive candidiasis in selected critically ill patients. Clin Microbiol Infect 18(7):680–687

246. Betts RF, Nucci M, Talwar D, Gareca M, Queiroz-Telles F, Bedimo RJ et al (2009) A multicenter, double-blind trial of a high-dose caspofungin treatment regimen versus a standard caspofungin treatment regimen for adult patients with invasive candidiasis. Clin Infect Dis 48(12):1676–1684
247. Maertens JA, Raad II, Marr KA, Patterson TF, Kontoyiannis DP, Cornely OA et al (2016) Isavuconazole versus voriconazole for primary treatment of invasive mould disease caused by Aspergillus and other filamentous fungi (SECURE): a phase 3, randomised-controlled, non-inferiority trial. Lancet 387(10020):760–769
248. Marty FM, Ostrosky-Zeichner L, Cornely OA, Mullane KM, Perfect JR, Thompson GR et al (2016) Isavuconazole treatment for mucormycosis: a single-arm open-label trial and case-control analysis. Lancet Infect Dis 16:828–837
249. Centers for Disease Control and Prevention (2013) Antibiotic resistance threats in the United States. 1-114. 16-9-2013. 1600 Clifton Rd. Atlanta, GA 30333, USA, Centers for Disease Control and Prevention. Ref Type: Internet Communication
250. Tacconelli E, Cataldo MA, Dancer SJ, De AG, Falcone M, Frank U et al (2014) ESCMID guidelines for the management of the infection control measures to reduce transmission of multidrug-resistant Gram-negative bacteria in hospitalized patients. Clin Microbiol Infect 20(Suppl 1):1–55
251. Pittet D (2001) Compliance with hand disinfection and its impact on hospital-acquired infections. J Hosp Infect 48(Suppl A):S40–S46
252. Zingg W, Imhof A, Maggiorini M, Stocker R, Keller E, Ruef C (2009) Impact of a prevention strategy targeting hand hygiene and catheter care on the incidence of catheter-related bloodstream infections. Crit Care Med 37(7):2167–2173
253. Clark TA, Slavinski SA, Morgan J, Lott T, rthington-Skaggs BA, Brandt ME et al (2004) Epidemiologic and molecular characterization of an outbreak of Candida parapsilosis bloodstream infections in a community hospital. J Clin Microbiol 42(10):4468–4472
254. Strausbaugh LJ, Sewell DL, Ward TT, Pfaller MA, Heitzman T, Tjoelker R (1994) High frequency of yeast carriage on hands of hospital personnel. J Clin Microbiol 32(9):2299–2300
255. Climo MW, Yokoe DS, Warren DK, Perl TM, Bolon M, Herwaldt LA et al (2013) Effect of daily chlorhexidine bathing on hospital-acquired infection. N Engl J Med 368(6):533–542
256. MacDougall C, Polk RE (2005) Antimicrobial stewardship programs in health care systems. Clin Microbiol Rev 18(4):638–656
257. Ruhnke M (2014) Antifungal stewardship in invasive Candida infections. Clin Microbiol Infect 20(Suppl 6):11–18
258. Jones TM, Drew RH, Wilson DT, Sarubbi C, Anderson DJ (2017) Impact of automatic infectious diseases consultation on the management of fungemia at a large academic medical center. Am J Health Syst Pharm 74(23):1997–2003
259. Ostrosky-Zeichner L (2003) New approaches to the risk of Candida in the intensive care unit. Curr Opin Infect Dis 16(6):533–537
260. Penk A, Pittrow L (1998) Status of fluconazole in the therapy of endogenous Candida endophthalmitis. Mycoses 41(Suppl 2):41–44
261. Breit SM, Hariprasad SM, Mieler WF, Shah GK, Mills MD, Grand MG (2005) Management of endogenous fungal endophthalmitis with voriconazole and caspofungin. Am J Ophthalmol 139(1):135–140
262. Nasser RM, Melgar GR, Longworth DL, Gordon SM (1997) Incidence and risk of developing fungal prosthetic valve endocarditis after nosocomial candidemia. Am J Med 103(1):25–32
263. Cornely OA, Lasso M, Betts R, Klimko N, Vazquez J, Dobb G et al (2007) Caspofungin for the treatment of less common forms of invasive candidiasis. J Antimicrob Chemother 60(2):363–369
264. Kujath P, Lerch K, Kochendorfer P, Boos C (1993) Comparative study of the efficacy of fluconazole versus amphotericin B/flucytosine in surgical patients with systemic mycoses. Infection 21(6):376–382
265. Abele-Horn M, Kopp A, Sternberg U, Ohly A, Dauber A, Russwurm W et al (1996) A randomized study comparing fluconazole with amphotericin B/5-flucytosine for the treatment of systemic Candida infections in intensive care patients. Infection 24(6):426–432
266. Penk A, Pittrow L (1998) Fungal arthritis--a rare complication of systemic candidiasis or orthopedic intervention. Review of therapeutic experience with fluconazole. Mycoses 41(Suppl 2):45–48
267. Mouas H, Lutsar I, Dupont B, Fain O, Herbrecht R, Lescure FX et al (2005) Voriconazole for invasive bone aspergillosis: a worldwide experience of 20 cases. Clin Infect Dis 40(8):1141–1147
268. Fan-Havard P, O'Donovan C, Smith SM, Oh J, Bamberger M, Eng RH (1995) Oral fluconazole versus amphotericin B bladder irrigation for treatment of candidal funguria. Clin Infect Dis 21(4):960–965

Clinical Syndromes: *Aspergillus* 5

Rosa Bellmann-Weiler and Romuald Bellmann

Invasive *Aspergillus* infection (IAI) is the second most common invasive fungal infection among patients with hematological malignancies [1]. Systemic infection with *Aspergillus* spp. is potentially life-threatening for patients suffering from severe diseases.

Persons at risk have severe and prolonged immunosuppression and may suffer from a hematological malignancy (in the first line patients with acute myeloid leukemia and recipients of allogeneic HSCT). Moreover solid organ transplant recipients and patients treated with corticosteroids for exacerbated COPD or with multiple myeloma are increasingly at risk for IAI [2, 3]. The most important risk factor is particularly severe granulocytopenia (<0.5 G/L), but other risk factors also include AIDS in a progressive stage and also intensive care patients with corticosteroid treatment, lung disease, and renal failure [4]. Additionally, patients who have to take immunosuppressive drugs other than corticosteroids or those suffering from inherited immunodeficiency may develop a severe *Aspergillus* infection [5]. IAI may result in a high mortality up to 90% in severely immunocompromised patients with involvement of the central nervous system [6–8]. The variance in epidemiological data may be due to the use of a variety of diagnostic tools. Most studies are based on autopsy results. In these studies *Aspergillus* species identification was rarely done. Although antemortem diagnosis of IAI has improved, some cases of IAI remain undetected. With the reduction in autopsies over time, a reliable estimate of the real prevalence of IAI in high-risk patients will not be available in the near future [9].

The four most common pathogenic species are *Aspergillus fumigatus*, *Aspergillus flavus*, *Aspergillus niger*, and *Aspergillus terreus*. However, there is a shift in the prevalence of the *Aspergillus* species in transplantation centers in the USA describing a decrease of *A. fumigatus* and an increase of *A. flavus*, *A. niger* and *A. terreus* [6, 10]. Thus, particularly in medical centers caring for patients with hemato-oncological diseases, stem cell, and solid organ transplantation, a specialized mycological laboratory service is pivotal for the modern diagnostic methods and exact identification plus susceptibility testing of pathogenic fungi (see Chap. 1). The knowledge of the locally predominant species is essential for the choice of therapy since, for example, *A. terreus* is resistant against amphotericin B (AMB) [11].

R. Bellmann-Weiler (✉)
Department of Internal Medicine II, Medical University of Innsbruck, Innsbruck, Austria
e-mail: rosa.bellmann-weiler@i-med.ac.at

R. Bellmann
Clinical Pharmacokinetics Unit, Division of Intensive Care and Emergency Medicine, Department of Internal Medicine I, Medical University of Innsbruck, Innsbruck, Austria

E. Presterl (ed.), *Clinically Relevant Mycoses*, https://doi.org/10.1007/978-3-319-92300-0_5

5.1 Diagnosis

The diagnosis of IAI is challenging. Diagnosis of IAI requires careful evaluation of the patient's history, clinical signs, and laboratory and microbiological work-up.

According to a review of the literature and the guidelines, invasive aspergillosis is defined as proven, probable, and possible [12]. The EORTC criteria classify IAI as proven, probable, and possible for clinical studies. These criteria were mainly defined for performing and comparing clinical studies but are also helpful in the diagnostic work-up and management in the clinical routine. IAI is proven by histopathology and positive culture of a specimen from a sterile site. IAI is defined as probable if there are clinical signs and symptoms of IAI but negative cultures and *Aspergillus* suggestive hyphae in histopathology, or negative cultures but positive galactomannan assay, or beta-D-glucan assay and typical radiologic signs (computed tomography). The sensitivity of chest radiography is low in the earliest stages of pulmonary infection. The radiographic manifestations are variable according to the host and the type of disease. There is a broad range of alterations from unspecific peribronchial infiltrations, nodules, or consolidations with or without cavitation. The mentioned lesions may be single or multiple. The next step in the workflow for diagnosis of IAI is the (high-resolution) computed tomography (CT) of chest and/or any other body site depending on the clinical sites and symptoms. To exclude systemic IAI, a full body CT including the brain is strongly recommended. CT scan is the diagnostic gold standard for imaging IAI. CT reveals alterations in lung tissue at an earlier stage and more precisely. The CT findings largely depend on the host. In patients with neutropenia, initial infiltrates and/or nodules with surrounding ground-glass infiltrates are described. These are called "halo signs," reflecting hemorrhages into the area surrounding the fungal infiltration. In a typical course of the disease, the nodules enlarge; they may cavitate. This cavitation of the former solid nodule is called "air-crescent sign." The appearance of the air-crescent sign is supposed to be linked with reconstitution of the immune response but independent of appropriate therapy. The material inside is infarcted lung tissue containing *Aspergillus*, but it may also be another fungus. This is also called a mycotic lung sequestrum. Any nodules or abscesses at any site in patients at risk for IAI may be caused by *Aspergillus* sp. To prove or to exclude IAI, a needle biopsy with mycological and with histology work-up is recommended [13]. Blood cultures hardly show positive results, even in invasive infection.

Therefore, for the diagnosis of pulmonary IAI, the acquisition of a specimen by bronchoalveolar lavage, CT-assisted transthoracic percutaneous needle aspiration, or even thoracoscopic biopsy is the diagnostic options. These procedures assume that the patient is hemodynamically stable, has sufficient platelet counts, and has normal or only slight-altered coagulation values. For cytological and histopathologic examinations and fungal culture and identification, presentative specimens of bronchial fluid or tissue are required. Hemato-oncological centers have specialized laboratories, where molecular diagnostic methods and antifungal susceptibility testing are available. The identification of the *Aspergillus species* is also recommended in the recently published guidelines of the IDSA [14].

Microscopy and histology are conclusive for IAI, if the specimen is gained from a sterile body site ("relevant specimen"). This diagnostic method allows exclusion of contamination and differentiation between septate and non-septate hyphae and pseudohyphae and is available within a short time. However, microscopy and culture of specimen from BAL which is not considered to be "relevant" display a sensitivity of about 50% in high-risk patients suffering from a hematologic disease. Culture results are available only a few days after the onset and do not assure the differentiation between contamination, colonization, or infection. Advantages of cultures are that they facilitate the identification of *Aspergillus species* and determination of susceptibility testing to antifungal agents for therapy guidance.

Biomarkers like the surface galactomannan (GM) and β-D-glucan (BDG) or molecular (PCR) techniques are considered to be helpful for a reliable diagnosis of IAI in the absence of positive culture results. Information and details for both, GM and BDG, are given in Chap. 1. Briefly, whether a positive GM result justifies initiation of preemptive therapy for suspected IAI can only be answered in context with the patient's risk factors for IAI and the clinical presentation. But, in case of suspected infection of the central nervous system, this test is also of diagnostic value. Therapeutic monitoring may be facilitated by serial determination of the GM in blood.

Detection of *Aspergillus* nucleic acid in the different specimens is still a challenge. Validated and commercially available assays are a precondition for application in the clinical microbiology lab. The advantage of a PCR in the obtained specimen is the timely delivery of a specific result. However, molecular detection methods, such as PCR, are more sensitive than culture. Again, it is important to consider the particular patient's clinical situation and risk factors for IAI. The presence of fungal nucleic acid in relevant material alone is not the proof of infection but may have the consequence of further diagnostic procedures. For details of molecular fungal diagnostics, see also in Chap. 1.

According to experts' opinion, the *interpretation of the microbiological results* requires several items to be considered, particularly in case of strong suspicion of IAI but negative culture results:

- Was antifungal therapy started before diagnostic samples were taken?
- Is the quality of the specimen relevant, i.e., sterile site of the needle biopsy, bronchoalveolar lavage, superficial swabs, or any respiratory tract secretions?

For example in severely immunocompromised patients with hematological malignancy, the interpretation of the radiological films (preferentially CT-scan) is of utmost importance. An intrapulmonary lesion with halo sign or air-crescent sign is characteristic though not diagnostic for invasive pulmonary aspergillosis. However, similar radiological signs may be described in infections with other fungi like *Zygomycetes*, *Fusarium* spp., or *Scedosporium* spp. but also with bacteria like *Pseudomonas aeruginosa* or *Nocardia* spp. These typical radiological signs are only described for patients with severe neutropenia and hematological malignancies but cannot be extrapolated on other immunocompromised patients [15]. Because of the high risk for invasive *Aspergillus* infection in immunocompromised patients, guidelines for the diagnosis and treatment have been published and are continuously updated [14, 16]. Nevertheless, the diagnostic pathways have to be tailored to patient groups at risk as well as the availability of a microbiological laboratory familiar with mycology and of radiological services optimally equipped with an interventional unit for needle biopsies.

5.1.1 Clinical Presentations of IAI

Aspergillus sp. may enter the body through the lower respiratory tract, the sinuses, or the skin. From there either direct continuation of invasive growth or hematogenous dissemination may follow. Spread of *Aspergillus* infection to the central nervous system (CNS), the thyroid gland, the skin, the cardiovascular tissue, and each possible organ can potentially occur.

5.1.2 Clinical Presentation

On the assumption that the conidia of *Aspergillus* are inhaled into the lungs or sinuses, IAI most frequently presents with respiratory symptoms. Less common ways of inoculation of *Aspergillus* are the ingestion via the gastrointestinal tract or direct inoculation via skin lesions.

Invasive pulmonary *Aspergillus infection* is the most common invasive fungal infection in patients with hematological malignancies, second only to invasive Candida infection. However, in the times of antifungal prophylaxis, invasive fungal infection caused by other fungi may emerge in this distinct patient population. Patients usually present with fever not responsive to broad-spectrum antibacterial therapy, pleuritic chest pain, shortness of breath, cough, and sometimes hemoptysis. Even if antifungal prophylaxis has been administered, the next diagnostic steps will be the CT scan of the lungs, the acquisition of respiratory samples for fungal culture preferentially by needle biopsy and only second by BAL, and the determination of biomarkers (GM, BDG).

For hemoptysis symptomatic treatment is sufficient for mild hemoptysis, whereas embolization may be required with this severe complication with bleeding from vascular nexus of small vessels of the systemic circulation. With a skilled interventional radiologist, the chance of a successful embolization is high, though up to 50% of the patients can develop recurrent hemoptysis. A successful long-term antifungal therapy can help to minimize the rate of relapses.

Tracheobronchitis occurs most commonly in patients with severe COPD, lung transplantation, hematological malignancies, and bone marrow transplantation and may be obstructive, ulcerative, or pseudomembranous. In lung transplant recipients, *Aspergillus* tracheobronchitis may develop in the bronchial stump due to infection of the suture material. In this concern nylon sutures should be preferred to silk material [17]. Though immunocompromised patients and patients at risk may only report fever but no pulmonary symptoms. Performing high-resolution CT scan is mandatory when invasive aspergillosis is suspected because conventional x-rays have poor sensitivity.

Disseminated invasive Aspergillus infection refers to IAI with metastatic lesions in many organs including the brain, bone, skin, eyes, thyroid gland, liver, kidneys, and any other body sites. The pathogenesis is either by direct invasive growth when the fungus invades the vessels or most probably via dissemination by macrophages which take up the conidia but are incompetent to kill the fungus [18]. The prognosis of generalized disease is very poor.

Invasive Aspergillus infection of the central nervous system involves the brain, the meninges, or the myelon either by dissemination or continuous infection from local extension from the paranasal sinuses or by dissemination [19]. The clinical symptoms of *Aspergillus* infection of the CNS include focal neurological signs or even generalized seizures. Cerebral mycotic aneurysm is a severe complication because it may rupture and cause a hemorrhage [20].

Invasive Aspergillus infection of the eye includes corneal infection by direct inoculation after trauma with presentation of pain in the eye and visual alterations. The outcome may be poor with loss of vision, and sometimes progression of disease may necessitate enucleation of the usually totally destroyed eye ball [18, 21].

Invasive Aspergillus infection of the heart may present as endocarditis, predominantly as prosthetic valve endocarditis or as invasive *Aspergillus* myopericarditis. The time of inoculation infection may be during or shortly after the surgical intervention. However, the presence of ill-kept central vascular catheters or intravenous drug abuse are risk factors for *Aspergillus* endocarditis. The symptoms are usually fever and septic embolism. In case of *Aspergillus* endocarditis, blood cultures may be positive for *Aspergillus* sp. To exclude contamination more than two sets of blood cultures should be taken. However, negative blood cultures do not exclude *Aspergillus* endocarditis if there are vegetations or paravalvular abscesses, and no other pathogen isolated and GM in serum is repeatedly positive. The demonstration of invasive *Aspergillus* hyphae in the tissue and the growth of *Aspergillus* sp. of the culture of excised valves are the proof of infection. Therapy includes antifungal treatment and surgical therapy. However, the prognosis of cardiac involvement is poor.

The skin may be involved directly via inoculation, by trauma, burns, or during operation. Otherwise the skin may be involved in disseminated IAI particularly in patients with hematological malignancies or allogenic stem cell transplantation. Lesions in skin level may be reddish at first but then get blue to dark gray color (see also cutaneous aspergillosis). Later there may develop ulceration in severe cases. Deep skin biopsy for microscopy and microbiology is the diagnostic method of choice.

Gastrointestinal IAI may present as focal neutropenic enterocolitis, appendicitis, colonic ulcers with gastrointestinal hemorrhage, and abdominal pain. Mucositis in patients with neutropenia and in patients receiving high doses of corticosteroids allow direct invasion of ingested *Aspergillus* cells [22].

Chronic pulmonary aspergillosis (CPA) is a rare pulmonary *Aspergillus* infection and is caused by *Aspergillus fumigatus*, although patients have been described with *A. niger* or *A. flavus* infection. Occasionally, *A. fumigatus* isolates may be atypical, growing slowly with poor sporulation, delaying identification. It is still not clear how chronic pulmonary aspergillosis develops. Patients with chronic *Aspergillus* infection do not have these risk factors and may be considered immunocompetent, but they may have either preexisting pulmonary damage or disease. Patients are not immunocompromised by malignoma, HIV, cytotoxic chemotherapy, or any immunosuppressive therapy but may be malnourished and underweight. Previous infections, e.g., tuberculosis or atypical mycobacterial disease, severe COPD, allergic bronchopulmonary aspergillosis, COPD, precedent pneumothorax, or treated lung cancer, are the predominant risk factors for development of CPA.

CPA starts with nodules containing *Aspergillus*. They appear single or multiple at a size smaller than 3 cm. The lesions contain fungus balls consisting of *Aspergillus* hyphae and of cellular debris and of mucus maintaining chronic inflammation. Most commonly, the lesions remain solid but may progress into cavitary pulmonary aspergillosis as the late manifestation of CPA. The fungus balls and the cystic lesion are morphologically similar to the aspergilloma and consist of fungal hyphae and extracellular matrix. It is formed by collapse of the superficial fungal growth inside its cavity [23, 24].

The clinical signs and symptoms are cough, recurrent pneumonia, and/or exacerbation of asthma or chronic obstructive pulmonary disease. The duration of the symptoms usually persists for at least 3 months. The disease is usually progressing despite of adequate antifungal treatment. Complex genetic factors are supposed to be underlying to CPA [25].

Advanced diagnostic work-up is required to differentiate the nodules from metastases, lung carcinoma, or infiltrations caused by rare fungi or pathogens. Even in rheumatoid arthritis, nodules may occur, and in summary the definite diagnosis on the entity of pulmonary nodules can only be secured by histology. The diagnosis of CPA is done using a combination of procedures: CT scan, a direct evidence of *Aspergillus* infection by culture of relevant (biopsy) material, and immune response to *Aspergillus* spp.

Radiological findings in the CT scan are a sum of the preexisting lung disease and the alterations secondary to CPA with nodular infiltrates, alveolar consolidations, preexisting bronchopulmonary or pleural cavities, and the formation of new cavities, nodules or alveolar consolidations. Positron-emission tomography (PET) shows an isometabolic halo or nodule pattern but does not distinguish between malignancy and CPA.

Aspergillus IgG or a precipitin test will be positive in more than 90% of the patients with CPA. Tissue sections of biopsy material showing hyphae invading lung parenchyma indicate acute or subacute invasive aspergillosis. In summary, the diagnostic criteria for CPA are the detection of *Aspergillus* IgG, IgE, or precipitins in the serum; the detection of galactomannan, *Aspergillus* antigen, or *Aspergillus* DNA in respiratory specimens, a percutaneous or excision biopsy showing fungal hyphae in the tissue section, and/or a growth of *Aspergillus* spp.

Persistent lesions and cavities in the lung are also a breeding place for commensal bacteria present in the respiratory tract. Thus, *Streptococcus pneumoniae*, *Haemophilus influenzae*, *Staphylococcus aureus*, *Pseudomonas aeruginosa*, and anaerobic bacteria can cause serious bacterial infections on the basis of CPA [26].

Aspergilloma is a generally single fungus ball in a usually preformed single pulmonary cavity and is called a single pulmonary aspergilloma. Pulmonary or systemic symptoms and serological or microbiological proof of *Aspergillus* are usually negative. Progression of the disease is observed for months. Usually, the diagnosis of aspergilloma is incidentally in a chest x-ray or a CT scan done for another purpose. Rarely the patients present with asthma (allergic bronchopulmonary aspergillosis) or even more rarely with hemoptysis. In patients with adequate pulmonary function presenting a single aspergilloma, resection is a promising therapy option. It is very important that the aspergilloma can be completely resected and that no fungal material can spread into the pleural space. In patients with hemoptysis, embolization of respective arteries is indicated before surgical resection of an aspergilloma. The patient's condition should be carefully observed because a good cardiopulmonary function correlates with the outcome, i.e., fewer complications and lower risk of death.

Allergic bronchopulmonary aspergillosis (ABPA) is a complex hypersensitivity reaction in response to colonization of the airways with *Aspergillus fumigatus*. Tissue sections characteristically show mucoid impaction of the bronchi or eosinophilic pneumonia and bronchial granulomas in addition to histologic features of asthma. In the mucus-filled bronchial lumina, there are septate hyphae, but the fungi do not invade the mucosa.

ABPA occurs in 2% of all asthma patients, particularly in those with frequent exacerbations and corticosteroid treatment and in up to 14% in patients with cystic fibrosis. Chronic ABPA develops after repeated episodes of bronchial obstruction, inflammation, and mucoid impaction which lead to bronchiectasis and respiratory compromise. ABPA may also occur in chronic granulomatous diseases, in hyperimmunoglobulinemia E, and in lung transplant recipients.

Patients with ABPA present with asthma exacerbations, recurrent episodes of bronchial obstruction, malaise, fever, pleuritic chest pain and occasional hemoptysis, or episodic wheezing and expectoration of sputum containing brown plugs. Some patients with ABPA also have allergic *Aspergillus* rhinosinusitis and report nasal obstruction or sinus pressure.

The diagnosis is confirmed by radiological and serological testing. Growth of *Aspergillus* spp. in respiratory samples is only detected in up to 60% of ABPA patients with *Aspergillus*. The skin prick test with *Aspergillus* antigen is positive. Blood tests show a significant elevation of blood eosinophils (>0.5 G/L in patients not receiving corticosteroids) and the serum IgE (>1000 U/L) as well as precipitating IgG antibodies to *Aspergillus*. The immunoassay reveals positive results for IgG antibodies to *Aspergillus* that are diagnostic for ABPA.

The chest x-ray shows consolidations in the upper or middle lobes, central bronchiectasis, parenchymal opacities, and/or mucoid impaction with atelectasis. The CT scan shows bronchiectasis, thickening of the bronchial wall, mucus plugging, or air trapping. The skin prick test with *Aspergillus* antigen is positive. Pulmonary function tests typically reveal reduced forced expiratory volume in 1 second (FEV1) and increased residual volume of the lung.

A negative prick skin test and the absence of precipitins to *Aspergillus* virtually exclude ABPA and should prompt evaluation of other diagnostic possibilities. Differential diagnosis of allergic bronchopulmonary aspergillosis (ABPA) comprises asthma with *Aspergillus* sensitization, bronchocentric granulomatosis, eosinophilic granulomatosis with polyangiitis, and pulmonary eosinophilia due to drugs or parasitic infection and chronic pulmonary aspergillosis [14, 27].

5.2 Superficial Aspergillus Infection

Primary cutaneous aspergillosis can develop at sites of skin injury, near intravenous catheter insertion sites, at areas of traumatic skin lesions and subsequent *Aspergillus* inoculation, and in burn or surgical wounds. Secondary cutaneous aspergillosis may occur during disseminated *Aspergillus* infection through hematogenous spread or through continuous growth. Cutaneous aspergillosis is a rare complication described in AIDS and in non-HIV-infected severely immunocompromised patients or patients with extensive burn wounds. The most common fungus in HIV-associated cutaneous aspergillosis is *Aspergillus fumigatus*, whereas in non-HIV-infected or in burn patients, *A. flavus* and *A. fumigatus* were detected more often.

Initial lesions display a variable picture with macules, papules, nodules, plaques, or pustules. A hemorrhagic bulla may develop under an occlusive tape, whereas at the catheter insertion site, erythema and induration are the first manifestations which progress to necrosis. These lesions are preceded by fever, swelling, and tenderness. Diagnosis is made by skin biopsy of a lesion. The biopsy should reach the subcutaneous fat to rule out invasion of the blood vessels of the dermis and subcutis. A part of the biopsy should be put into saline and sent to the microbiology for microbiologic culture, and the other part should be sent in formalin to perform histopathology.

5.2.1 Case Presentation

An 84-year-old female patient presents with falls and vertigo. In her history she has a fibrosis of the lung, and she has been treated for Waldenström macroglobulinemia since 2001; due to progression of the disease, therapy was intensified with prednisolone 60 mg/day and rituximab. The patient reports fever, cough, dyspnea, and weakness. Because of her clinical presentation and the need of oxygen therapy and the reduced general condition, antibiotic therapy is started immediately. In the x-ray already a node in the lung raises suspicion for a fungal infection. The additional diagnostic investigations result in a positive galactomannan test, sputum microscopy, and culture with proof of *Aspergillus fumigatus*. As the fungus is sensitive to voriconazole, therapy is initiated. The question of a single aspergilloma potentially offering the opportunity for surgical resection arises. Therefore, a CT scan is performed which shows multiple bilateral cavities with central accumulation of soft tissue consistent with a fungus ball.

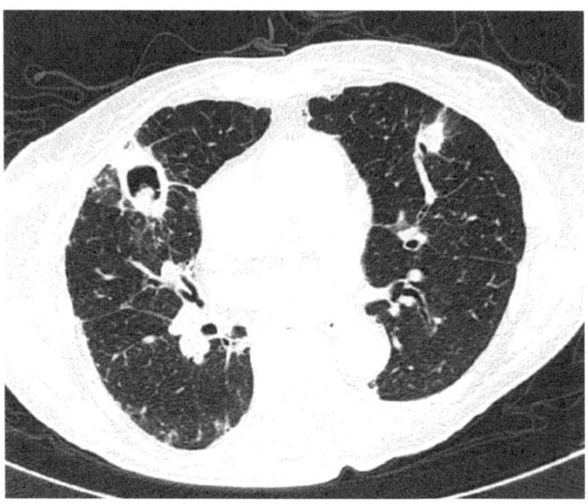

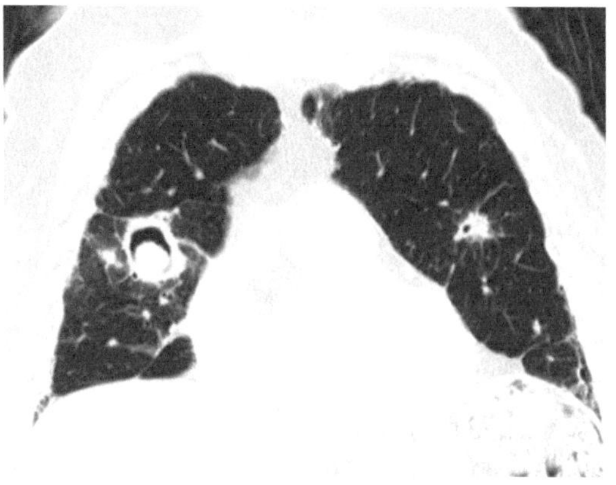

CT scan of pulmonary aspergillosis with fungus ball inside the cavity

Due to multiple infiltrations and cavities, surgical resection is not indicated, and the antifungal therapy is continued for 12 weeks (images with kind permission of Prof W. Jaschke, Department of Radiology, Medical University Innsbruck).

5.3 Strategies to Prevent and to Treat IAI

5.3.1 Prevention

Regarding the patients at risk, protective measures have to be provided. After an allogeneic hematopoietic stem cell transplantation (HSCT), exposure to the fungus should be avoided, i.e., especially construction and renovation sites and plants and/or flowers in patients' rooms. Consequently, outpatients are instructed to avoid these places as well as gardening.

5.3.2 Antifungal Prophylaxis

Primary antifungal prophylaxis is the use of antifungal agents before any evidence of fungal colonization or infection starts at the initiation of cytotoxic chemotherapy and immunosuppression in every patient at risk.

Secondary antifungal prophylaxis is the use of antifungal agents after recovery from a proven and documented fungal infection prior to additional and necessary immunosuppressive therapy or cytotoxic chemotherapy.

The challenge of antifungal prophylaxis is to target the patient population at risk while not overusing antifungal agents that may have toxic side effects, interfere with other medications, foster the emergence of resistant fungi, and, at last, are not needed. Thus prophylaxis strategies are restricted to patients at the highest risk of fungal infections. To avoid overuse of antifungal prophylaxis, the decision to give prophylaxis should be risk-adjusted. Risk adjustment should be based on the incidence and the severity of invasive fungal infections (>10%) [28]. Local epidemiology of invasive fungal infection may be helpful to guide and evaluate the efficacy of antifungal prophylaxis and is therefore recommended in centers caring for patients with hemato-oncological malignancies. Patients at highest risk for IAI are (1) allogenic stem cell recipients (10–20%) with an age >40 years, hematological diseases other than chronic myeloid leukemia, graft failure, long-term steroids, and graft-versus-host disease, and (2) in patients with AML (10%) with an age >40 years, high-dose cytarabine and in an advanced state of the disease without remission [29]. These patient populations should receive antifungal prophylaxis according to current international guidelines, i.e., IDSA and ECIL-6 guidelines [14, 16].To minimize the high risk of IAI, antifungal agents with good efficacy against *Aspergillus* spp. are recommendable. First-line antifungal agents for prophylaxis are posaconazole and voriconazole. Posaconazole (dose, oral suspension 3 × 200 mg po; tablet and intravenous solution, day 1: 2 × 300 mg, following days 1 × 300 mg) is licensed for antifungal prophylaxis in selected hematological high-risk patients, i.e., allogeneic stem cell transplant recipients with graft-versus-host disease and patients with acute myeloid leukemia or myelodysplastic syndrome based on two randomized controlled trials [30, 31]. Voriconazole and micafungin are additional options for prophylaxis in severely immunocompromised patients at high risk [32–34]

Itraconazole is effective for prophylaxis too, but there are problems with absorption and tolerance. It is important to know that itraconazole should not be coadministered with other drugs that might get toxic levels due to metabolic interference with triazoles. Micafungin or caspofungin is recommended as second-line prophylactic agents [14].

5.3.3 Empirical Antifungal Therapy

In patients with prolonged (>10 days) severe neutropenia (<0.5 G/L), hemato-oncological malignancy, and no response to broad-spectrum antibacterial therapy, empirical therapy with antifungal agents may be used. The recommended antifungals are liposomal amphotericin B, caspofungin, micafungin, or voriconazole [14].

5.3.4 Preemptive Antifungal Therapy

Taking an even more refined approach is to initiate treatment only upon positive identification of biomarkers of infection together with appropriate clinical signs and symptoms and/or the presence of lesions in the CT that are suggestive for IAI in patients at risk. Biomarkers that should be continuously determined in patients at high risk for IAI are galactomannan and/or 1,3-beta-D-glucan, both parts of the *Aspergillus* cell wall. This strategy is called preemptive or presumptive therapy. There is excellent evidence that this strategy is effective and safe with the advantage that there are more documented IAI cases [35].

5.3.5 Antifungal Treatment of IAI

Antifungal treatment of strongly suspected IAI should be initiated as soon as possible. However, samples for fungal cultures should be best taken before the administration of antifungal therapy. Voriconazole is the antifungal drug of choice for treatment of IAI according to current guidelines [14, 16]. Voriconazole achieved a better clinical outcome than amphotericin B deoxycholate in an open-label randomized trial in patients with IAI. For intravenous infusion of voriconazole, a loading dose of 2 × 6 mg/kg on day 1 followed by

2 × 4 mg/kg (maintenance dose) is recommended. Although the enteral absorption of voriconazole depends on the clinical condition, oral administration is justified as a step-down therapy in stable patients. The oral standard dose is 2 × 400 mg on day 1 followed by a maintenance dose of 2 × 200 mg daily. Numerous drug-drug interactions have to be considered, as voriconazole undergoes hepatic metabolism involving CYP2C9, CYP2C19, and CYP3A4 [36]. Enhanced exposition to immunosuppressants can be particularly harmful. Therefore, the doses of cyclosporine A and of tacrolimus have to be reduced and closely monitored during concomitant voriconazole treatment. There are ultrarapid and poor voriconazole metabolizers due to genetic polymorphisms of CYP2C9. Close therapeutic drug monitoring of immunosuppressants is indispensable to avoid excessive immunosuppression and renal damage. Renal impairment at any stage appears to have no relevant influence on voriconazole pharmacokinetics and does not require dose adjustment for the oral voriconazole preparations. However, when the intravenous formulation had been applied, accumulation of the solvent SBECD was reported from patients with renal impairment. Preclinical and available clinical data as well as autopsy studies have shown favorable penetration of voriconazole into the majority of relevant tissues (Table 5.1). However, its complex, nonlinear pharmacokinetics requires therapeutic drug monitoring. The central nervous system, the eye, and the liver are the major targets of voriconazole toxicity with dizziness and hallucinations, visual disturbances, and increase of the liver enzymes [37].

Amphotericin B has been introduced in therapy already in 1958 and has been the standard therapy of invasive aspergillosis for decades. However, the use of its conventional deoxycholate formulation is discouraged now because of poor tolerability. Infusion-related adverse events such as chills, rigors, fever, nausea, hypotension or hypertension, and renal deterioration have been observed in almost 50% of the patients on treatment with this preparation. Lipid formulations of amphotericin B, particularly liposomal amphotericin B, are an alternative to voriconazole for treatment of IAI, particularly, when azole resistance is a concern. The recommended standard dose is 3–5 mg/kg per day. Although the toxicity of liposomal amphotericin B is much lower than that of the conventional formulation, renal safety is a concern, and close monitoring of renal function is strongly advised.

Posaconazole (dose, oral suspension 3 × 200 mg/day; tablet and intravenous solution, day 1: 2 × 300 mg, following days 1 × 300 mg) is licensed for second-line treatment of invasive aspergillosis, because it achieved a response rate of 42% in an open-label, multicenter study on salvage therapy for invasive aspergillosis and other mycoses in comparison to 26% response rate in a retrospective control group [38].

In the current guidelines, posaconazole is mentioned as an option for salvage therapy. If an azole (e.g., voriconazole) had been previously tried, salvage therapy should be performed with an antifungal belonging to a different class [14].

Recently the new broad-spectrum azole isavuconazole with a 5-day half-life has been licensed for treatment of invasive aspergillosis, as it had shown clinical efficacy similar to that of voriconazole in a randomised controlled double-blind trial of 516 patients with invasive aspergillosis and other mold infections [39]. Less severe interactions than voriconazole are expected when isavuconazole is

Table 5.1 Tissue penetration of antifungals for treatment of invasive aspergillosis

	Liver	Spleen	Lung	Kidney	Heart	CNS	Samples
Amphotericin B and its lipid formulations	+++	+++	+++	+/++	+/–	+/–	Autopsy epithelial lining fluid
Voriconazole	++	++	++ +++	++	++	+	Autopsy, biopsy, epithelial lining fluid
Caspofungin	+++	+	+	++	+/–	+/–	Rat, rabbit

+++, favorable penetration; ++, probably sufficient penetration, modest penetration; +/–, poor tissue penetration, probably insufficient for antifungal eradication

administered with drugs being metabolized by CYP. Monitoring of serum drug levels is recommended [14]. Isavuconazole is mentioned as an alternative to voriconazole in the recent guidelines.

Echinocandins are fungistatic to *Aspergillus* spp. Caspofungin is licensed for salvage therapy of IAI based on an open non-comparative trial with failure or toxicity of first-line treatment with lipid-formulated amphotericin B, itraconazole, or voriconazole [40]. However, the clinical response to caspofungin was found to be modest in this condition. As poor outcome was achieved in two studies on first-line treatment of invasive aspergillosis with caspofungin [41–43], it is not licensed for this indication. Caspofungin, however, is a therapeutic option in empirical antifungal treatment of patients with febrile neutropenia [44].

Because of the high morbidity and mortality caused by IAI, antifungal combination therapy has been investigated in numerous preclinical and in several clinical studies. The combination of azoles with amphotericin B yielded variable and contradictory results. Because of a potential mechanism-based antagonism, this combination is discouraged for treatment of invasive aspergillosis. In a small randomised trial, the administration of liposomal amphotericin B combined with caspofungin achieved an improved outcome in comparison with high-dose liposomal amphotericin B monotherapy [45]. The combination of voriconazole with caspofungin was promising as salvage therapy of IAI [46]. In a large randomised clinical trial, however, the benefit of the combination of voriconazole with anidulafungin over voriconazole monotherapy failed its significance [47]. Therefore, the current guidelines advise against routine administration of antifungal combination. It should be considered in proven IAI on a case-by-case analysis as well as for salvage therapy.

The duration of medical treatment of invasive aspergillosis depends on the immunological condition of the patient and on the site of the infection (Table 5.1). Treatment for 6–12 weeks is required in most of the cases. *Aspergillus* endophthalmitis should be treated with a combination of systemic and intravitreal voriconazole. Surgical debridement along with intravenous treatment plays an important role in cardiac manifestation of aspergillosis, as well as in sinusitis, osteomyelitis, and septic arthritis caused by *Aspergillus*. For renal aspergillosis, urological decompression is required. When the renal parenchyma is affected, voriconazole therapy must be administered; otherwise local amphotericin B instillation might be helpful. However, fungus balls within the renal pelvis will have to be surgically removed.

Overall, for those patients with IAI who fail prophylaxis or therapy, it is recommended that antifungal therapy has to be switched to antifungals of another class [14, 48].

5.3.6 Treatment of CPA

Symptomatic patients with pulmonary and/or general symptoms and/or loss of lung funtions should be treated for at least 6 months. Oral voriconazole or itraconazole are the preferred treatment. Itraconazole can be used as well as intravenous therapy with caspofungin, micafungin, or amphotericin B in the intolerability or resistance to triazoles. Hemorrhage has been treated locally in bronchoscopy, arterial embolisation, or even with surgical intervention. Surgical resection may be considered if there is persistent hemoptysis or a resistant *Aspergillus* species. However, the outcome is moderate. Asymptomatic patients may be observed and followed every 3–6 months [26].

5.3.7 Treatment of ABPA

Treatment of ABPA aims to control the exacerbation of asthma episodes and to avoid progressive lung damage. Systemic glucocorticoids and antifungal agents are applied depending on the activity of the disease. Antifungal therapy is able to decrease episodes of exacerbations, whereas inhaled glucocorticoids improve symptoms of asthma. For acute ABPA, prednisone at an initial dose of 0.5 mg/kg/day for 2 weeks is recommended, following a tapering with intermittent dosing over 3 months. Success of therapy can be measured by decrease of IgE. Usually patients report clinical improvement, in radiography the opacities resolve, and total serum IgE is reduced by about 35%. At the same time, antifungal therapy for acute or recurrent exacerbated ABPA in combination with corticosteroids is recommended. Itraconazole, alternatively voriconazole or isavuconazole, and possibly posaconazole are effective antifungal drugs against *Aspergillus* spp. However, until now are only studies using itraconazole or voriconazole [48, 49]. The dosage of itraconazole in adults is 200 mg thrice a day for 3 days and twice a day from day 4 onward. Concomitant antifungal therapy is considered to help reduce the glucocorticoid dose. The duration of antifungal therapy is at least 16 weeks. For severe cases there are also therapeutic regimens of up to 6 months described. To assure adequate serum levels of the antifungal drug, the monitoring of the drug levels in the blood should be done: voriconazole is recommended with 400 mg twice on day 1, followed by 200 mg twice daily. After 5 days serum concentration should be measured, and throughout the therapy duration liver function tests should be taken. Though as a rare complication under the treatment with itraconazole and systemic glucocorticoids, acute invasive pulmonary aspergillosis may occur, stressing the need of regular controls [14].

5.3.8 Treatment of Cutaneous Aspergillosis

Treatment of cutaneous aspergillosis depends on the general clinical state of the patient [50]. Diagnosis of aspergillosis in the skin should imply the differentiation of primary or secondary fungal infection due to IAI. Secondary cutaneous aspergillosis and complicated and disseminated cases of primary cutaneous aspergillosis are treated as IAI. For primary cutaneous aspergillosis only, itraconazole has been shown to successfully eradicate *Aspergillus* in most cases [51].

In patients with extensive burns, cutaneous aspergillosis occurs as primary disease, which should be treated surgically. Also in AIDS patients, organism directed antifungal medication and surgical therapy are successful. In immunocompromised patients after cytotoxic chemotherapy and with vascular catheter exit sites or tunnel infections due to *Aspergillus* spp., surgical resection followed by antifungal therapy are recommended.

References

1. Kontoyiannis DP, Marr KA, Park BJ, Alexander BD, Anaissie EJ, Walsh TJ et al (2010) Prospective surveillance for invasive fungal infections in hematopoietic stem cell transplant recipients, 2001-2006: overview of the Transplant-Associated Infection Surveillance Network (TRANSNET) Database. Clin Infect Dis 50(8):1091–1100
2. Meersseman W, Lagrou K, Maertens J, Van Wijngaerden E (2007) Invasive aspergillosis in the intensive care unit. Clin Infect Dis 45(2):205–216
3. Herbrecht R, Bories P, Moulin JC, Ledoux MP, Letscher-Bru V (2012) Risk stratification for invasive aspergillosis in immunocompromised patients. Ann N Y Acad Sci 1272:23–30
4. Meersseman W, Vandecasteele SJ, Wilmer A, Verbeken E, Peetermans WE, Van Wijngaerden E (2004) Invasive aspergillosis in critically ill patients without malignancy. Am J Respir Crit Care Med 170:621–625
5. Wojtowicz A, Gresnigt MS, Lecompte T, Bibert S, Manuel O, Joosten LA et al (2015) IL1B and DEFB1 polymorphisms increase susceptibility to invasive mold infection after solid-organ transplantation. J Infect Dis 211(10):1646–1657
6. Gregg KS, Kauffman CA (2015) Invasive aspergillosis: epidemiology, clinical aspects, and treatment. Semin Respir Crit Care Med 36(5):662–672
7. Klingspor L, Saaedi B, Ljungman P, Szakos A (2015) Epidemiology and outcomes of patients with invasive mould infections: a retrospective observational study from a single centre (2005-2009). Mycoses 58(8):470–477
8. Wingard JR, Ribaud P, Schlamm HT, Herbrecht R (2008) Changes in causes of death over time after treatment for invasive aspergillosis. Cancer 112(10):2309–2312
9. Lewis RE, Cahyame-Zuniga L, Leventakos K, Chamilos G, Ben-Ami R, Tamboli P et al (2013) Epidemiology and sites of involvement of invasive fungal infections in patients with haematological malignancies: a 20-year autopsy study. Mycoses 56(6):638–645
10. Pappas PG, Alexander BD, Andes DR, Hadley S, Kauffman CA, Freifeld A et al (2010) Invasive fungal infections among organ transplant recipients: results of the Transplant-Associated Infection Surveillance Network (TRANSNET). Clin Infect Dis 50(8):1101–1111

11. Johnson EM, Oakley KL, Radford SA, Moore CB, Warn P, Warnock DW et al (2000) Lack of correlation of in vitro amphotericin B susceptibility testing with outcome in a murine model of Aspergillus infection. J Antimicrob Chemother 45(1):85–93
12. De Pauw B, Walsh TJ, Donnelly JP, Stevens DA, Edwards JE, Calandra T et al (2008) Revised definitions of invasive fungal disease from the European Organization for Research and Treatment of Cancer/Invasive Fungal Infections Cooperative Group and the National Institute of Allergy and Infectious Diseases Mycoses Study Group (EORTC/MSG) Consensus Group. Clin Infect Dis 46(12):1813–1821
13. Liss B, Vehreschild JJ, Bangard C, Maintz D, Frank K, Gronke S et al (2015) Our 2015 approach to invasive pulmonary aspergillosis. Mycoses 58(6):375–382
14. Patterson TF, Thompson GR, Denning DW, Fishman JA, Hadley S, Herbrecht R et al (2016) Practice guidelines for the diagnosis and management of aspergillosis: 2016 update by the Infectious Diseases Society of America. Clin Infect Dis 63(4):e1–e60
15. Maertens J, Groll AH, Cordonnier C, de la Camara R, Roilides E, Marchetti O (2011) Treatment and timing in invasive mould disease. J Antimicrob Chemother 66(Suppl 1):i37–i43
16. Tissot F, Agrawal S, Pagano L, Petrikkos G, Groll AH, Skiada A et al (2017) ECIL-6 guidelines for the treatment of invasive candidiasis, aspergillosis and mucormycosis in leukemia and hematopoietic stem cell transplant patients. Haematologica 102(3):433–444
17. Parry MF, Coughlin FR, Zambetti FX (1982) Aspergillus empyema. Chest 81(6):768–770
18. Hoenigl M, Krause R (2013) Antifungal therapy of aspergillosis of the central nervous system and aspergillus endophthalmitis. Curr Pharm Des 19(20):3648–3668
19. McCarthy M, Rosengart A, Schuetz AN, Kontoyiannis DP, Walsh TJ (2014) Mold infections of the central nervous system. N Engl J Med 371(2):150–160
20. Endo T, Tominaga T, Konno H, Yoshimoto T (2002) Fatal subarachnoid hemorrhage, with brainstem and cerebellar infarction, caused by Aspergillus infection after cerebral aneurysm surgery: case report. Neurosurgery 50(5):1147–1150 discussion 50-1
21. Levin LA, Avery R, Shore JW, Woog JJ, Baker AS (1996) The spectrum of orbital aspergillosis: a clinicopathological review. Surv Ophthalmol 41(2):142–154
22. Gonzalez-Vicent M, Diaz MA, Colmenero I, Sevilla J, Madero L (2008) Primary gastrointestinal aspergillosis after autologous peripheral blood progenitor cell transplantation: an unusual presentation of invasive aspergillosis. Transpl Infect Dis 10(3):193–196
23. Denning DW (2001) Chronic forms of pulmonary aspergillosis. Clin Microbiol Infect 7(Suppl 2):25–31
24. Patterson TF, Thompson GR, Denning DW, Fishman JA, Hadley S, Herbrecht R et al (2016) Executive summary: practice guidelines for the diagnosis and management of aspergillosis: 2016 update by the Infectious Diseases Society of America. Clin Infect Dis 63(4):433–442
25. Vinh DC (2011) Insights into human antifungal immunity from primary immunodeficiencies. Lancet Infect Dis 11(10):780–792
26. Andes DR, Safdar N, Baddley JW, Alexander B, Brumble L, Freifeld A et al (2016) The epidemiology and outcomes of invasive Candida infections among organ transplant recipients in the United States: results of the Transplant-Associated Infection Surveillance Network (TRANSNET). Transpl Infect Dis 18(6):921–931
27. Muldoon EG, Strek ME, Patterson KC (2017) Allergic and noninvasive infectious pulmonary aspergillosis syndromes. Clin Chest Med 38(3):521–534
28. O'Brien SN, Blijlevens NM, Mahfouz TH, Anaissie EJ (2003) Infections in patients with hematological cancer: recent developments. Hematology Am Soc Hematol Educ Program 2003:438–472
29. Leather HL, Wingard JR (2006) New strategies of antifungal therapy in hematopoietic stem cell transplant recipients and patients with hematological malignancies. Blood Rev 20(5):267–287
30. Cornely OA, Maertens J, Winston DJ, Perfect J, Ullmann AJ, Walsh TJ et al (2007) Posaconazole vs. fluconazole or itraconazole prophylaxis in patients with neutropenia. N Engl J Med 356(4):348–359
31. Ullmann AJ, Lipton JH, Vesole DH, Chandrasekar P, Langston A, Tarantolo SR et al (2007) Posaconazole or fluconazole for prophylaxis in severe graft-versus-host disease. N Engl J Med 356(4):335–347
32. Wingard JR, Carter SL, Walsh TJ, Kurtzberg J, Small TN, Baden LR et al (2010) Randomized, double-blind trial of fluconazole versus voriconazole for prevention of invasive fungal infection after allogeneic hematopoietic cell transplantation. Blood 116(24):5111–5118
33. Cordonnier C, Rovira M, Maertens J, Olavarria E, Faucher C, Bilger K et al (2010) Voriconazole for secondary prophylaxis of invasive fungal infections in allogeneic stem cell transplant recipients: results of the VOSIFI study. Haematologica 95(10):1762–1768
34. van Burik JA, Ratanatharathorn V, Stepan DE, Miller CB, Lipton JH, Vesole DH et al (2004) Micafungin versus fluconazole for prophylaxis against invasive fungal infections during neutropenia in patients undergoing hematopoietic stem cell transplantation. Clin Infect Dis 39(10):1407–1416
35. Maertens J, Theunissen K, Verhoef G, Verschakelen J, Lagrou K, Verbeken E et al (2005) Galactomannan and computed tomography-based preemptive antifungal therapy in neutropenic patients at high risk for invasive fungal infection: a prospective feasibility study. Clin Infect Dis 41(9):1242–1250
36. Nivoix Y, Leveque D, Herbrecht R, Koffel JC, Beretz L, Ubeaud-Sequier G (2008) The enzymatic basis of drug-drug interactions with systemic triazole antifungals. Clin Pharmacokinet 47(12):779–792
37. Malani AN, Kerr LE, Kauffman CA (2015) Voriconazole: how to use this antifungal agent and what to expect. Semin Respir Crit Care Med 36(5):786–795

38. Walsh TJ, Raad I, Patterson TF, Chandrasekar P, Donowitz GR, Graybill R et al (2007) Treatment of invasive aspergillosis with posaconazole in patients who are refractory to or intolerant of conventional therapy: an externally controlled trial. Clin Infect Dis 44(1):2–12
39. Maertens JA, Raad II, Marr KA, Patterson TF, Kontoyiannis DP, Cornely OA et al (2016) Isavuconazole versus voriconazole for primary treatment of invasive mould disease caused by Aspergillus and other filamentous fungi (SECURE): a phase 3, randomised-controlled, non-inferiority trial. Lancet 387(10020):760–769
40. Heinz WJ, Buchheidt D, Ullmann AJ (2016) Clinical evidence for caspofungin monotherapy in the first-line and salvage therapy of invasive Aspergillus infections. Mycoses 59(8):480–493
41. Kartsonis NA, Saah AJ, Joy LC, Taylor AF, Sable CA (2005) Salvage therapy with caspofungin for invasive aspergillosis: results from the caspofungin compassionate use study. J Infect 50(3):196–205
42. Maertens J, Raad I, Petrikkos G, Boogaerts M, Selleslag D, Petersen FB et al (2004) Efficacy and safety of caspofungin for treatment of invasive aspergillosis in patients refractory to or intolerant of conventional antifungal therapy. Clin Infect Dis 39(11):1563–1571
43. Hiemenz JW, Raad II, Maertens JA, Hachem RY, Saah AJ, Sable CA et al (2010) Efficacy of caspofungin as salvage therapy for invasive aspergillosis compared to standard therapy in a historical cohort. Eur J Clin Microbiol Infect Dis 29(11):1387–1394
44. Walsh TJ, Teppler H, Donowitz GR, Maertens JA, Baden LR, Dmoszynska A et al (2004) Caspofungin versus liposomal amphotericin B for empirical antifungal therapy in patients with persistent fever and neutropenia. N Engl J Med 351(14):1391–1402
45. Caillot D, Thiebaut A, Herbrecht R, de Botton S, Pigneux A, Bernard F et al (2007) Liposomal amphotericin B in combination with caspofungin for invasive aspergillosis in patients with hematologic malignancies: a randomized pilot study (Combistrat trial). Cancer 110(12):2740–2746
46. Maertens J, Glasmacher A, Herbrecht R, Thiebaut A, Cordonnier C, Segal BH et al (2006) Multicenter, noncomparative study of caspofungin in combination with other antifungals as salvage therapy in adults with invasive aspergillosis. Cancer 107(12):2888–2897
47. Marr KA, Schlamm HT, Herbrecht R, Rottinghaus ST, Bow EJ, Cornely OA et al (2015) Combination antifungal therapy for invasive aspergillosis: a randomized trial. Ann Intern Med 162(2):81–89
48. Stevens DA, Schwartz HJ, Lee JY, Moskovitz BL, Jerome DC, Catanzaro A et al (2000) A randomized trial of itraconazole in allergic bronchopulmonary aspergillosis. N Engl J Med 342(11):756–762
49. Camuset J, Nunes H, Dombret MC, Bergeron A, Henno P, Philippe B et al (2007) Treatment of chronic pulmonary aspergillosis by voriconazole in nonimmunocompromised patients. Chest 131(5):1435–1441
50. van Burik JA, Colven R, Spach DH (1998) Cutaneous aspergillosis. J Clin Microbiol 36(11):3115–3121
51. van Burik JA, Colven R, Spach DH (1998) Itraconazole therapy for primary cutaneous aspergillosis in patients with AIDS. Clin Infect Dis 27(3):643–644

6 Clinical Syndromes: Mucormycosis

Aigner Maria and Lass-Flörl Cornelia

6.1 Epidemiology

Mucormycosis has emerged as an important fungal infection with high morbidity and mortality. The genera *Rhizopus*, *Lichtheimia*, and *Mucor* are most often recovered from clinical specimens and are ubiquitous in nature, but their precise ecology remains to be determined. Cases with mucormycosis have been reported from all over the world, and seasonal variation is possible. Israel reported that 16 of 19 rhino-orbitocerebral mucormycosis cases occurred in autumn [1], and in Japan, 6 of 7 pulmonary mucormycosis cases developed from August to September [2]. However, others report invasive cases all of the year [3–7]. There are several factors that limit our ability to accurately determine the exact incidence of mucormycosis. First, these infections are not reportable; the risk varies widely in different populations, and the proof of diagnosis is extremely difficult to obtain. Mucormycosis remains an uncommon disease, even in high-risk patients, and represents between 4 and 23% of all fungal infections in patients at risk [3–5]. Postmortem evaluation showed mucormycosis being 10–50-fold less frequent than candidiasis or aspergillosis with a frequency of 1–5 cases per 10,000 autopsies [3–7]. The epidemiology of mucormycosis varies between developed and developing countries. In developed countries the disease is most often seen in patients with hematological malignancies undergoing chemotherapy or who received allogeneic stem cell transplants (HSCT) [8]. Roden et al. compiled 929 cases of mucormycosis and displayed an increasing proportion of immunocompromised patients with mucormycosis in the 1980s and 1990s [9]. The registry of the European Confederation of Medical Mycology Working Group recorded 230 cases between 2005 and 2007 and found patients with hematological malignancies (44%), trauma (15%), HSCT (9%), and diabetes mellitus (9%) being infected [10]. Similar data were obtained by a French analysis comprising 101 cases of mucormycoses (60 proven and 41 probable cases), mostly in men (58%) older than >50 years (mean age, 50.7 ± 19.9 years). The incidence increased from 0.7 cases per 1 million in 1997 to 1.2 cases per 1 million in 2006 ($P < 0.001$) [11]. An active population-based surveillance study from California calculated an annual incidence of mucormycosis of 1.7 cases per 1 million individuals (~500 cases per year) [12]. An incidence of 0.43 cases per 1 million inhabitants or 0.62 cases per 100,000 hospital admissions was rated for Spain [13]. In developing countries, especially in India, mucormycosis occurs mainly in patients with uncontrolled diabetes or trauma [14, 15].

A. Maria · L.-F. Cornelia (✉)
Division of Hygiene and Medical Microbiology, Medical University of Innsbruck, Innsbruck, Austria
e-mail: cornelia.lass-floerl@i-med.ac.at

E. Presterl (ed.), *Clinically Relevant Mycoses*, https://doi.org/10.1007/978-3-319-92300-0_6

6.2 The Pathogen

Mucormycoses, previously termed zygomycoses, are infections due to fungi within the order Mucorales. Invasive infections are marked by invasion of blood vessels causing thrombosis, tissue infarction, and necrosis and are rapidly progressing and frequently lethal. The most important genera are *Rhizopus*, *Mucor*, *Lichtheimia* (previously termed *Absidia*), *Rhizomucor*, *Apophysomyces*, *Cunninghamella*, and *Saksenaea*. Human infections are mainly caused through inhalation of aerosolized spores leading to rhinocerebral and pulmonary mucormycosis. Estimating that humans inhale more than 170,000 airborne fungal spores per day [16], invasive infection is infrequent. Moreover gastrointestinal infections as well as infections of the skin through direct traumatic inoculation have been described; subsequently fungal disease can disseminate throughout the body, and any organ can be involved. By now, several risk factors for invasive infection have been described: most prevalent predisposing conditions are immunosuppression, especially granulocytopenia, organ transplant recipient, poorly controlled/uncontrolled diabetes mellitus, and burns.

6.3 Predisposing Conditions

The most important conditions predisposing to mucormycosis include malignant hematological disease with or without stem cell transplantation, prolonged and severe neutropenia, poorly controlled diabetes mellitus with or without diabetic ketoacidosis, iron overload, major trauma, prolonged use of corticosteroids, illicit intravenous drug use, neonatal prematurity, malnourishment, and antifungals with no activity against Mucormycetes, such as voriconazole and echinocandins [8–10, 17]. Nosocomial cases have been associated with construction work, contaminated air filters, wound dressings, transdermal nitrate patches, intravenous catheters, tongue depressors, and even allopurinol pills [18–20].

Mucorales are vasotropic, causing tissue infarctions resulting from angioinvasion and subsequent thrombosis. The infection is rapidly progressive and results in death unless underlying risk factors are corrected and aggressive treatment with antifungal agents and surgical excision is initiated. The mucormycosis spectrum ranges from cutaneous, rhinocerebral, and sinopulmonary to disseminated and frequently fatal infections, especially in immunocompromised hosts [21, 22]. Any of the Mucorales may cause infection at the various sites [23–25]. Commonly affected are the sinuses (39%), lungs (24%), and skin (19%), with an overall dissemination of 23% [13]. The overall mortality rate is 66% in patients with malignancies, 44% in diabetics, and 35% in patients without underlying conditions. The skin and gut are affected more frequently in children than in adults [26].

6.4 Pulmonary Mucormycosis

Most often pulmonary infection occurs in neutropenic patients with cancer undergoing induction chemotherapy and those with HSCT and graft-versus-host disease [27]. The clinical presentation is nonspecific and usually may not be distinguished from pulmonary aspergillosis. Patients usually present with nonproductive cough and fever (>38 °C) that is unresponsive to broad-spectrum antibiotics. Airway obstruction due to endobronchial fungal masses may cause a lung collapse, following invasion of hilar blood vessels and massive hemoptysis [28–30]. The mediastinum, pericardium, and chest wall may be affected [31].

Chest images are also nonspecific and include infiltration, consolidation, nodules, cavitations, air-crescent sign, atelectasis, effusion, posterior tracheal band thickening, hilar or mediastinal lymphadenopathy, and even normal findings [32–36]. Multiple lung nodules (≥10) and pleural effusion on initial CT scans was an independent predictor of pulmonary mucormycosis [37]. A reversed halo sign and a focal round area of ground-glass attenuation enclosed by a ring of consolidation seem to be more specific for mucormycosis than for other fungal infections [38].

6.5 Rhinocerebral Mucormycosis

Most often rhinocerebral mucormycosis occurs in patients with diabetes mellitus [9, 10], underlying malignancies, and recipients of hematopoietic stem cell or solid organ transplants, and in individuals with other risk factors [39]. The infection rapidly extends into adjacent tissues and may spread to the palate, sphenoid and cavernous sinus, orbits, or brain [40]. Vascular cerebral invasion may lead to dissemination with or without the development of mycotic aneurysms [41]. The initial symptoms are consistent with those of sinusitis and periorbital cellulitis [17]. A black necrotic eschar is the hallmark of mucormycosis. Fever may be absent in 50% of cases, and the white blood cell count is typically elevated. CT scan [42] magnetic resonance imaging is nonspecific, and diagnosis requires evidence of fungal tissue invasion [26, 43].

6.6 Cutaneous Mucormycosis

Most often cutaneous mucormycosis results from direct inoculation of fungal spores in the skin, which may lead to disseminated disease [8, 9]. Infections present as localized (skin or subcutaneous tissue), deep (muscle, tendons, or bone), and disseminated [44]. The clinical manifestations vary, may progress slowly or fulminant, and may lead to gangrene and hematogenous dissemination [45–47]. A necrotic eschar is typical of cutaneous mucormycosis; lesions may mimic pyoderma gangrenosum [48] or other fungal infections [46].

6.7 Gastrointestinal Mucormycosis

Gastrointestinal mucormycosis is uncommon and has been reported in premature neonates, malnourished children, and individuals with hematological malignancies, diabetes mellitus, and corticosteroid use [49–54]. The use of fungal-contaminated herbal and homeopathic drugs and tongue depressors was linked with gastrointestinal mucormycosis [50, 54, 55]. Most often the stomach is affected, followed by the colon and ileum [53, 56, 57]. Symptoms are nonspecific and may include appendiceal, cecal, or ileac masses or gastric perforations with bleeding [51, 54, 56–61]. In premature neonates, gastrointestinal mucormycosis presents as necrotizing enterocolitis [17, 62]. Infections may disseminate and be a common cause of death [58, 62].

6.8 Disseminated Mucormycosis

Mucormycosis may spread hematogenously [63–68] and most commonly associated is the lung. Patients with iron overload (especially those receiving deferoxamine) and profound immunosuppression or neutropenia and active leukemia are at risk for dissemination [14, 21, 69, 70]. The clinical signs and symptoms vary widely and are reflected by the immune status of the host, without appropriate treatment, the infection is fatal [67].

6.9 Uncommon Forms of Mucormycosis

Unilateral or bilateral renal mucormycosis has been reported during fungemia, and patients may present with unexplained anuric renal failure. Risk factors include intravenous catheters, intravenous drug use, or AIDS [71–75]. Cases of isolated renal mucormycosis have been reported from developing countries such as India, Egypt, Saudi Arabia, Kuwait, and Singapore [25, 76, 77]. Other forms cover the endocarditis, brain, osteomyelitis, peritonitis, and pyelonephritis [66, 68, 70, 78–85].

6.10 Diagnosis and Applications of Diagnostics

Early diagnosis of mucormycosis is a major challenge in daily clinical and laboratory work. Prognostic clinical symptoms and radiographic signs indicating mucormycosis are lacking. Laboratory diagnosis is based on conventional methods, such as the direct microscopic examination and fungal culture from clinical specimens. The detection of characteristic hyphae from sterile body sites considers the proof of diagnosis. However, secretions from the upper and lower respiratory tract, i.e., paranasal sinuses and bronchoalveolar lavage fluids, are also appropriate. Molecular assays aim to close the gap between microscopic examination and culture.

6.10.1 Conventional Methods

6.10.1.1 Microscopic Examination

Direct microscopic examination using optical brighteners such as calcofluor-white is an important step in diagnosing mucormycoses. Optical brighteners bind to chitin, and subsequently fungal elements fluoresce in ultraviolet light. Hyphae of Mucorales are presenting non- or pauci-septate, irregular with variable width (6–25 μm), ribbon-like with wide-angle branched bifurcations (>90°). This basic and rapid examination gives a first orientation of diagnosis and provides essential information for guiding treatment. Notably, direct microscopic examination allows no species identification. Histopathology is highly recommended as well. Characteristic are prominent infarcts, perineural invasion, and angioinvasion; the latter tends to be more extensive in neutropenic patients [87]. Scrapings cannot reliably proof invasive infection. Due to the lack of monoclonal antibodies, clinical validation immunohistochemistry is of minor importance [88].

6.10.1.2 Culture

Fungal culture supports the identification of fungal agents to species level and susceptibility testing. Mucorales grow rapidly (3–5 days) and well on both nonselective and fungus-selective media at 25–30 °C, typically covering the lid of the agar plate [89, 90]. Cultures are essential, but sensitivity is low; only one-third of microscopically positive specimens end up with positive cultures [91]. Especially aggressive specimen processing seems to correlate with sterile cultures [89]. The nonseptate mycelia are fragile and vulnerable to sample processing. Microaerophilic conditions, which aim to mimic infarcted tissues, have shown to improve the growth of the genera *Cunninghamella* and *Rhizopus* [92]. Nutrient-poor medium (e.g., water agar with 0.1% yeast extract) enhances the sporulation of *Apophysomyces* and *Saksaena* [93].

Microscopic species identification of Mucorales requires expertise and experience; species are distinguished by their sporangiospores, the columella, the apophysis, the appearance and branching of the stolons, and the presence or absence of rhizoids. A failure rate of 20% is typically for morphological identification when compared to molecular identification [94]. Matrix-assisted laser desorption ionization time-of-flight mass spectrometry (MALDI-TOF MS) has shown to be useful for identification of *Rhizopus* species [95]; although promising, adequate reference databases are missing, hence limiting the wide application for identification. Internal transcribed spacer (ITS)—sequencing may be a good way for appropriate species identification. However, up to now, there is no strong evidence that genus/species identification may be important to guide treatment [96].

For antifungal susceptibility testing, the broth microdilution reference method of the European Committee on Antimicrobial Susceptibility Testing (EUCAST) and Clinical and Laboratory Standards Institute (CLSI) is recommended. However, clinical breakpoints are lacking; hence minimal inhibitory concentrations (MICs) obtained may be difficult to be clinically interpreted. MICs obtained by the ETest® should be handled cautiously, as the overall agreement between the ETest® and EUCAST was 75% [96].

6.11 Diagnostic Add-Ons

Standardized assays for the detection of Mucorales-specific antigens are lacking. Molecular-based assays may be used for the detection of Mucormycetes from clinical specimens as well as identification of the species from positive cultures. Conventional PCR methods, analysis of restriction fragment length polymorphisms (RFLP) of specific genome regions, and DNA sequencing of defined gene regions, and melt curve analysis of PCR products are commonly used [97–102]. The majority of molecular-based assays focus on the ITS region of the genome ("pan-fungal barcode"). However, any of these methods is marked by limitations depending on their commercial availability, the lack of clinical studies and validation, restriction in application on only specific species, and/or pure cultures and cross-reactivity, respectively.

6.12 Treatment

Treatment of mucormycosis involves a combination of antifungal therapy and surgical intervention [103, 104]. Early initiation of antifungal therapy improves the outcome, and first-line treatment is intravenous amphotericin B (lipid formulation) [105], followed by posaconazole or isavuconazole as salvage treatment. Aggressive surgical debridement of involved tissues is of most importance [27, 106, 107]. In addition, the elimination of predisposing factors such as hyperglycemia, metabolic acidosis, deferoxamine therapy, immunosuppressive treatment, and neutropenia is critical.

Usually, the dose is 5 mg/kg daily of liposomal amphotericin B; a combination therapy is not recommended. Posaconazole and isavuconazole have activity against the Mucorales and are available in parenteral and oral formulations [108–111]. For patients who have responded to a lipid formulation of amphotericin B, posaconazole or isavuconazole may be used as oral step-down therapy. The use of posaconazole delayed-release tablets (300 mg every 12 h on the first day, then 300 mg once daily) is recommended [112], and a serum trough concentration of >1 mcg/mL should be attained 1 week after therapy. Limited data are available for isavuconazole, which has been evaluated in a multicenter open-label single-arm study including 37 patients with proven or probable mucormycosis [113]. Patients were treated with isavuconazole IV or orally; a case-control analysis compared patients who received isavuconazole for primary therapy of mucormycosis with control patients who received amphotericin B. Here, all-cause mortality on day 42 was similar in both groups [113].

Posaconazole or isavuconazole may be used as salvage therapy for patients who do not respond to or cannot tolerate amphotericin B [112, 114]. However, only limited data are available. Posaconazole (both IV and delayed-release formulations) should be given as a loading dose of 300 mg every 12 h on the first day, followed by a maintenance dose of 300 mg every 24 h thereafter. Isavuconazole should be given as a loading dose of 200 mg IV or orally every 8 h for the first 6 doses followed by 200 mg IV or orally every 24 h thereafter.

Generally, antifungal therapy should continue until there is clinical resolution of infection, including radiographic signs; therapy should also continue until reversal of underlying immunosuppression [115]; therapy extends for months.

The use of deferasirox as an adjunctive therapy for mucormycosis has been evaluated in few studies but with mixed results. Hence, no clear recommendations can be drawn. Hyperbaric oxygen has been used in some patients with mucormycosis, but a clear benefit has not been shown [116–118].

6.13 Case Presentation

A 56-year-old female patient was admitted to the emergency department complaining about weakness, shortness of breath, coughing, and hemoptysis. Three months before admission, systemic lupus erythematosus (SLE) was diagnosed, fulfilling the criteria serositis, fibrotic lung disease, renal failure, and Raynaud's syndrome; a rapidly progressive membranous glomerulonephritis was diagnosed by renal biopsy, and treatment with methylprednisolone (1 mg/kg) and cyclophosphamide (500 mg/kg every 2 weeks) was started. At the time of admission, laboratory data were as follows: leucocytes 0.5 G/l, erythrocytes 3.21 T/l, hemoglobin 88 g/l, thrombocytes 105 G/l, serum creatinine 4.03 mg/dl, and CRP 8.43 mg/dl. Beside pneumonia, which was treated with piperacillin/tazobactam and levofloxacin, the patient is presented with melena and a continuously decreasing hemoglobin. In order to locate and stop the site of bleeding, a gastroscopy was performed. Macroscopically

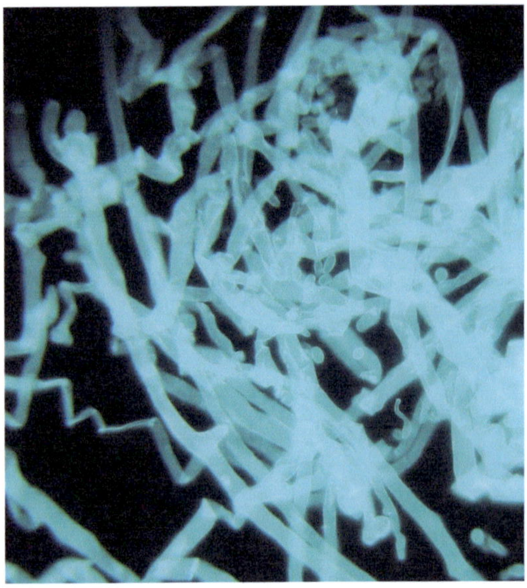

Fig. 6.1 Calcofluor-white staining of gastric fluid showing Mucorales-characteristic non- or pauci-septate hyphae, irregular with variable width, ribbon-like with wide-angle branched bifurcations

suspicious lesions for gastric cancer/lymphoma were identified, and after platelets' transfusion, a biopsy was taken. Direct microscopic examination showed fungal elements, suspicious for mucormycoses. Subsequently, gastric fluid was retrieved via a nasogastric tube for further microbiological diagnostics; calcofluor-white staining showed Mucorales-characteristic hyphae (Fig. 6.1). Fungal culture yielded *Rhizomucor pusillus*. Treatment with amphotericin B colloidal dispersion 5 mg/kg intravenously combined with amphotericin B oral suspension was initiated. Two weeks after, microscopic and culture results remained negative in further samples. The patient died of respiratory failure in the context of her fibrotic lung disease after 2 further weeks.

References

1. Talmi YP, Goldschmied-Reouven A, Bakon M et al (2002) Rhino-orbital and rhino-orbitocerebral mucormycosis. Otolaryngol Head Neck Surg 127:22–31
2. Funada H, Matsuda T (1996) Pulmonary mucormycosis in a hematology ward. Intern Med 35:540–544
3. Kume H, Yamazaki T, Abe M et al (2003) Increase in aspergillosis and severe mycotic infection in patients with leukemia and MDS: comparison of the data from the Annual of the Pathological Autopsy Cases in Japan in 1989, 1993 and 1997. Path Intern 53:744–750
4. Chamilos G, Luna M, Lewis RE et al (2006) Invasive fungal infections in patients with hematologic malignancies in a tertiary care cancer center: an autopsy study over a 15-year period (1989-2003). Haematologica 91:986–989
5. Hotchi M, Okada M, Nasu T (1980) Present state of fungal infections in autopsy cases in Japan. Am J Clin Pathol 74:410–416
6. Tietz HJ, Brehmer D, Janisch W, Martin H (1998) Incidence of endomycoses in the autopsy material of the Berlin Charité Hospital. Mycoses 41:81–85
7. Yamazaki T, Kume H, Murase S et al (1999) Epidemiology of visceral mycoses: analysis of data in annual of the pathological autopsy cases in Japan. J Clin Microbiol 37:1732–1738
8. Spellberg B, Edwards J Jr, Ibrahim A (2005) Novel perspectives on mucormycosis: pathophysiology, presentation, and management. Clin Microbiol Rev 18:556–569
9. Roden MM, Zaoutis TE, Buchanan WL et al (2005) Epidemiology and outcome of mucormycosis: a review of 929 reported cases. Clin Infect Dis 41:634–653
10. Skiada A, Pagano L, Groll A et al (2007) Zygomycosis in Europe: analysis of 230 cases accrued by the registry of the European Confederation of Medical Mycology (ECMM) Working Group on Zygomycosis between 2005 and 2007. Clin Microbiol Infect 17:1859–1867
11. Bitar D, Van Cauteren D, Lanternier F et al (2009) Increasing incidence of zygomycosis (mucormycosis), France 1997-2006. Emerg Infect Dis 15:1395–1401
12. Rees JR, Pinner RW, Hajjeh RA et al (1998) The epidemiological features of invasive mycotic infections in the San Francisco Bay area 1992-1993: results of population-based laboratory active surveillance. Clin Infect Dis 27:1138–1147
13. Torres Narbona M, Guinea J, Martinez-Alarcon J et al (2007) Impact of mucormycosis on microbiology overload: a survey study in Spain. J Clin Microbiol 45:2051–2053
14. Prabhu RM, Patel R (2004) Mucormycosis and entomophthoramycosis: a review of the clinical manifestations, diagnosis and treatment. Clin Microbiol Infect 10:31–47
15. Chakrabarti A, Das A, Mandal J et al (2006) The rising trend of invasive mucormycosis in patients with uncontrolled diabetes mellitus. Med Mycol 44:335–342
16. Buzina W, Braun H, Freudenschuss K et al (2003) Fungal biodiversity – as found in nasal mucus. Med Mycol 41:149–161
17. Ribes JA, Vanover-Sams CL, Baker DJ (2000) Zygomycetes in human diseases. Clin Microbiol Rev 13:236–301

18. Petrikkos GL, Skiada A, Sambatakou H et al (2003) Mucormycosis: ten year experience in a tertiary-care centre in Greece. Eur J Clin Microbiol Infect Dis 22:753–756
19. Antoniadou A (2009) Outbreaks of mucormycosis in hospitals. Clin Microbiol Infect 15:55–59
20. Cheng VC, Chan JF, Ngan AH et al (2009) Outbreak of intestinal infection due to Rhizopus microsporus. J Clin Microbiol 47:2834–2843
21. Gonzalez CE, Rinaldi MG, Sugar AM (2002) Mucormycosis. Infect Dis Clin N Am 16:895–914
22. Rogers TR (2008) Treatment of mucormycosis: current and new options. J Antimicrob Chemother 61:35–39
23. Goodman NL, Rinaldi MG (1991) Agents of mucormycosis. In: Balows A, Hausler WJ, Herrmann KL, Isenberg HD, Shadoomy HJ (eds) Manual of clinical microbiology, 5th edn. ASM Press, Washington, pp 674–692
24. Lopes JO, Pereira DV, Streher LA et al (1995) Cutaneous mucormycosis caused by Absidia corymbifera in a leukemic patient. Mycopathologia 130:89–92
25. Stas KJF, Louwagie GLH, Van Damme BJC et al (1996) Isolated mucormycosis in a bought living unrelated kidney transplant. Transpl Int 9:600–602
26. Zaoutis TE, Roilides E, Chiou CC et al (2007) Mucormycosis in children: a systematic review and analysis of reported cases. Pediatr Infect Dis J 26:723–727
27. Tedder M, Spratt JA, Anstadt MP et al (1994) Pulmonary mucormycosis: results of medical and surgical therapy. Ann Thorac Surg 57:1044–1050
28. Gupta KL, Khullar DK, Behera D et al (1998) Pulmonary mucormycosis presenting as fatal massive haemoptysis in a renal transplant recipient. Nephrol Dial Transplant 13:3258–3260
29. Kitabayashi A, Hirokawa M, Yamaguchi A, Takatsu H, Miura AB (1998) Invasive pulmonary mucormycosis with rupture of the thoracic aorta. Am J Hematol 58:326–329
30. Passamonte PM, Dix JD (1985) Nosocomial pulmonary mucormycosis with fatal massive hemoptysis. Am J Med Sci 289:65–68
31. Connor BA, Anderson RJ, Smith JW (1979) Mucor mediastinitis. Chest 75:525–526
32. Hsu JW, Chiang CD (1996) A case report of novel roentgenographic finding in pulmonary mucormycosis: thickening of the posterior tracheal band. Kaohsiung J Med Sci 12:595–600
33. Rubin SA, Chaljub G, Winer-Muram HT, Flicker S (1992) Pulmonary mucormycosis: a radiographic and clinical spectrum. J Thorac Imaging 7:85–90
34. McAdams HP, Rosado de Christenson M, Strollo DC, Path EF Jr (1997) Pulmonary mucormycosis: radiologic findings in 32 cases. Am J Roentgenol 168:1541–1548
35. Dykhuizen RS, Kerr KN, Soutar RL (1994) Air crescent sign and fatal haemoptysis in pulmonary mucormycosis. Scand J Infect Dis 26:498–501
36. Funada H, Misawa T, Nakao S et al (1984) The air crescent sign of invasive pulmonary mucormycosis in acute leukemia. Cancer 53:2721–2723
37. Chamilos G, Marom EM, Lewis RE, Lionakis MS, Kontoyiannis DP (2005) Predictors of pulmonary mucormycosis versus invasive pulmonary aspergillosis in patients with cancer. Clin Infect Dis 41:60–66
38. Wahba H, Truong MT, Lei X, Kontoyiannis DP, Marom EM (2008) Reversed halo sign in invasive pulmonary fungal infections. Clin Infect Dis 46:1733–1737
39. Meyer RD, Rosen P, Armstrong D (1972) Phycomycosis complicating leukemia and lymphoma. Ann Intern Med 77:871–879
40. Hosseini SM, Borghei P (2005) Rhinocerebral mucormycosis: pathways of spread. Eur Arch Otorhinolaryngol 262:932–938
41. Orguc S, Yuceturk AV, Demir MA, Goktan C (2005) Rhinocerebral mucormycosis: perineural spread via the trigeminal nerve. J Clin Neurosci 12:484–486
42. Franquet T, Gimenez A, Hidalgo A (2004) Imaging of opportunistic fungal infections in immunocompromised patient. Eur J Radiol 51:130–138
43. Garces P, Mueller D, Trevenen C (1994) Rhinocerebral mucormycosis in a child with leukemia: CT and MR findings. Pediatr Radiol 24:50–51
44. Oliveira-Neto MP, Da Silva M, Monteiro PCF et al (2006) Cutaneous mucormycosis in a young, immunocompetent girl. Med Mycol 44:567–570
45. Hampson FG, Ridgway EJ, Feeley K, Reilly JT (2005) A fatal case of disseminated mucormycosis associated with the use of blood glucose self-monitoring equipment. J Infect 51:e269–e272
46. Hocker TL, Wada DA, Bridges A, El-Azhary R (2010) Disseminated mucormycosis heralded by a subtle cutaneous finding. Dermatol Online J 16:3
47. Rubin AI, Grossman ME (2004) Bull's-eye cutaneous infarct of mucormycosis: a bedside diagnosis confirmed by touch preparation. J Am Acad Dermatol 51:996–1001
48. Kerr OA, Bong C, Wallis C, Tidman MJ (2004) Primary cutaneous mucormycosis masquerading as pyoderma gangrenosum. Br J Dermatol 150:1212–1234
49. Diven SC, Angel CA, Hawkins HK, Rowen JL, Shattuck KE (2004) Intestinal mucormycosis due to Absidia corymbifera mimicking necrotizing enterocolitis in a preterm neonate. J Perinatol 24:794–796
50. Mitchell SD, Gray J, Morgan ME et al (1996) Nosocomial infection with Rhizopus microsporus in preterm infants: association with wooden tongue depressors. Lancet 348:441–443
51. Michalak DM, Cooney DR, Rhodes KH, Telander RL, Kleinberg F (1980) Gastrointestinal mucormycoses in infants and children: a cause of gangrenous intestinal cellulitis and perforation. J Pediatr Surg 15:320–324
52. Garg PK, Gupta N, Gautam V, Hadke NS (2008) Gastric mucormycosis: unusual cause of gastric per-

foration in an immunocompetent patient. South Med J 101:449–450
53. Bittencourt AL, Ayala MA, Ramos EA (1979) A new form of abdominal mucormycosis different from mucormycosis: report of two cases and review of the literature. Am J Trop Med Hyg 28:564–569
54. Oliver MR, Van Voorhis WC, Boeckh M et al (1996) Hepatic mucormycosis in a bone marrow transplant recipient who ingested naturopathic medicine. Clin Infect Dis 22:521–524
55. Ismail MH, Hodkinson HJ, Setzen G, Sofianos C, Hale MJ (1990) Gastric mucormycosis. Trop Gastroenterol 11:103–105
56. Geramizadeh B, Modjalal M, Nabai S et al (2007) Gastrointestinal mucormycosis: a report of three cases. Mycopathologia 164:35–38
57. Echo A, Hovsepian RV, Shen GK (2005) Localized cecal mucormycosis following renal transplantation. Transpl Infect Dis 7:68–70
58. Virk SS, Singh RP, Arora AS, Grewal JS, Puri H (2004) Gastric mucormycosis – an unusual cause of massive upper gastrointestinal bleed. Indian J Gastroenterol 23:146–147
59. Azadeh B, McCarthy DO, Dalton A, Campbell F (2004) Gastrointestinal mucormycosis: two case reports. Histopathology 44:298–300
60. Park YS, Lee JD, Kim TH et al (2002) Gastric mucormycosis. Gastrointest Endosc 56:904–905
61. Siu KL, Lee WH (2004) A rare cause of intestinal perforation in an extreme low birth weight infant – gastrointestinal mucormycosis: a case report. J Perinatol 24:319–321
62. Cherney CL, Chutuape A, Fikrig MK (1999) Fatal invasive gastric mucormycosis occurring with emphysematous gastritis: case report and literature review. Am J Gastroenterol 94:252–256
63. Liu MF, Chen FF, Hsiue TR, Liu CC (2000) Disseminated mucormycosis simulating cerebrovascular disease and pulmonary alveolar haemorrhage in a patient with systemic lupus erythematosus. Clin Rheumatol 19:311–314
64. Tomita T, Ho H, Allen M, Diaz J (2005) Mucormycosis involving lungs, heart and brain, superimposed on pulmonary edema. Pathol Int 55:202–205
65. Fujii T, Takata N, Katsutani S, Kimura A (2003) Disseminated mucormycosis in an acquired immunodeficiency syndrome (AIDS) patient. Intern Med 42:129–130
66. Richardson MD, Warnock DW (2003) Mucormycosis. In: Richardson MD, Warnock DW (eds) Fungal infection diagnosis and management. Blackwell, Oxford, pp 230–240
67. Ingram CW, Sennesh J, Cooper JN, Perfect JR (1989) Disseminated mucormycosis: report of four cases and review. Rev Infect Dis 11:741–754
68. Virmani R, Connor DH, McAllister HA (1982) Cardiac mucormycosis: a report of five patients and review of 14 previously reported cases. Am J Clin Pathol 78:42–47
69. McNab AA, McKelvie P (1997) Iron overload is a risk factor for mucormycosis. Arch Ophthalmol 115:919–921
70. Sanchez-Recalde A, Merino JL, Dominguez F et al (1999) Successful treatment of prosthetic aortic valve mucormycosis. Chest 116:1818–1820
71. Levy E, Bia MJ (1995) Isolated renal mucormycosis: case report and review. J Am Soc Nephrol 5:2014–2019
72. Nagy-Agren SE, Chu P, Smith GJ et al (1995) Zygomycosis (mucormycosis) and HIV infection: report of three cases and review. J Acquir Immune Defic Syndr Hum Retrovirol 10:441–449
73. Weng DE, Wilson WH, Little R, Walsh TJ (1998) Successful medical management of isolated renal zygomycosis: case report and review. Clin Infect Dis 26:601–605
74. Langston C, Roberts DA, Porter GA, Bennett WM (1973) Renal phycomycosis. J Urol 109:941–944
75. Melnick JZ, Latimer J, Lee EI, Heinrich WL (1995) Systemic mucormycosis complicating acute renal failure: case report and review of the literature. Ren Fail 17:619–627
76. Chkhotua A, Yussim A, Tovar A et al (2001) Mucormycosis of the renal allograft: case report and review of the literature. Transpl Int 14:438–441
77. Weng DE, Wilson WH, Little R, Walsh TJ (1998) Successful medical management of isolated renal mucormycosis: case report and review. Clin Infect Dis 26:601–605
78. Mishra B, Mandal A, Kumar N (1992) Mycotic prosthetic-valve endocarditis. J Hosp Infect 20:122–125
79. Solano T, Atkins B, Tambosis E, Mann S, Gottlieb T (2000) Disseminated mucormycosis due to Saksenaea vasiformis in an immunocompetent adult. Clin Infect Dis 30:942–943
80. Zhang R, Zhang JW, Szerlip HM (2002) Endocarditis and hemorrhagic stroke caused by Cunninghamella bertholletiae infection after kidney transplantation. Am J Kidney Dis 40:842–846
81. Kalayjian RC, Herzig RH, Cohen AM, Hutton MC (1988) Thrombosis of the aorta caused by mucormycosis. South Med J 81:1180–1182
82. Mehta NN, Romanelli J, Sutton MG (2004) Native aortic valve vegetative endocarditis with Cunninghamella. Eur J Echocardiogr 5:156–158
83. Gubarev N, Separovic J, Gasparovic V, Jelic I (2007) Successful treatment of mucormycosis endocarditis complicated by pulmonary involvement. Thorac Cardiovasc Surg 55:257–258
84. Burke WV, Zych GA (2002) Fungal infection following replacement of the anterior cruciate ligament: a case report. J Bone Joint Surg 84A:449–453
85. Pierce PP, Wood MB, Roberts GD et al (1987) Saksenaea vasiformis osteomyelitis. J Clin Microbiol 25:933–935
86. Holtom PD, Obuch AB, Ahlmann ER, Shepherd LE, Patzakis MJ (2000) Mucormycosis of the tibia: a case report and review of the literature. Clin Orthop 381:222–228

87. Ben-Ami R, Luna M, Lewis RE, Walsh TJ, DP Kontoyiannis DP (2009) A clinicopathological study of pulmonary mucormycosis in cancer patients: extensive angioinvasion but limited inflammatory response. J Infect 59:134–138
88. Cornely OA, Arikan-Akdagli S, Dannaoui E et al (2014) ESCMID and ECMM joint clinical guidelines for the diagnosis and management of mucormycosis 2013. Clin Microbiol Infect 20:5–26
89. Ribes JA, Vanover-Sams CL, Baker DJ (2000) Zygomycetes in human disease. Clin Microbiol Rev 13:236–301
90. Lass-Flörl C (2009) Zygomycosis: conventional laboratory diagnosis. Clin Microbiol Infect 5:60–65
91. Lass-Flörl C, Resch G, Nachbaur D et al (2007) The value of computed tomography-guided percutaneous lung biopsy for diagnosis of invasive fungal infection in immunocompromised patients. Clin Infect Dis 45:e101–e104
92. Kontoyiannis DP, Chamilos G, Hassan SA et al (2007) Increased culture recovery of zygomycetes under physiologic temperature conditions. Am J Clin Pathol 127:208–212
93. Padhye AA, Ajello L (1988) Simple method of inducing sporulation by Apophysomyces elegans and Saksenaea vasiformis. J Clin Microbiol 26:1861–1863
94. Kontoyiannis DP, Lionakis MS, Lewis RE et al (2005) Zygomycosis in a tertiary-care cancer center in the era of Aspergillus-active antifungal therapy: a case–control observational study of 27 recent cases. J Infect Dis 191:1350–1360
95. Dolatabadi S, Kolecka A, Versteeg M, de Hoog SG, Boekhout T (2015) Differentiation of clinically relevant Mucorales Rhizopus microsporus and R. arrhizus by matrix-assisted laser desorption ionization time-of-flight mass spectrometry (MALDI-TOF MS). J Med Microbiol 64:694–701
96. Caramalho R, Maurer E, Binder U et al (2015) Etest cannot be recommended for in vitro susceptibility testing of Mucorales. Antimicrob Agents Chemother 59:3663–3665
97. Hsiao CR, Huang L, Bouchara J-P et al (2005) Identification of medically important molds by an oligonucleotide array. J Clin Microbiol 43:3760–3768
98. Nagao K, Ota T, Tanikawa A et al (2005) Genetic identification and detection of human pathogenic Rhizopus species, a major mucormycosis agent, by multiplex PCR based on internal transcribed spacer region of rRNA gene. J Dermatol Sci 39:23–31
99. Larché J, Machouart M, Burton K et al (2005) Diagnosis of cutaneous mucormycosis due to Rhizopus microsporus by an innovative PCR-restriction fragment-length polymorphism method. Clin Infect Dis 41:1362–1365
100. Machouart M, Larché J, Burton K et al (2006) Genetic identification of the main opportunistic mucorales by PCR-restriction fragment length polymorphism. J Clin Microbiol 44:805–810
101. Nyilasi I, Papp T, Csernetics Á et al (2008) High-affinity iron permease (FTR1) gene sequence-based molecular identification of clinically important Zygomycetes. Clin Microbiol Infect 14:393–397
102. Kasai M, Harrington SM, Francesconi A et al (2008) Detection of a molecular biomarker for zygomycetes by quantitative PCR assays of plasma, bronchoalveolar lavage, and lung tissue in a rabbit model of experimental pulmonary zygomycosis. J Clin Microbiol 46:3690–3702
103. Spellberg B, Walsh TJ, Kontoyiannis DP et al (2009) Recent advances in the management of mucormycosis: from bench to bedside. Clin Infect Dis 48:1743–1751
104. Farmakiotis D, Kontoyiannis DP (2016) Mucormycoses. Infect Dis Clin N Am 30:143–163
105. McCarthy M, Rosengart A, Schuetz AN et al (2014) Mold infections of the central nervous system. N Engl J Med 371:150–160
106. Brown RB, Johnson JH, Kessinger JM, Sealy WC (1992) Bronchovascular mucormycosis in the diabetic: an urgent surgical problem. Ann Thorac Surg 53:854–855
107. Gonzalez CE, Couriel DR, Walsh TJ (1997) Disseminated zygomycosis in a neutropenic patient: successful treatment with amphotericin B lipid complex and granulocyte colony-stimulating factor. Clin Infect Dis 24:192–196
108. Spanakis EK, Aperis G, Mylonakis E (2006) New agents for the treatment of fungal infections: clinical efficacy and gaps in coverage. Clin Infect Dis 43:1060–1068
109. Sun QN, Fothergill AW, McCarthy DI et al (2002) In vitro activities of posaconazole, itraconazole, voriconazole, amphotericin B, and fluconazole against 37 clinical isolates of zygomycetes. Antimicrob Agents Chemother 46:1581–1582
110. Thompson GR, Wiederhold NP (2010) Isavuconazole: a comprehensive review of spectrum of activity of a new triazole. Mycopathologia 170:291–313
111. Arendrup MC, Jensen RH, Meletiadis J (2015) In vitro activity of isavuconazole and comparators against clinical isolates of the mucorales order. Antimicrob Agents Chemother 59:7735–7742
112. Noxafil (posaconazole). Highlights of prescribing information. https://www.merck.com/product/usa/pi_circulars/n/noxafil/noxafil_pi.pdf. Accessed 18 March 2014
113. Marti FM, Ostrosky-Zeichner L, Cornely OA et al (2016) Isavuconazole treatment for mucormycosis: a single-arm open-label trial and case-control analysis. Lancet Infect Dis 16:828–837
114. Cresemba (isavuconazonium sulfate). Highlights of prescribing information. http://www.accessdata.fda.gov/drugsatfda_docs/label/2015/207500Orig1s000lbl.pdf. Accessed 9 March 2015

115. Kontoyiannis DP, Lewis RE (2011) How I treat mucormycosis. Blood 118:1216–1224
116. Yohai RA, Bullock JD, Aziz AA, Markert RJ (1994) Survival factors in rhino-orbital-cerebral mucormycosis. Surv Ophthalmol 39:3–22
117. Ferguson BJ, Mitchell TG, Moon R et al (1988) Adjunctive hyperbaric oxygen for treatment of rhinocerebral mucormycosis. Rev Infect Dis 10:551–559
118. Bentur Y, Shupak A, Ramon Y et al (1998) Hyperbaric oxygen therapy for cutaneous/soft-tissue zygomycosis complicating diabetes mellitus. Plast Reconstr Surg 102:822–824

Clinical Syndromes: Cryptococcosis

7

Romain Guery, Fanny Lanternier, and Olivier Lortholary

7.1 Epidemiology Overview

Human cryptococcosis corresponds to an invasive fungal disease caused by the encapsulated yeast *Cryptococcus* spp. Historically, cryptococcal meningitis was strongly associated with HIV epidemics in 1980s. Though incidence decreased in developed countries with cART (combination anti-retroviral therapy, formerly called highly active antiretroviral therapy) availability, cryptococcosis remains an important concern in low-resource countries. In 2014, incidence of cryptococcal meningitis was estimated to be 220,000 cases per year in the world with 73% of cases occurring in sub-Saharan Africa. Despite recent access to cART in many African countries with high HIV prevalence, there is no decrease of cryptococcal meningitis incidence. Without treatment, cryptococcosis is always fatal. Early global mortality approaches 20% in developed countries and up to 70% in low-resource countries where cART and "mandatory" antifungal agents of cryptococcosis (i.e., amphotericin B, flucytosine, fluconazole) are not available. Cryptococcosis still accounts for 15% of AIDS-related mortality.

R. Guery · F. Lanternier · O. Lortholary (✉)
Université Paris Descartes, Sorbonne Paris Cité, Assistance Publique-Hôpitaux de Paris, Hôpital Necker Enfants Malades, Centre d'Infectiologie Necker-Pasteur and Institut Imagine, Paris, France
e-mail: olivier.lortholary@aphp.fr

In HIV-negative individuals, cryptococcosis occurs in patients with primary or acquired impaired cell-mediated immunity including solid organ transplant recipient (Table 7.1). Cryptococcosis is the third most frequent fungal infection in solid organ transplant patients (SOT). As up to 20% of patients in non-HIV/non-transplant cohorts of cryptococcosis had no apparent immunodeficiency, immunogenetic investigation should be performed. Autoantibodies against GM-CSF, for example, have been recently detected in cryptococcosis in otherwise healthy individuals. Moreover, emergences of *C. gattii* throughout the tropics in patients with no known risk factors were observed during an outbreak in Pacific Norwest in 1999 and some sporadic cases in the USA and Europe. Regarding these recent findings, all patients including apparently immunocompetent ones with unexplained acute or chronic meningitis should be tested for cryptococcosis if common differential diagnoses have been excluded.

7.2 Pathogen

Cryptococcus spp. belong to the group of Basidiomycetes. *C. neoformans* and *C. gattii* are the two main species complexes that cause cryptococcosis in humans (Fig. 7.1). Less commonly rare emerging pathogenic species are *C. laurentii* and *C. albidus*. *Cryptococcus* spp. identification

E. Presterl (ed.), *Clinically Relevant Mycoses*, https://doi.org/10.1007/978-3-319-92300-0_7

at species complex level (*C. neoformans* and *C. gattii*) is sufficient in clinical context. Both species are now ubiquitous and reside in a wide range of ecological niches such as decaying material from trees and their surrounding or avian excreta for *C. gattii* and *C. neoformans*, respectively. Initially confined to tropical regions including South America, Australia, and New Zealand, *C. gattii* has now emerged in temperate zones during the British Columbia/Pacific Northwest outbreak. There is also a significant increase of *C. gattii* infections in humans and animals outside Pacific Northwest region in Europe, Africa, and Asia, while mechanisms of its recent widespread remain unclear. Acquired infection by *C. neoformans* occurs via airway transmission, but direct cutaneous inoculation or organ-transmitted diseases have also been described. *C. neoformans* infects humans after inhalation mostly during childhood as seroepidemiological surveys indicate that 70% of children below 5 years have antibodies against *C. neoformans* proteins. This step is followed by yeast dormancy which can persist for years. In some individuals reactivation occurs upon immunosuppression and conducts to dissemination in blood and central nervous system. However, de novo acquisition from the environment rather than reactivation is a possible route of invasive infection especially for clonal strains of *C. gattii* responsible of outbreaks. Major virulence factors of *C. neoformans* include a capsule that confers resistance to phagocytosis, ability to grow at 37 °C, and melanization providing protection from reactive oxygen molecules. However virulence of this encapsulated yeast is quite complex and variable among different strains but also for a same strain depending of the environment.

Table 7.1 Risk factors for cryptococcosis

Risk factors of cryptococcosis
HIV infection +++
Solid organ transplantation[a] ++ Hematological malignancies[a] (mostly chronic lymphoid disorders) HTLV-1 carriers and ATLL
Immunosuppressive therapy
Corticosteroids ++
Fludarabine
Alemtuzumab (anti-CD52)
Anti-TNF-alpha agents Fingolimod Ibrutinib
Connective tissue disease[a]
Sarcoidosis
Systemic lupus erythematosus
Rheumatoid arthritis
Primary immunodeficiencies
Idiopathic CD4 lymphopenia
GATA 2 deficiency IL12Rβ1 deficiency
X-linked CD40L deficiency
STAT3 mutated hyper IgE syndrome
Autoantibodies against IFN-γ Autoantibodies against GM-CSF STAT 1 gain-of-function
Diabetes mellitus
Renal failure or peritoneal dialysis
Chronic pulmonary disease or lung cancer
Cirrhosis
Pregnancy

Abbreviations: *ATLL* acute T-cell leukemia/lymphoma, *GM-CSF* granulocyte macrophage colony-stimulating factor, *IFN-γ* interferon gamma, *HIV* human immunodeficiency virus, *HTLV-1* human T-cell leukemia virus type 1, *TNF* tumor necrosis factor

[a]Often associated with concomitant immunosuppressive therapy

7.3 Clinical Presentation: Major Syndrome

By contrast with *C. neoformans* incubation that could last for more than several decades, median

Fig. 7.1 Simplified classification of *Cryptococcus* spp. according to serotypes and molecular types (PCR-fingerprinting/RFLP-genotype). RFLP: restriction fragment length polymorphism

Species complex	Varieties	Serotypes	Molecular types
Cryptococcus neoformans	*Grubii*	A	VNI, VNII, VNB
	Neoformans	D	VNIV
	-	A/D (diploid hybrid)	VNIII
Cryptococcus gattii	-	B/C	VGI, VGII, VGIII, VGIV

C. gattii incubation is 6 months (from 6 weeks to 2 years) according to studies of travelers returning from Vancouver Island during the outbreak. The lung and/or central nervous system (CNS) is the predilection site of infection. Symptoms usually develop over several weeks, but clinical manifestations may be acute.

7.3.1 Neurological Presentation

As cryptococcal meningitis can be diagnosed in HIV patients with only cephalalgia and/or fever, degree of suspicion should be extremely high especially if CD4 count is below 100/mm^3. Fever can be absent in half of cases. Seizures and focal neurological signs are inconstant. Altered level of consciousness is a strong prognosis factor. Outside HIV context, common causes of chronic meningitis are tuberculosis, cryptococcosis, carcinomatous meningitis, and coccidioidomycosis in endemic areas. Clinicians should actively search for these etiologies that imply large volume of CSF (at least 7 ml–120 drops) and exhaustive microbiological work-up (Fig. 7.2). Inaugural hearing or visual losses are more prevalent in non-HIV/non-transplant patients. Cryptococcomas are defined as abscesses caused by *Cryptococcus* spp. It has been reported more frequently with *C. gattii*.

7.3.2 Pulmonary Presentation

During Vancouver outbreak of *C. gattii*, lung involvement was the most common site of disease in 87% of patients. In Australia, isolated lung and combined lung and CNS diseases were reported in 12% and 51% of cases, respectively. During HIV-associated cryptococcal meningitis, pulmonary involvement occurs in 10–55% of the cases, while true incidence of cryptococcal pneumonia in absence of meningitis remains partially unknown due to lack of facilities for investigation in developing countries. Spectrum of clinical manifestation ranges from asymptomatic to acute respiratory distress syndrome. No particular findings are associated with pulmonary cryptococcosis which is undistinguishable from other causes of pneumonia. Large pulmonary cryptococcomas are sometimes misdiagnosed as tumor. Thoracic imaging shows most commonly solitary or multiple nodules from 5 to 30mm, but consolidation, interstitial infiltration, pleural effusion, mediastinal lymphadenopathy, and cavities may be seen.

7.3.3 Fungemia

Fungemia commonly precedes CNS involvement. One positive blood culture should lead to exhaustive work-up for *C. neoformans* dissemination and start specific therapy. HIV patients have more frequently bloodstream infection compared to non-HIV patients.

7.3.4 Cutaneous Involvement

Molluscum contagiosum-like lesions are highly suggestive of disseminated disease in immunocompromised patients. By contrast, primary

Exhaustive work-up for *Cryptococcus* spp. diagnosis
Lumbar puncture with a minimum of 3ml (50-60 drops) of CSF for India-ink testing, fungal cultures, LFA, CRAG titres
Measure of CSF opening pressure
Brain imaging (MRI or CT) (before lumbar puncture if focal signs or altered vigilance (GCS<8))
Urine sample for direct examination and cultures (at least in male patients)
Blood sample for culture
Skin biopsy of any suspect lesion
LFA and/or CRAG testing in serum
Chest imaging +/- cultures of sputum or bronchoalveolar lavage if clinic-radiological signs
Work-up for risk factors: testing for HIV, HTLV-1 status and measure of CD4 count
Identification of species complex (*C. gattii* or *C. neoformans*)
Start antifungal therapy after sampling

Fig. 7.2 Exhaustive work-up for *Cryptococcus* spp. diagnosis. Abbreviations: *CRAG* cryptococcal antigen, *CSF* cerebrospinal fluid, *GCS* Glasgow coma scale, *LFA* lateral flow assay

cryptococcosis occurs by direct inoculation and has been reported in apparently immunocompetent individuals. Nodules, ulcers, or cellulitis are reported in patients living in rural areas reporting outdoor activities and exposition to contaminated source such as avian excreta, wood debris, and soil.

7.3.5 Other Involvement

Genitourinary tract can be involved. Some relapse may result from *Cryptococcus* reservoir in the prostate. Other localizations of cryptococcosis have been described including lymph nodes, muscle, bones and joints, heart valve, and peritoneum.

7.4 Diagnosis

7.4.1 Microbiology Pathology

7.4.1.1 Cerebrospinal Fluid (CSF) Findings

A normal CSF profile does not rule out cryptococcosis. White cell count is generally low below 100 cells per mm^3 with a predominance of lymphocytes. CSF glucose is low or normal. CSF protein level is generally elevated below 1.5 g/L. CSF findings depend on host immunity and species of *Cryptococcus* spp. Spectrum varies from normal CSF with high fungal burden in immunocompromised hosts to elevated pleocytosis (>100 mm^3) with high protein concentration (>2 g/L) in apparently immunocompetent host infected by *C. gattii*. A limited inflammatory reaction (<20 cells/mm^3) is associated with poor prognosis in HIV patients.

7.4.1.2 Microscopic Testing

India ink staining of CSF sample with centrifugation has nearly 80% of sensitivity in HIV-related cryptococcosis, but it can be lower in HIV-negative patients because of low fungal burden (Fig. 7.3). Sensitivity of microscopic examination may increase in case of staining of CSF sediments with at least 1 ml of CSF.

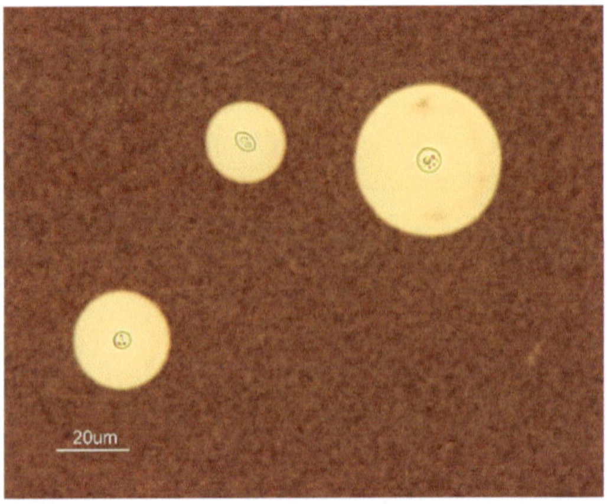

Fig. 7.3 Ink india staining of *Cryptococcus* yeasts with large capsule

7.4.1.3 Cultures

Cultures of CSF, urine, blood, as well as sputum or bronchoalveolar lavage samples are the gold standard for diagnosis. *Cryptococcus* spp. grows well at 30 °C rather than 37 °C on usual media used for bacteria and fungi except those with cycloheximide. Large volumes of CSF (3–5 ml) are required (for optimal recovery of *Cryptococcus* spp.) as well as prolonged fungal cultures up to 3 weeks (especially during antifungal therapy). Use of quantitative CSF yeast count in management is so far not routinely done.

7.4.1.4 Antigen Detection (CRAG)

Detection of capsule antigen (CRAG) is carried out using latex agglutination (LA) and/or enzyme-linked immunoassays (EIA) in fresh samples such as serum and CSF. Performances are better in HIV patients compared to non-HIV patients even in case of disseminated disease. Low fungal burden or very high fungal burden due to prozone phenomenon and absence of pronase use could explain false-negative tests in serum or CSF sample. Thus, high degree of clinical suspicion needs to repeat LA and/or EIA with different kits as sensitivity between two kits is sometimes different for *C. gattii* species. In contrast, false positive of CRAG includes the presence of rheumatoid factor, use of hydroxyethyl starch fluid, cross-reaction with *Trichosporon* spp. antigen, and nonpathogenic *Cryptococcus* species.

Cryptococcal antigen lateral flow assay (LFA) is a rapid and reliable method based on dipstick sandwich immunochromatographic assay which is more sensitive than LA in HIV patients. Two kits are available: (1) LFA IMMY (Norman, Oklahoma) and (2) LFA Biosynex (Biosynex and Institut Pasteur, Paris). LFA IMMY could be performed on serum, whole blood, and CSF. Its use with urine is not approved as false positive has been reported by Longley et al. in a prospective study conducted in South Africa and by Magambo et al. in Tanzania. Results are available in 15 min, and 40 μl of body fluid (serum, plasma, CSF) are generally sufficient for testing. Samples do not require pronase pretreatment. A second lateral flow test (LFA Biosynex) is recently available; it permits a semiquantitative approach with one (low fungal burden) or two positive bands (high fungal burden). Compared to CRAG, performances of LFA IMMY on serum or CSF could be excellent in non-HIV patients but still require evaluations. LFA cross-react with *C. gattii* (serotype B and C) and could also be as useful tool for diagnosis of *C. gattii* infection, but sufficient data are lacking so far.

7.4.1.5 Pathology

In some settings such as unusual localization of cryptococcosis or in apparently immunocompetent patients, samples are not commonly sent to mycology unit because cryptococcosis is not suspected. In this case, pathology findings with special stains remain the cornerstone of cryptococcosis diagnosis. Yeast measures 5–10μ and is surrounded by a clear space corresponding to a capsule in tissue section colored by HES. Alcian Blue or Southgate's mucicarmine stains color the capsule. Fontana-Masson stain is positive and detects production of melanin by *Cryptococcus* spp. Spectrum of pathological findings encompasses well-formed necrotizing granulomas with intracellular yeasts to abundant extracellular yeasts without any inflammation depending on host immunity.

7.4.1.6 Antifungal Susceptibility Testing

There are currently no breakpoints for antifungals against *C. neoformans* and *C. gattii*. No controlled trial has actually demonstrated any correlation between MICs and clinical outcome. High MICs for any antifungal agents should be interpreted with caution despite interlaboratory variability and technical issues of susceptibility testing of *Cryptococcus* spp.

7.4.1.7 Species Complex Identification

C. gattii can be easily identified using a colorimetric culture on cavanine glycine bromothymol blue agar. MaldiTOF has been shown to be a promising tool for species complex identification. However, large capsule of *Cryptococcus* spp. isolated from fresh patient sample can interfere with spectra identification. In vitro capsule-reduction protocol could increase rate of identification at species level by MaldiTOF. Some simple PCR protocols emerge as reliable method for species identification in low-resource settings but still require standardization.

7.4.2 Is a Correct Identification of *Cryptococcus* at Species Complex Level Relevant or Not in Clinical Practice?

C. gattii affects more frequently apparently immunocompetent individuals. While lung involvement is more frequent in the USA, *C. gattii* neurological manifestations are more frequent and severe in Australasia, Asia, and Europe. Neurological sequelae such as blindness and deafness are more frequent compared with *C. neoformans* infections and depend on other factors such as sporadic or outbreak infection, *C. gattii* genotypes, and hosts factors. Despite the lack of randomized trials, patients with *C. gattii* may be treated longer with antifungal treatment. A 6 weeks induction course of amphotericin B and flucytosine (5-FC) followed by fluconazole consolidation may be necessary. Moreover, shunting or placement of CSF drains should be considered earlier in management of raised intracranial pressure. Whereas corticosteroid are deleterious in HIV-related cryptococcal meningitis, it could be beneficial in some patients infected by *C. gattii* especially those with severe inflammatory response. Finally, *C. gattii* strains exhibit commonly higher fluconazole MICs than *C. neoformans* strains, but no data correlate this finding with clinical outcome. However there remain controversies about the need for species identification as guidelines show no treatment differences between *C. neoformans* infection in apparently immunocompetent host and *C. gattii* infection. In addition, few laboratories outside endemic areas of *C. gattii* are able to identify both species complex. IDSA guidelines recommend up to 6 weeks of induction therapy in non-transplant/non-HIV patients whatever the identified *Cryptococcus* species. Chen et al. support these recommendations and suggest treating *C. gattii* VGI infection involving the lung and/or the CNS with induction therapy with amphotericin B plus 5-flucytosine for 6 weeks for CNS disease and for 2 weeks for severe isolated lung disease. Shorter induction courses may be effective in patients with mild CNS disease, but current data are insufficient to definitively support this proposal.

7.4.3 Imaging

Cryptococcosis pulmonary imaging is non-specific (*see pulmonary presentation*). Conversely, it is useful to be aware of some imaging-specific CNS cryptococcosis findings. MRI is more sensitive at baseline than CT in HIV patients (abnormal imaging in 92% versus 53%). Dilated Virchow-Robin spaces, masses, pseudocysts, and meningitis are the most frequent patterns in HIV patients. Dilated Virchow-Robin spaces correspond to accumulation of *Cryptococcus* gelatinous material along the wall of theses spaces that surround vessels from subarachnoid space through the brain parenchyma (Fig. 7.4). In apparent immunocompetent, leptomeningeal enhancement and hydrocephalus are more common, but dilated Virchow-Robin spaces and pseudocysts near to basal ganglia may be seen. Cryptococcomas and other masses are sometimes mistaken as tumor especially in otherwise healthy patients.

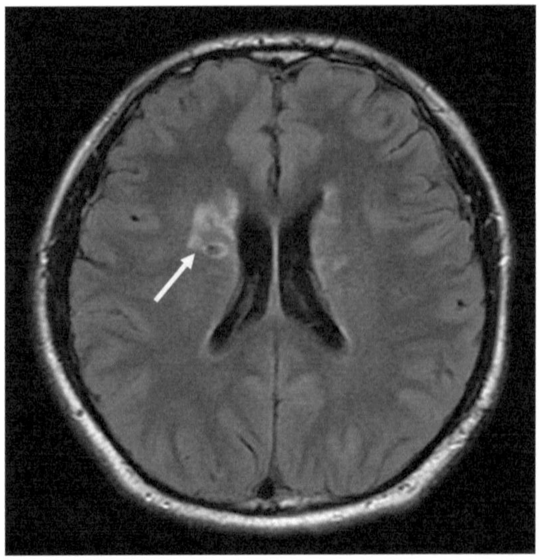

Fig. 7.4 MR imaging of brain showing hyperintense lesions on T2-FLAIR sequences corresponding to dilated perivascular Virchow-Robin spaces (*white arrow*)

7.5 Treatment

7.5.1 Principles of Antifungal Treatment

Patients with mild-to-moderate localized forms (cutaneous, bones and joints, or urine) without evidence of disseminated disease can be treated with fluconazole monotherapy (fluconazole 400 mg/day for 6–12 months). In other situations, amphotericin B (AmB) + flucytosine (5-FC) association for a minimum of 14 days remains the cornerstone of induction therapy of cryptococcosis. In high-resource countries, liposomal AmB rather than deoxycholate AmB should be preferred (opinion of the authors) regarding a better profile of tolerance (Table 7.2).

Three phases of cryptococcosis treatment (Table 7.2):

- Induction phase with liposomal amphotericin B (3 mg/kg/day) and flucytosine (100 mg/kg/day in four divided doses) for at least 2 weeks and up to 6 weeks depending on host and clinical/mycological response to therapy. Guidelines recommend 4–6 weeks of induction therapy in non-HIV/non-transplant

Table 7.2 Cryptococcosis treatment adapted from IDSA guidelines, WHO recommendations, and recent ACTA trial results

	Meningoencephalitis *recommended therapy*	Meningoencephalitis *alternatives adapted from WHO guidelines and ACTA trial*				Mild to moderate isolated pulmonary disease or skin disease	Severe extra CNS forms or fungemia
Induction[a] (2–6 weeks)	Liposomal amphotericin B[b] (3 mg/kg/day) + 5-FC (100 mg/kg/day per os given in four divided doses)	5-FC + FCZ[c] (1200 mg/day) *preferred alternative*	AmB 14 days + FCZ[d] (800–1200 mg/day)	AmB 7 days + FCZ[d] (1200 mg/day)	FCZ[e] (1200 mg/day)	FCZ (400 mg/day) 6–12 months	Treat as CNS disease
Consolidation[f] (8–10 weeks)	FCZ (400-800 mg/day)[c]	ITZ (400 mg/day) *VCZ not evaluated* *PSZ not evaluated*				/	Treat as CNS disease
Maintenance[f] (6–12 months minimum until stable immune reconstitution)	FCZ (200–400 mg/day)[f]	ITZ (400 mg/day) *VCZ not evaluated* *PSZ not evaluated*				/	Treat as CNS disease

Abbreviations: *AmB* amphotericin B, *CNS* central nervous system, *FCZ* fluconazole, *ITZ* itraconazole, *VCZ* voriconazole, *PSZ* posaconazole, *5-FC* flucytosine)

[a]In HIV-associated cryptococcal meningitis (African setting), 1 week of deoxycholate AmB + 5-FC as first-line induction therapy followed by FCZ 1200 mg/day (7 days) is non-inferior to 2 weeks regimen of AmB + 5-FC regarding recent ACTA trial results [1]

[b]Authors proposition: only deoxycholate AmB given at doses reaching 1 mg/kg (most commonly accepted daily dosage) has been prospectively evaluated in combination with 5-FC, but from our opinion, L-AmB is a preferable alternative less nephrotoxic with similar outcome, as it has been observed in three studies but unfortunately not in combination with 5-FC in both HIV patients and SOT recipients [2–4]

[c]If amphotericin B is not available. Best effective alternative regarding recent ACTA trial results [1]

[d]If flucytosine is not available. FCZ 1200 mg/day was the chosen dosage for ACTA trial

[e]If flucytosine and amphotericin B are not available. Fluconazole monotherapy is discouraged due to poor effectiveness (approximately 70% of mortality)

[f]FCZ dose and duration of each phase during consolidation and maintenance therapy should be adapted on host immunity (see text)

patients as well as patients with *C. gattii* meningitis. The second phase should begin only if there is a global improvement and ideally CSF sterile cultures at day 14.
- Consolidation phase with fluconazole (400–800 mg/day) for 8–10 weeks. We and others suggest using fluconazole (FCZ) at a dose of 800 mg/day in non-HIV patients and in HIV patients until cART introduction.
- A maintenance phase is indicated and depends on host immunity. Maintenance phase should begin after microbiological assessment in CSF at week 10. A minimum of 6–12 months of FCZ (200–400 mg/day) is required. Long-term maintenance therapy with FCZ (200 mg/day) is indicated in HIV patients until immune reconstitution (CD4 >100/mm^3, undetectable viral load for at least 3 months, cryptococcal antigen <1/512) and after a minimum of 12 months of antifungal therapy. FCZ (200–400 mg/day) maintenance is indicated in non-HIV patients for 6–12 months.

There are currently no specific guidelines on *C. gattii* cryptococcosis, but as mentioned above, induction therapy phase should be prolonged up to 6 weeks regardless of host immunity status. Eradication phase with FCZ (400 mg/day) rather than concept of consolidation/maintenance phase should be continued up to 18 months in CNS disease caused by *C. gattii*.

7.5.1.1 New Strategies in Developing Countries

As amphotericin B (deoxycholate or liposomal form) and flucytosine are not widely available, new treatment strategies are urgently needed. A phase III randomized non inferiority trial in Africa (AMBITION study) will evaluate the efficacy and safety of a short course of high dose of liposomal AmB (10 mg/kg at day one) versus deoxycholate AmB 1 mg/kg/day for 14 days. In the same vein, the ACTA (Advancing Cryptococcal Meningitis Treatment for Africa) study has compared 3 strategies in 680 HIV patients: FCZ (1200 mg/day) plus 5-FC (100 mg/kg/day) for 2 weeks, AmB deoxycholate (1 mg/kg/day) plus FCZ (1200 mg/day) or 5-FC (100 mg/kg/day) for 7 days, or AmB deoxycholate (1 mg/kg/day) plus FCZ (1200 mg/day) or 5-FC (100 mg/kg/day) for 14 days. Preliminary results [1] showed that a short course of 1 week combined AmB-based therapy and oral combination (FCZ+5FC) was non-inferior to 2 weeks AmB-based therapy. 5-FC appears to be the best adjunctive therapy with AmB compared to FCZ.

7.5.2 Supportive Treatment

7.5.2.1 Surgery

Surgery is sometimes indicated in large cryptococcomas (>3 cm) with or without mass effect or large empyemas. A stereotaxic debulking procedure or surgical resection may be performed especially for CNS or pulmonary lesions not responding to antifungal therapy.

7.5.2.2 Treatment of Intracranial Hypertension

Opening pressure (OP) should be measured at baseline. Every 24–48 h, lumbar puncture drainage are required if OP is above 25 cmH20. Brain imaging should be performed before lumbar puncture if presence of focal neurological signs seriously altered vigilance. We and others recommend to repeat pressure measure after 10 ml of CSF drained and then stop if OP is below 20 cmH20 or 50% of initial opening pressure. A maximum of 30 ml (500–600 drops) of CSF daily drained seems to be safe. If this strategy is not sufficient to control OP, the situation should prompt neurosurgical evaluation for temporary drain or permanent ventricular or lumbar shunt. As CNS imaging or fundoscopy may be normal even in the case of severe intracranial hypertension, indication of drainage should be based on opening pressure. Positive CSF fungal cultures are not a contra-indication for shunting.

7.5.2.3 Treatment of Hydrocephalus

True hydrocephalus is quite rare in cryptococcal meningitis but occurs in apparently immunocompetent patients and/or those infected with *C. gattii*. Hydrocephalus requires early neurosurgical evaluation for shunt or drains.

7.5.2.4 Corticosteroid

Corticosteroid as adjunctive therapy is not recommended in HIV-associated cryptococcosis outside IRIS-related severe manifestations. A recent double-blind, randomized, placebo-controlled trial conducted in Asia and Africa has shown no effect on mortality and more adverse event and disability in patients with HIV-associated cryptococcal meningitis. However one retrospective study conducted in Papua New Guinea suggests a benefit on visual outcome in *C. gattii* meningitis in non-HIV/non-transplant patients. In addition, some cases report described substantive effect of corticosteroids in management of refractory cases of *C. gattii* meningitis but does not support its use in routine clinical practice or during non-*C. gattii* CNS disease.

7.5.2.5 Gamma Interferon

Recombinant gamma interferon could be considered in selected refractory cases as salvage therapy if combined with antifungals

7.5.2.6 Management of IRIS and/or Relapse

IRIS corresponds to a sterile granulomatous process induced by the restoration of Th1 response following initiation of HAART in HIV patients or reduction of immunosuppressive drugs in SOT patients. In a practical way, symptomatic relapse of cryptococcal meningitis or IRIS are indistinguishable. Thus, adherence to fluconazole therapy and other opportunistic infections should be investigated. A lumbar puncture must be obtained with measure of opening pressure, routine investigations, and fungal and mycobacterial cultures with large volume of CSF (3–5 ml). While fungal cultures are pending, induction therapy with amphotericin B and flucytosine must be restarted. If cultures of CSF are positive, fluconazole susceptibility compared to initial isolates should be obtained to detect secondary resistance. If cultures of CSF are negative, IRIS should be considered if other opportunistic infections have been excluded. IRIS with minor symptoms does not require specific treatment. In contrast, IRIS with major complications (CNS inflammation) often requires corticosteroids (0.5 mg/kg/day for 2–6 weeks) and aggressive management of raised intracranial pressure in addition to antifungal treatment. Some studies suggest a role for thalidomide or anti-TNF agents in steroid resistant/dependent IRIS.

7.5.3 Host Specificities

7.5.3.1 HIV Patients

Introduction of cART should be deferred until 4–5 weeks after cryptococcal meningitis diagnosis as early introduction is associated with increased mortality. Virtually all cART regimens could be used. Physicians need to be vigilant considering a drug-drug interaction between fluconazole and cART. Hepatitis and overdosing of nevirapine are reported in this case.

7.5.3.2 Solid Organ Transplant Patients

Reducing the degree of immunosuppression is highly recommended in a multistep process. Occurrence of severe IRIS has been described in transplant patients with increased risk of graft dysfunction or loss. We recommend starting with corticosteroid reduction and not tapering or discontinuing calcineurin inhibitors. Drug-drug interaction between fluconazole and calcineurin inhibitors implies therapeutic monitoring of tacrolimus and ciclosporin.

7.5.3.3 Non-transplant/Non-HIV Patients

As mentioned above and according to old studies, this heterogeneous group may require a prolonged induction phase (4–6 weeks) because poor outcomes attributed to delayed diagnosis in these patients. However, some patients respond successfully to a 2 weeks induction phase with 5-FC (100 mg/kg/day) and AmB at conventional dosage (1 mg/kg/day). A consolidation and maintenance phases decrease the risk of relapse. Resolution of symptoms and at least 1 year of antifungal therapy are prerequisites for stopping therapy if no patent immunodeficiency has been proved. Large cryptococcomas without surgical removal often require prolonged antifungal consolidation therapy with high doses of fluconazole (400–800 mg/day) for 6–18 months.

7.5.3.4 Pregnant Women

Liposomal amphotericin B (3 mg/kg/day) is the only approved antifungal in cryptococcosis occurring in pregnant woman. Data on 5-FC are lacking to justify its use outside life-threatening cryptococcosis. However it is worth noting that AmB monotherapy is a less effective alternative to the combination of 5-FC and AmB. Fluconazole is highly teratogenic (total FCZ dose >300 mg) and should be only considered after delivery.

7.5.3.5 Children

Children are treated as adults with induction therapy with L-AmB and 5-FC. Fluconazole is prescribed at a dose of 10–12 mg/kg/day for consolidation therapy and at a dose of 6 mg/kg/day for maintenance therapy.

7.5.4 Follow-up

The primary objectives at week 2 of induction phase are clinical improvement, resolving of intracranial hypertension, and CSF sterility. Quantitative cultures are not routinely done in a clinical context. As mentioned above, antigen CSF and serum decrease is often difficult to monitor and to correlate to outcome. A microbiological assessment on CSF should be done at week 2 and at week 10.

7.5.5 Prognosis

Despite cART therapy, global mortality of cryptococcosis approaches 20% in developed countries and much over 50% in low-resource countries lacking of antiretroviral therapy and/or antifungal agents. Concerning determinants of early and late mortality during cryptococcal meningitis, a study enrolling 230 patients in France reported a death rate of 6.5% and 18% at day 14 and week 10, respectively. Predictive factor of mortality at baseline were abnormal neurological status and abnormal brain imaging. Another study conducted in low-resource countries (Thailand, Uganda, Malawi, and South Africa) has followed 501 HIV-patients for a minimum of 10 weeks between 2002 and 2010. Mortality rates were 17% and 34% at 2 weeks and 10 weeks, respectively. High CSF fungal burden, altered mental status, age >50 years, and reduction of rate of clearance of infection were predictors of early mortality at week 2. The median time to death was 13 days suggesting that early management is critical during cryptococcal meningitis. According to recent reports, non-HIV/non-transplant patients may have an increased risk of mortality due to delayed diagnosis and treatment.

7.5.6 Prevention

Positive cryptococcal antigenemia precedes cryptococcal disease in asymptomatic HIV patients with CD4 below 100/mm^3. Cryptococcal LFA should be done in HIV patients with CD4 below 100/mm^3. In case of positivity, a lumbar puncture must rule out cryptococcal meningitis. In the absence of meningitis, patients should receive fluconazole (800 mg/day) as preemptive treatment. cART can be deferred 2 weeks after fluconazole beginning. Routine screening is not recommended in transplant patients. At the present time, no vaccine has been evaluated in human clinical trials.

7.6 Common Mistakes to Avoid in Cryptococcosis Management

One serious mistake to avoid is stopping flucytosine because of high MICs. In fact, resistance to 5-FC can occur by mutation on cytosine permease or cytosine deaminase, but AmB can restore 5-FC activity if there is a defect for cytosine permease. Actual techniques cannot distinguish these mechanisms of resistance. For clinical practice, we therefore recommend to use 5-FC even if high MICs were found during susceptibility testing which has sometimes technical issues. Concerning fluconazole resistance, high MICs of *C. neoformans* in absence of prior azole exposure is classically reported. Again, no study has proven that high fluconazole MICs at baseline correlates with clinical outcome.

A second mistake is to use monitoring of serum CRAG during follow-up of cryptococcal meningitis. Almost two studies from Powderly et al. [5] and Aberg et al. [6] did not show any correlations between CRAG titers changes over time and outcome (relapse or persistent disease). However, serum CRAG measurement is of major importance when decision of interrupting maintenance therapy is raise. Indeed, we evidenced that high LA titers (>1/512) were associated with relapse in patients for whom fluconazole maintenance has been interrupted. Thus, maintenance therapy with fluconazole should not be stopped if CRAG titers are above 1/512 in HIV patients treated for cryptococcal meningitis.

A third mistake is to delay shunting in case of incontrollable elevated opening pressure because brain imaging shows no hydrocephalus and no radiological signs of intracranial hypertension. Severity of cranial hypertension should be especially evaluated on clinical findings and opening pressure.

As discussed above, last mistakes to avoid in HIV-related cryptococcal meningitis due to increased mortality include the use of corticosteroid as adjunctive therapy outside IRIS-related severe manifestations and the beginning of cART before 4 weeks of antifungal therapy.

Suggested Readings

Beardsley J, Wolbers M, Kibengo FM et al (2016) Adjunctive dexamethasone in HIV-associated cryptococcal meningitis. N Engl J Med 374:542–554

Boulware DR, Meya DB, Muzoora C et al (2014) Timing of antiretroviral therapy after diagnosis of cryptococcal meningitis. N Engl J Med 370:2487–2498

Chen SC-A, Meyer W, Sorrell TC (2014) Cryptococcus gattii infections. Clin Microbiol Rev 27:980–1024

Day JN, Chau TTH, Wolbers M et al (2013) Combination antifungal therapy for cryptococcal meningitis. N Engl J Med 368:1291–1302

Guery R, Lanternier F, Pilmis B, Lortholary O Cryptococcus neoformans (cryptococcosis) - infectious disease and antimicrobial agents. In: antimicrobe.org. http://www.antimicrobe.org/new/f04.asp. Accessed 27 Apr 2017

Kwon-Chung KJ, Bennett JE, Wickes BL et al (2017) The case for adopting the "species complex" nomenclature for the etiologic agents of cryptococcosis. mSphere 2:e00357–e00316

May RC, Stone NRH, Wiesner DL, Bicanic T, Nielsen K (2016) Cryptococcus: from environmental saprophyte to global pathogen. Nat Rev Microbiol 14:106–117

Perfect JR, Dismukes WE, Dromer F et al (2010) Clinical practice guidelines for the management of cryptococcal disease: 2010 update by the Infectious Diseases Society of America. Clin Infect Dis 50:291–322

Sun H-Y, Alexander BD, Huprikar S et al (2015) Predictors of immune reconstitution syndrome in organ transplant recipients with cryptococcosis: implications for the management of immunosuppression. Clin Infect Dis 60:36–44

Williamson PR, Jarvis JN, Panackal AA, Fisher MC, Molloy SF, Loyse A, Harrison TS (2016) Cryptococcal meningitis: epidemiology, immunology, diagnosis and therapy. Nat Rev Neurol. doi: https://doi.org/10.1038/nrneurol.2016.167

References

1. Molloy SF, Kanyama C, Heyderman RS, Loyse A, Kouanfack C, Chanda D et al (2018) Antifungal combinations for treatment of cryptococcal meningitis in Africa. N Engl J Med 378(11):1004–1017
2. Hamill RJ, Sobel JD, El-Sadr W, Johnson PC, Graybill JR, Javaly K et al (2010) Comparison of 2 doses of liposomal amphotericin B and conventional amphotericin B deoxycholate for treatment of AIDS-associated acute cryptococcal meningitis: a randomized, double-blind clinical trial of efficacy and safety. Clin Infect Dis Off Publ Infect Dis Soc Am 51(2):225–232
3. Leenders AC, Reiss P, Portegies P, Clezy K, Hop WC, Hoy J et al (1997) Liposomal amphotericin B (AmBisome) compared with amphotericin B both followed by oral fluconazole in the treatment of AIDS-associated cryptococcal meningitis. AIDS Lond Engl 11(12):1463–1471
4. Sun H-Y, Alexander BD, Lortholary O, Dromer F, Forrest GN, Lyon GM et al (2009) Lipid formulations of amphotericin B significantly improve outcome in solid organ transplant recipients with central nervous system cryptococcosis. Clin Infect Dis Off Publ Infect Dis Soc Am 49(11):1721–1728
5. Powderly WG, Cloud GA, Dismukes WE, Saag MS (1994) Measurement of cryptococcal antigen in serum and cerebrospinal fluid: value in the management of AIDS-associated cryptococcal meningitis. Clin Infect Dis Off Publ Infect Dis Soc Am 18(5):789–792
6. Aberg JA, Watson J, Segal M, Chang LW (2000) Clinical utility of monitoring serum cryptococcal antigen (sCRAG) titers in patients with AIDS-related cryptococcal disease. HIV Clin Trials 1(1):1–6

Clinical Syndromes: Rare Fungi

8

Dunja Wilmes and Volker Rickerts

Besides the more prevalent deep fungal infections covered in individual chapters, additional fungi are regularly described as human pathogens. Typical attributes of human pathogenic fungi include the ability to grow at human body temperature and mechanisms to resist host defenses. Human pathogenic fungi are found in all major fungal lineages. Therefore, this chapter is predominantly organized by clinical syndromes covering important infections.

Fungal pathogens causing the so-called *endemic mycoses* can be cultivated from the environment, typically from soil in restricted geographic areas. After inhalation of spores, these fungi cause localized, in non-immunocompromised subjects mostly self-limiting infections. However, they may persist in the body or can disseminate leading to life-threatening infections mostly in immunocompromised hosts. These infections, including histoplasmosis, coccidioidomycosis blastomycosis, and paracoccidioidomycosis, can mimic several infectious and noninfectious medical conditions and may be lethal if not recognized early and treated. In endemic areas, these infections can be highly prevalent. Outside endemic areas, travel history is frequently a trigger for specific diagnostic tests establishing the diagnosis.

Implantation mycoses occur after traumatic inoculation by environmental fungi. Most of these infections have a subacute to chronic course and remain restricted to subcutaneous tissues. However, they can become recalcitrant to antifungal therapy and lead to physical disabilities. Although many of the causative fungi are found worldwide, infections are more prevalent in tropical climates.

Phaeohyphomycosis and *hyalohyphomycosis* are terms used to classify mold infections according to the appearance of fungal hyphae documented by histopathology as either melanized or non-melanized hyaline hyphae, irrespective of the mode of infection, the regional distribution, or the causative agent. These terms are used in an attempt to avoid the generation of separate names for infections by rare fungi. The clinical presentation is often not different from the more prevalent mold infections such as aspergillosis or mucormycosis.

Rare yeast and yeast-like infections include diseases caused by opportunistic yeasts and non-fungal agents with tissue forms resembling yeasts. Infections are typically diagnosed after cultivation from sterile sites such as blood or after biopsies demonstrate suggestive tissue forms. The clinical presentation is often not different from the more prevalent mycoses including candidiasis.

8.1 Endemic Systemic Fungal Infections

The term endemic mycosis is used for systemic fungal infections caused by obligate pathogenic environmental fungi with restricted areas of

D. Wilmes · V. Rickerts (✉)
Robert Koch Institute, Berlin, Germany
e-mail: RickertsV@rki.de

E. Presterl (ed.), *Clinically Relevant Mycoses*, https://doi.org/10.1007/978-3-319-92300-0_8

Table 8.1 Endemic, systemic fungal infections: causative agents, distribution, tissue forms, and clinical presentations

Disease	Fungus	Main endemic areas	Tissue forms	Typical presentation
Histoplasmosis	*Histoplasma capsulatum*	USA (Mississippi, Ohio River Valley) South-Central America Caribbean Africa Australia Asia	Small (2–5 μm) yeasts with narrow-based budding, intra- and extracellular	Flu-like illness Acute pneumonia Chronic pneumonia Disseminated infection
Coccidioidomycosis	*Coccidioides immitis* *Coccidioides posadasii*	USA (Southwest, Eastern Washington) Central-South Americas	Spherules (5–100 μm) and endospores (2–5 μm)	Flu-like illness Acute pneumonia Chronic pneumonia Disseminated infection Meningitis
Blastomycosis	*Blastomyces dermatitidis* *Blastomyces gilchristii* *Blastomyces percursus*	USA (Mississippi, Ohio River Valley) Canada Africa India Israel	Thick-walled yeast-like cells (3–30 μm) with broad-based budding	Acute pneumonia Chronic pneumonia Cutaneous infections Disseminated infection
Paracoccidioidomycosis	*Paracoccidioides brasiliensis* *Paracoccidioides lutzii*	From the south of Mexico to the north of Argentina	Yeast cells (3–30 μm) with multiple buds ("ship's wheel")	Juvenile form Adult form
Adiaspiromycosis	*Emmonsia crescens* *Emmonsia parva*	Worldwide	Adiaspores 200–400 μm	Pulmonary infections
Emergomycosis	*Emergomyces pasteurianus* *Emergomyces africanus* *Emergomyces orientalis*	South Africa China Other locations likely	Small (2–5 μm) yeasts with narrow-based budding, intra-, extracellular	Pulmonary infections disseminated infections with skin lesions
Talaromycosis (formerly known as penicilliosis)	*Talaromyces (Penicillium) marneffei*	India Southeast Asia Southern China Hong Kong Taiwan	Non-budding yeast cells (3–5 μm) with transverse septum, intra-, extracellular	Pulmonary infections Disseminated infection with skin lesions

endemicity. These fungi are thermally dimorphic; they grow as molds at environmental temperatures but develop specialized tissue forms including yeast cells (histoplasmosis, blastomycosis, and emergomycosis) or cysts (coccidioidomycosis, adiaspiromycosis) at mammalian body temperature.

After inhalation of infectious propagules from environmental sources, most encounters between non-immunocompromised humans and these fungi result in subclinical or self-limiting, localized infections, but these fungi may persist in the host and cause reactivation. They may also cause potentially life-threatening disseminated infections predominantly in immunocompromised hosts. As clinical symptoms of these infections are nonspecific, the diagnosis requires a high index of suspicion, especially in non-endemic areas where these infections are diagnosed mainly in immigrants or after travel to endemic regions. Except for rare transmission with transplanted organs, person-to-person spread has not been documented. Typical infections, their causative agents, endemic regions, and frequent clinical presentations of these infections are summarized in Table 8.1.

The diagnostic workup of these infections includes antibody and antigen testing, the detection of characteristic tissue forms by microscopy in secretions or tissue samples, and the cultivation of the fungi. As specific culture conditions and prolonged incubation periods are needed; microbiology laboratories need to be informed when these infections are suspected. Presumptive identification of these fungi may be achieved by macro- and micromorphology of the cultivated fungi and in some by demonstration of a switch from the mold phase that grows at 25–30 °C to the yeast phase after incubation at 37 °C. Many of these fungi need to be handled in biosafety level 3 laboratories to prevent laboratory infections. Sequencing of barcoding genes is necessary for an exact identification of these pathogens, as phylogenetic studies suggest they represent species complexes of separate species with differing environmental niches and potentially clinically relevant physiologic differences that cannot be distinguished by culture morphology alone.

Antifungal therapy is often not prescribed in otherwise healthy hosts with localized, self-limiting infections. However, patients with persistent symptoms, or at increased risk for dissemination, including immunocompromised subjects, are treated with systemic antifungal agents to prevent progressive infections potentially leading to lethal outcome.

8.2 Histoplasmosis

Histoplasmosis refers to infections caused by *Histoplasma capsulatum*. Following inhalation, these fungi cause a variety of clinical manifestations ranging from asymptomatic pulmonary infections, acute or chronic pneumonia, to disseminated infections. While most infections are asymptomatic, high inoculum exposure or host characteristics including immunodeficiencies may predispose to clinical disease.

Histoplasma capsulatum is found in the soils of river valleys especially when enriched with bird or bat droppings and in places such as bat caves. Traditionally, three varieties have been distinguished:

- *H. capsulatum* var. *capsulatum* is the most prevalent agent of histoplasmosis in most countries.
- *H. capsulatum* var. *duboisii,* the causative agent of so-called African histoplasmosis, is found in Central and in West Africa. This variety may be differentiated by larger, thicker-walled yeasts in tissue. Infections often manifest with disseminated skin and bone lesions not typically found in histoplasmosis in other regions.
- *H. capsulatum* var. *farciminosum* has been described as an agent of superficial infections of animals such as horses in North Africa.

More recently, the application of molecular typing data suggests that the differentiation of these varieties may not be accurate. Instead, seven and potentially more phylogenetic species can be differentiated with differing geographic distribution and potentially differences in clinical manifestations. After inhalation of spores present in the environment, *H. capsulatum* transforms into yeast cells. The infection may be asymptomatic in most cases or present as flu-like illness after an incubation period from 1 to 3 weeks and as acute to chronic pneumonia or disseminated infections with the involvement of the skin, mucous membranes, and bone marrow among other organs. Fungi may also persist in the body to cause disease subsequently.

Acute pulmonary histoplasmosis may present with high-grade fever, chills, myalgia, headache, cough, and pleuritic chest pain. Additional symptoms include arthralgia and erythema nodosum in a minority of patients. Chest X-rays may demonstrate nodular infiltrates and mediastinal lymphadenopathy. Most otherwise healthy people recover within 3 weeks, but constitutional symptoms can persist for months. Lung infiltrates heal as calcified lesions. In the absence of calcification, these nodules resemble neoplasm and may be diagnosed incidentally. In immunosuppressed patients or after massive exposure, the infection can present with diffuse infiltrates associated with respiratory distress syndrome. In some patients, massive enlargement of single or multiple lymph nodes occurs due to granulomatous inflammation leading to caseating necrosis (granulomatous mediastinitis). Lymph node enlargement may lead to tracheal, bronchial, or esophageal compression or pericarditis. Resulting symptoms including cough and chest pain usually resolve spontaneously over months. Mediastinal fibrosis is an uncommon, late complication of pulmonary histoplasmosis that may lead to the occlusion of central blood vessels or bronchi.

Chronic pulmonary histoplasmosis typically occurs in patients with chronic lung conditions such as chronic obstructive lung disease. Here, pneumonic infiltrates may slowly progress to tissue destruction leading to cavitation and fibrosis resulting in progressive worsening of lung function if untreated. Clinical manifestations include productive cough, chest pain, hemoptysis, and potentially constitutional symptoms.

8.2.1 Disseminated Histoplasmosis

Hematogenous dissemination from pulmonary lesions occurs early in the course of most acute infections. However, after specific immunity develops, most lesions are not symptomatic, and radiography may demonstrate calcified lesions subsequently. Symptomatic disseminated infections occur in about 1 in 2000 exposed individuals, often subjects with impaired T-cell immunity such as HIV infection, in children or older patients. In elderly (>54 years) patients without immunosuppression, disseminated infection manifests as a progressive disease and may be fatal in weeks to months if untreated. Presenting symptoms include mucosal ulcers of the gastrointestinal tract (60%), mostly the mouth, the genitourinary tract, or other sites. Hepatosplenic enlargement and adrenal gland destruction are frequently found, while skin lesions are unusual. Often, chest X-rays are unremarkable. CNS involvement may present as chronic meningitis or brain abscess. In AIDS patients and infants, the course is often more acute and is even with specific treatment often fatal within several weeks. Unspecific symptoms including high fever, fatigue, weight loss, hepatosplenomegaly, anemia, leukocytopenia, and thrombocytopenia may be present with or without pulmonary infiltrates and mucocutaneous lesions. If the diagnosis of disseminated histoplasmosis is missed, the infection can progress to a sepsis-like syndrome and may be associated with a hemophagocytic syndrome and high mortality rate.

African histoplasmosis takes a more indolent course and rarely manifests with pulmonary lesions but with papular skin lesions, soft tissue, and bone involvement. Involvement of the liver, the spleen, and other organs is possible and manifests with a wasting syndrome. The infection is fatal within weeks to months if left untreated. Besides these infections caused by the variety *duboisii*, infections resembling histoplasmosis in other regions caused by classic *H. capsulatum* also occur in endemic African regions.

Differential diagnosis of acute pulmonary histoplasmosis includes atypical pneumonias, other endemic mycoses, and cryptococcosis. The presentation of chronic pulmonary histoplasmosis is similar to tuberculosis, sarcoidosis, blastomycosis, and coccidioidomycosis. The mucocutaneous lesions of the disseminated form are similar to the lesions of other infections including tuberculosis, emergomycoses, paracoccidioidomycosis, syphilis, viral infections, and noninfectious diseases.

Diagnosis of histoplasmosis requires a high index of suspicion and often involves a combination of different laboratory techniques. Microscopic examinations of respiratory secretions, pus, and even blood smears stained with fungal stains such as Grocott or calcofluor may show small yeast cells (<5 μm) with narrow-based buds typically clustering within phagocytes. These cells may not always be differentiated from other small yeasts such as *Candida glabrata*, *Talaromyces marneffei*, *Emergomyces*, or acapsular *Cryptococci*. Larger, thick-walled yeasts are suggestive for African histoplasmosis. Cultivation of *Histoplasma capsulatum* is required for definitive proof of the infection. Mold colonies can be cultivated on standard mycological media containing cycloheximide for inhibition of other fungi at 25–30 °C for 4–6 weeks. As colony morphology may be difficult to distinguish from other molds, the conversion to yeast form at 37 °C on rich media or sequencing of barcoding genes is needed for confirmation. Multiple samples from the respiratory tract may be cultivated to increase sensitivity. In disseminated infections, fungi can be cultivated from bloodcultures and bone marrow aspirates. Cerebrospinal fluid is a valuable first sample to confirm CNS infection. Antibody testing is most useful for subacute and chronic pulmonary histoplasmosis, granulomatous mediastinitis, and pericarditis. Antibodies detected with the immunodiffusion (ID) test appear 4–8 weeks after exposure in up to 75% of patients with acute pulmonary histoplasmosis. The complement fixation (CF) test becomes positive after 2–6 weeks and is more sensitive but less specific than the ID test. Titers of 1:8 or greater are considered as presumptive evidence for histoplasmosis. Titers above 1:32 or a fourfold rise in paired samples offer strong evidence for active infection. Titers decrease with successful therapy and increase in chronic progressive disease. Cross-reactions may be observed with blastomycosis and coccidioidomycosis. Both tests may be applied to CSF if CNS disease is suspected. Antigen detection by ELISA is useful for the diagnosis of disseminated infections in immunocompromised patients that often do not produce antibodies. Sensitivity is greatest in urine where it is detected in over 90% of AIDS patients with disseminated disease. Antigen levels decline with successful antifungal therapy. Cross-reactions may be observed with blastomycosis, paracoccidioidomycosis, and coccidioidomycosis.

Antifungal treatment is indicated for moderately severe acute pulmonary histoplasmosis with symptoms such as fever, fatigue, or weight loss persisting for more than 3 weeks with itraconazole 2 × 200 mg for 6–12 weeks. In severe pulmonary infections with diffuse infiltrates, therapy is started with conventional (0.7–1 mg/kg per day) or liposomal amphotericin B (3–5 mg/kg/day). After patients show improvement, treatment may be continued with itraconazole (3 × 200 mg for 3 days, than 2 × 200 mg daily) to complete a 12-week course. In patients with hypoxemia, prednisone may be added. Chronic pulmonary infection is treated with itraconazole for at least 12 months with therapeutic drug monitoring to assure adequate drug exposure. Treatment of disseminated and CNS infections is started with amphotericin B for 1–2 weeks and later switched to itraconazole with a 3-day loading dose and control of serum levels for a total of 12 months or newer azoles with better CNS exposure such as voriconazole or posaconazole. AIDS patients may require suppressive therapy with itraconazole (1 × 200 mg) after completion of treatment until CD4 count is above 200/μl for at least 6 months. Mild disseminated infections may be treated with itraconazole alone. If itraconazole is not tolerated, it may be switched to posaconazole or voriconazole. If these are not available, fluconazole 400–800 mg may be used.

8.3 Coccidioidomycosis

The infection is caused by fungi of the genus *Coccidioides*. These fungi can be found in alkaline soils in regions with arid climate, hot summers, and mild winters. The endemic region of *Coccidioides immitis* includes the San Joaquin Valley of California, Utah, and as recently discovered the eastern part of Washington State in the USA. *Coccidioides posadasii* has a much larger and dispersed geographic distribution including Arizona, New Mexico, and Texas in the USA, Mexico, and Central and South America, where it occurs in isolated pockets. Infection is acquired after inhalation of aerosolized arthroconidia often in the context of natural or human-induced soil disruption. After inhalation, arthroconidia enlarge and transform into immature spherules in host tissue. Spherules undergo nuclear division to develop endospores. After 3–4 days, mature spherules rupture and release 100–300 endospores, which can each transform into a new spherule. In certain regions of Arizona, about a quarter of community-acquired pneumonias are caused by *Coccidioides*. Based on earlier coccidioidal skin test studies, it is thought that most infections are subclinical. In the general population, only 1% of exposed individuals will develop disseminated infections. However, that percentage may be higher in immunosuppressed patients (HIV patients with a CD4 count <250/μl, allogenic transplant recipients, patients treated by TNF-α inhibitors or high doses of corticosteroids), people of certain ethnicities (Afro-Americans and Filipino), and pregnant women.

Acute pulmonary coccidioidomycosis develops about 1–3 weeks after exposure. Symptoms are nonspecific and may include fever, weight loss, malaise, nonproductive cough, dyspnea and pleuritic chest pain, and peripheral blood eosinophilia. Chest X-ray shows hilar adenopathy and pneumonic infiltrates. A generalized maculopapular rash may be present. These symptoms can be accompanied in 5% of the cases by the classical "valley fever" or "desert rheumatism," consisting of fever, arthralgia, and erythema nodosum or erythema multiforme. Most of the affected adults will recover spontaneously over 6–8 weeks. In HIV-infected persons with a CD4 count <100 cells/μl, the disease can be much more fulminant with diffuse pneumonia, potentially resulting in respiratory failure.

Chronic pulmonary coccidioidomycosis develops in 5–10% of infected individuals, many of whom suffer from previous lung conditions including COPD over weeks to months. Patients present with cough and hemoptysis. Chest X-ray findings include nodules, cavities, abscesses, or infiltrates. Potential complications include bronchopleural fistula, empyema, and pulmonary hemorrhage.

Disseminated coccidioidomycosis usually manifests 3–12 months after the primary infection. The presentation can range from an acute illness which may be fatal within a few weeks if left untreated to an indolent chronic disease, which may progress during months and even years. The most common symptoms at presentation include fever, cough, night sweats, and chills. Hematogenous spread may affect the skin, the bones, and the central nervous system. Cutaneous and subcutaneous lesions are the most common manifestations of disseminated disease. They may appear as verrucous nodules, papules, or subcutaneous abscesses. Often, these lesions occur in the face of the patients. Bone and joint disease is a common complication. Asymmetric arthritis regularly involves the knees, the joints of the hands and wrists, the feet and ankles, and the pelvis. Although long bones may be infected, the most affected bones are the vertebrae. On radiographs, osteolytic or osteosclerotic lesions may be seen. MRI is often necessary to exclude instability of the spine or a potential compression by an epidural abscess. The patients remain asymptomatic for a long time and develop often only a dull pain. Hematogenous spread to the leptomeninges almost always occurs within weeks to months following an initial untreated lower respiratory infection. Every patient with symptoms of CNS involvement, such as persistent headache, altered mental status, unexplained nausea, or new focal neurologic deficits, should undergo cerebral imaging and lumbar puncture with the analysis of the cerebrospinal fluid. Typically, CSF analysis will show pleocytosis, often with a lymphocytic predominance, but also a neutrophilic or an eosinophilic predominance is possible. Proteins may be normal or moderately elevated. The glucose may be normal but is often depressed.

8.3.1 Differential Diagnosis

The infection needs to be differentiated from viral and bacterial pneumonias and other respiratory and disseminated fungal or mycobacterial infections. Skin and bone lesions may resemble neoplasia.

8.3.2 Diagnosis

Microscopy of respiratory secretions may be positive in up to 30–40% of patients with pneumonia. Histopathological samples can show the characteristic spherules. If only endospores, which are 2–5 μm in size, are visualized, the diagnosis might be more difficult, requiring differentiation from small yeasts including *Histoplasma capsulatum* and *Candida*. Sometimes, hyphal forms are seen, especially in lung cavities. *Coccidioides* species are fast-growing molds and can be isolated from lower respiratory tract samples, blood cultures, and pus and sometimes from the CSF. After 2–7 days, this fungus will grow as an unpigmented mold on a variety of culture media at 35 °C. After 7–10 days, the mold will present a large number of infective arthroconidia. Laboratory-associated infections have occurred and cultures must be handled in BSL-3 laboratories. Serologic tests include antibody detection using immunodiffusion (ID) and complement fixation (CF). The ID test has the advantage to be more specific than the CF test and to be able to detect IgM response and to be useful in the diagnosis of recent infections. Generally IgM appears 1–3 weeks and IgG 2–6 weeks after onset of the first symptoms. The CF test is more sensitive and becomes positive 4–12 weeks after infection. The advantage of this serologic test is that it is semi-quantitative and that the testing of serial samples may give a clue about the evolution of the disease. Titers of 1:16 or above are indicative of a disseminated disease. A lateral flow device has recently introduced to detect antibodies. The test provides a bed side diagnosis with sensitivity and specificity comparable to the ID and CF tests.

8.3.3 Management

Medical follow-up should be assured for all patients, treated or not, for a minimum of 1–2 years. In previously healthy patients including nonpregnant woman without debilitating disease, acute pulmonary coccidioidomycosis doesn't require antifungal treatment. Treatment should be initiated in acute pulmonary coccidioidomycosis if the infection is severe, if the patient has comorbidities, or in pregnant woman. Severe primary infection is clinically defined as a disease in which the patient has lost >10% of his weight, has intense night sweats for >3 weeks, has symptoms that persist for >2 months, needs a hospital stay, or is unable to work. Radiological signs of severity include bilateral infiltrates or infiltrates which cover >50% of one lung. In addition, complement fixation (CF) titers of >1:16 are considered as a sign of severe, potentially disseminated disease. If treatment is required, current guidelines recommend for nonpregnant adults a treatment with azole antifungals, for example, itraconazole (400–800 mg/day), fluconazole (400–2000 mg/day), or voriconazole (4 mg/kg/12 h), for 3–6 months or longer depending on the clinical response. Reversal of underlying immunodeficiency should be considered if feasible. In pregnant women, treatment with intravenous amphotericin B (0.6–1 mg/kg/day) or liposomal amphotericin B (3–5 mg/kg/day) should be initiated. During the second or the third trimester, a treatment with azoles can be considered. No treatment is recommended in patients with asymptomatic pulmonary nodules and in immunocompetent patients with an asymptomatic coccidioidal cavity. Adults with symptomatic chronic cavitary coccidioidal pneumonia should be treated by fluconazole (at least 400 mg/day) or itraconazole (2 × 200 mg/day) for 1 year. Coccidioidal eradication may not be achieved and surgical treatment may be necessary in specific cases. The first-line therapy in soft-tissue involvement is itraconazole (2 × 200 mg/day) or fluconazole (400–800 mg/day). The minimum duration of treatment should be 6–12 months. Bone or joint infections are treated with itraconazole (2 × 200 mg/day) unless extensive or limb- threatening skeletal or vertebral disease is present. In this case a treatment by intravenous amphotericin B may be initiated, followed by oral azole therapy for a total of at least 3 years. Suspected vertebral disease should prompt spine imaging and surgical advice. The recommended treatment of coccidioidal meningitis is fluconazole 400–1200 mg/day or itraconazole 2–4 × 200 mg/day with a therapeutic drug monitoring. Sometimes high intracranial pressure will need repeated lumbar punctures or placement of a permanent shunt. The medical treatment should be continued for life. In pregnant patients during the first trimester, intrathecal amphotericin B may be used. During the rest of the pregnancy, a treatment by azoles can be considered. An alternative would be to treat the patient during all the pregnancy by intravenous amphotericin B.

8.4 Blastomycosis

Blastomycosis refers to infections caused by fungi of the genus *Blastomyces*. Following inhalation of fungi present in soil or traumatic inoculation, they can cause a wide spectrum of clinical manifestations including the respiratory tract, skin, bone, central nervous system, and urogenital infections. Most infections have been reported in regions surrounding the Mississippi and Ohio rivers, the midwestern states of the USA, and Canadian regions bordering the Great Lakes and the St. Lawrence River. Cases have also been documented in Africa, India, Israel, Central-, and

South America. Those at greatest risk include middle-aged men with outdoor occupations (construction or farming) or recreational activities (fishing, hunting). More aggressive diseases are seen in patients with AIDS, transplant recipients, and patients receiving corticosteroids.

8.4.1 Pulmonary Blastomycosis

After an incubation period of 4–6 weeks, patients manifest with a nonspecific, flu-like illness with nonproductive cough and pleuritic chest pain. Chest X-ray shows nonspecific infiltrates. Pleural effusions are uncommon. In contrast to histoplasmosis, hilar lymphadenopathy is uncommon. In the absence of recovery, chronic pulmonary infection resembling lung tuberculosis or cancer or disseminated infection may develop.

8.4.2 Cutaneous Blastomycosis

Skin lesions, starting as maculopapular lesions progressing to raised, crusted verrucous lesions or ulcers over subcutaneous abscesses, may develop on exposed sites such as the face (nose, mouth, oral and pharyngeal mucosa), neck, or scalp.

8.4.3 Disseminated Blastomycosis

Impaired T-cell immunity, such as advanced HIV infection, predisposes to hematogenous dissemination. Involved organs include the central nervous system with subacute meningitis or brain abscess manifesting as headache, confusion, or focal neurologic deficits. Additional affected organs include the skin, the adrenal glands, the liver, the spleen, the heart, the gastrointestinal tract, the genitourinary tract, and the eye. Osteomyelitis of the spine, the pelvis, the skull, the ribs, and the long bones manifests as osteolytic or osteoblastic lesions. They may remain clinically silent until adjacent joints become involved. AIDS patients may also present with a sepsis syndrome as in disseminated histoplasmosis.

Differential diagnosis of pulmonary blastomycosis includes bacterial pneumonia and fungal infections including histoplasmosis and cryptococcosis. Chronic pulmonary forms need to be differentiated from tuberculosis, histoplasmosis, and bronchogenic carcinoma. These infections are also indistinguishable from coccidioidomycosis and paracoccidioidomycosis, but their endemic regions have almost no overlap.

8.4.4 Diagnosis

The fungi may be visualized in wet mounts or stained specimens of pus, sputum, bronchial secretions, cerebrospinal fluid, urine, or tissue. Yeast cells vary in diameter from 3 to 30 μm, are oval to round with thick walls, and show characteristic broad-based single buds. Confirmation of blastomycosis depends on the cultivation of the fungi. Antibody testing is done by immunodiffusion (ID) using a purified surface antigen. This test is specific but remains negative in 10% of patients with disseminated infections and as much as 60% of patients with localized infections. Complement fixation tests lack specificity due to cross-reactions with *Histoplasma capsulatum* and *Coccidioides* sp.

8.4.5 Management

Patients with acute pulmonary infection are often treated to prevent dissemination. Mild to moderate pulmonary infections are treated with itraconazole (3 × 200 mg/day for 3 days, than 1–2 × 200 mg) for 6–12 months. Moderately severe to severe disease is treated with amphotericin B for 1–2 weeks until clinical improvement and then switched to itraconazole with control of serum levels. While fluconazole (400–800 mg) is less active, posaconazole and voriconazole may be effective. The treatment of disseminated infections depends on the presence of CNS lesions. In the presence of CNS infections, liposomal amphotericin B (5 mg/kg for 4–6 weeks) is followed by oral azoles such as fluconazole (800 mg/day) or voriconazole (2 × 200–400 mg) for at least 12 months until resolution of CSF abnormalities. In the absence of CNS lesions and mild-moderate disseminated disease, itraconazole is used, while more severe infections are treated with amphotericin B for 1–2 weeks, followed by itraconazole until resolution of symptoms and signs. Patients with osteoarticular disease should receive an azole for at least 12 months to prevent relapse. Surgical management may be needed for drainage of large abscesses and brain and epidural abscesses causing neurologic deficits. Debridement of bone lesions is only needed when refractory to antifungals.

8.5 Paracoccidioidomycosis

Paracoccidioidomycosis is a deep systemic mycosis caused by *Paracoccidioides brasiliensis* and *Paracoccidioides lutzii*. The disease is geographically restricted to subtropical areas of Latin America from the south of Mexico to the north of Argentina with a high prevalence in Brazil, Colombia, Venezuela, and Argentina. *Paracoccidioides lutzii* is predominantly found in the Central-West and Amazon Regions of Brazil and Ecuador. In Latin America, it is the second most prevalent endemic mycosis after histoplasmosis. Involvement in agriculture is an important risk factor for infection that occurs via inhalation of aerosolized spores from the soil. Symptomatic disease is predominantly diagnosed in males over 30 years as a chronic progressive granulomatous infection involving the skin and lymph nodes. Immunocompromised subjects are not at increased risk for infection, as are travelers spending less than 6 months in an endemic area.

8.5.1 Acute or Subacute Disseminated Paracoccidioidomycosis (Juvenile Type)

It is responsible for 5–25% of the cases and is mostly seen in children and adolescents. This may be related to specific phylogenetic clusters, as it is seen more frequently in certain endemic regions. Disease history is characterized by a short period of evolution and a more severe course. The most prominent symptoms and signs are linked to localized or generalized lymphadenopathy and hepatomegaly. The lumps may form fistulas or coalesce and exert compression on various organs. Systemic symptoms, such as fever, weight loss, and anorexia, are often present. A pulmonary (10–20%) or a mucocutaneous involvement (25%) in this form is uncommon. Eosinophilia occurs in 30–50% of the cases.

8.5.2 Chronic Disseminated Paracoccidioidomycosis (Adult Type)

The most often encountered type, which progresses slowly and often persists during months to years before the diagnosis is established. Besides the lungs, ulcerative mucocutaneous lesions of the face are present. Chest X-rays show bilateral infiltrates. Mucosal lesions may first involve the gums, evolve over weeks or months, and can lead to malnourishment. They can also involve other parts of the gastrointestinal tract, predominantly the ileocecal region. Skin involvement manifests as papular or nodular lesions that evolve to plaques, verrucous lesions, or ulcers. About 15% of the affected adults will develop adrenal gland insufficiency. CNS involvement is seen in a minority of patients leading to meningitis or encephalitis.

8.5.3 Differential Diagnosis

The differential diagnosis of the mucocutaneous lesions includes histoplasmosis, sporotrichosis, cryptococcosis, chromoblastomycosis, syphilis, leishmaniosis, leprosy, and tuberculosis. Pulmonary infections may be difficult to differentiate from tuberculosis, histoplasmosis, coccidioidomycosis, lymphoma, cancer, and cryptococcosis. The gastrointestinal symptoms and lesions may be misdiagnosed as amebiasis, balantidiasis, tuberculosis, cancer, or inflammatory bowel disease. The other etiologies to consider in case of CNS involvement are tuberculosis, cryptococcosis, cysticercosis, and neoplasia.

8.5.4 Diagnosis

The microscopic examination of KOH preparations or histopathology sections may be diagnostic. The typical findings include yeast cells at varying sizes (3–30 μm) with sometimes multiple budding. The definite diagnosis relies on the cultivation of the fungus which may take weeks to months. Serological tests can be helpful for the diagnosis of *P. brasiliensis* infection, but experience for the diagnosis *P. lutzii* infection is limited. The ID test is specific and has a good sensitivity. In contrast to the following antibody detection tests, cross-reactions with *Histoplasma capsulatum* antibody are uncommon with ID. The CF test has a comparable sensitivity but is less specific. A CF titer of 1:8 is considered as a presumptive evidence of the diagnosis.

8.5.5 Management

Patients with mild and moderate paracoccidioidomycosis are treated with itraconazole 200 mg/day for 9–18 months. Treatment with itraconazole is more advantageous than the treatment with cotrimoxazole (adults, TMP 160–240 mg/SMX 800–1200 mg 2×/day; children, TMP 8–10 mg/kg and SMX 40–50 mg/kg in two daily doses for 18–24 months), which is the second treatment option in endemic resource-limited regions. Although only a small number of patients have been treated with these drugs, voriconazole and posaconazole are potential alternatives. Amphotericin B deoxycholate (0.3–0.5 mg/kg/day, with a maximum of 50 mg/day) or lipid formulation (3–5 mg/kg/day) should be reserved for the induction period (for 2–4 weeks) of the treatment in severe cases, as well as for the treatment of pregnant women. Transition to oral medication should occur after clinical stabilization once the drug's oral absorption has been confirmed.

8.6 Talaromycosis (Penicilliosis)

Talaromycosis is an infection caused by *Talaromyces marneffei*, formerly known as *Penicillium marneffei*. The infection follows the inhalation of spores. Occupational exposure to plants and animals has been associated with human infection. The infection is diagnosed in India, Southeast Asia, Southern China, Hong Kong, and Taiwan. The disease affects primarily patients with impaired T-cell immunity such as AIDS patients. In addition, infections in organ or stem cell transplant recipients and patients with hematologic malignancy have been reported.

8.6.1 Clinical Manifestations

The infection is mostly diagnosed in HIV patients with a CD4 count below 100/μl. The lungs are the initial site of contact with the fungi but the infections may already be disseminated at the time of diagnosis. Presenting symptoms include fever and weight loss, nonproductive cough, generalized lymphadenopathy, and hepatosplenomegaly. Papulous skin lesions are among the most common symptoms of disseminated infections. They are often localized in the face, at the upper trunk, or the extremities. CNS involvement is uncommon and may present as altered mental state.

8.6.2 Differential Diagnosis

The skin lesions may be misdiagnosed as sporotrichosis, histoplasmosis, cryptococcosis, melioidosis, necrotic *Herpes zoster* infection, or *Molluscum contagiosum* or *Mycobacterium* sp. infection. The differential diagnosis of the lung lesions includes tuberculosis, histoplasmosis, bacterial pneumonia, and *Pneumocystis jirovecii* pneumonia.

8.6.3 Diagnosis

Microscopy from respiratory tract samples or tissue biopsies may reveal intra- or extracellulary located, non-budding yeast cells, with prominent transverse septum. *T. marneffei* cells can be confused with those of *Histoplasma capsulatum*, *Candida*, *Pneumocystis jirovecii*, *Toxoplasma gondii*, and *Leishmania* due to their size. Cultivation of *Talaromyces marneffei* mold colonies from bone marrow, blood, cutaneous, or respiratory tract specimens may be diagnostic.

Colonies produce a red pigment that diffuses into the agar. However, other nonpathogenic species of *Penicillium* may also produce red pigments. Therefore molecular tests are necessary to identify this organism. Antibody detection tests are not widely available. They are specific but less sensitive than culture in immunocompromised patients. Of note, the galactomannan antigen detection test for aspergillosis has been found to give false-positive results in HIV-infected patients with talaromycosis.

8.6.4 Management

In AIDS patients, deoxycholate amphotericin B (0.6–1 mg/kg/day) for 2 weeks, followed by itraconazole (400 mg/day) for 10 weeks, followed by low-dose itraconazole (200 mg/day) continued until CD4 counts >100/µl for 6 months minimum, is recommended. Induction therapy with itraconazole has been studied and is linked to higher mortality.

8.7 Other Infections Caused by Thermally Dimorphic Fungi and Close Relatives

Emergomycosis has been recently described as an emerging disseminated fungal infection in South African patients mostly with advanced HIV infection. Additional cases have been described in organ transplant recipients and non-immunocompromised hosts. Patients present with pulmonary involvement and disseminated skin lesions. The causative agent has been named *Emergomyces africanus*. The fungus is closely related to *Emmonsia* and *Histoplasma*, being thermally dimorphic. Closely related fungi have been isolated mostly from immunocompromised subjects in Canada, China, Italy, and Germany, suggesting a wide distribution of these fungal pathogens. Differential diagnosis includes other disseminated fungal infections such as histoplasmosis, tuberculosis, and other infections causing disseminated skin lesions. The diagnosis may be suggested by histopathology of skin lesions showing small budding yeast cells clustering in phagocytic cells resembling *Histoplasma capsulatum*. Therefore, cultivation of the fungi is necessary to establish the diagnosis. Fungi may be cultivated from skin and respiratory tract samples, from blood, or from bone marrow. Cross-reactivity with the *Histoplasma* urinary antigen detection test has been described. Good in vitro activity has been described for azoles and amphotericin B, while echinocandins and flucytosine are not active. Amphotericin B appears to be the most active agent clinically, while fluconazole therapy seems to be associated with worse outcome. Start of antiretroviral therapy has been linked to new and progressive skin lesions suggesting immune reconstitution inflammatory syndrome (IRIS) as described in cryptococcosis and other infections. Mortality of disseminated infections is up to 48% in case series from South Africa with half of the patients being diagnosed postmortem.

Adiaspiromycosis is a pulmonary fungal infection caused by *Emmonsia parva* and *Emmonsia crescens* present in soil. After inhalation, the fungi enlarge to form 40–500 µm large, non-replicating, not disseminating structures called adiaspores. They may induce a granulomatous tissue reaction associated with respiratory decline. Disease ranges from subclinical infections to diffuse pneumonia. The infection is common in small terrestrial mammals globally but has only rarely been diagnosed in humans. Diagnosis relies on the demonstration of characteristic adiaspores by histopathology. The fungi are not usually cultivated from human specimens. Steroids have been given as tissue destruction is mediated by the inflammatory response. The role of antifungals is not well defined.

8.8 Implantation Mycoses

Implantation mycoses are a diverse group of fungal infections that develop at the site of transcutaneous trauma with implantation of fungi present in environmental sources such as soil or on plant materials. These infections are also referred to as subcutaneous mycoses, but in some cases they

Table 8.2 Common implantation mycoses of the skin: etiologic agents, distribution, histopathological characteristics, and clinical presentation

Disease	Fungus	Distribution	Tissue form	Presentation
Sporotrichosis	*Sporothrix schenckii* *Sporothrix brasiliensis* *Sporothrix globosa* *Sporothrix luriei*	Worldwide	Cigar-shaped yeasts that may be surrounded by an asteroid body. Culture (3–5 days) is superior to histopathology	Papulonodular, ulcerating skin lesion with ipsilateral lesions following lymphatic vessels Pulmonary infection Disseminated infection
Chromoblastomycosis	*Fonsecaea pedrosoi* *Fonsecaea compacta* *Cladophialophora carrionii* *Phialophora verrucosa* *Rhinocladiella aquaspersa* *Exophiala jeanselmei* *Exophiala spinifera* *Fonsecaea monophora*	Worldwide (especially Brazil, Madagascar, and Costa Rica)	Muriform cells	Chronic skin infection with verrucous lesions
Eumycetoma	*Madurella mycetomatis* *Scedosporium apiospermum* *Diverse others*	Africa (worldwide)	Grains with fungal hyphae	Chronic painless soft-tissue swelling with draining sinuses

also involve adjacent structures such as the lymphatics, cartilage, fascia, joints, and bones.

Most affected individuals are otherwise healthy non-immunocompromised subjects with exposition to the fungi during outdoor activities including agriculture, hunting, and lumbering. These infections mostly occur in tropical or subtropical regions caused by fungi of diverse taxa. They represent subacute to chronic, slowly progressive infections that usually do not disseminate to distant organs. Typical disease entities are summarized in Table 8.2.

The diagnosis of particular entities within the implantation mycoses includes the clinical presentation, cultivation of the causative fungi, and demonstration of pathognomonic fungal elements such as muriform cells in chromoblastomycosis or grains in eumycetoma by microscopy or histopathology.

Although these infections may be cured with surgical resection of early, localized lesions, extensive infections may be difficult to control, requiring long-term antifungal therapy to prevent relapses. Surgical interventions may be needed in cases unresponsive to medical treatment.

8.9 Sporotrichosis

Sporotrichosis refers to subacute or chronic infections caused by thermally dimorphic fungi of the genus *Sporothrix*. The fungi are found in soil, on decomposing vegetation, and on plant materials. Infections occur worldwide after traumatic inoculation of the fungus, often by minor trauma afflicted by thorns or wood splinters. Sporotrichosis is the most prevalent implantation mycosis worldwide, mostly in tropical countries, especially in South America. Pulmonary infections may occur after inhalation of spores.

8.9.1 Lymphocutaneous Infections

This infection mostly occurs sporadically after outdoor work such as gardening or recreational activities. The disease may also be acquired as a zoonosis by scratches or bites from infected or colonized animals. Sporotrichosis should be suspected in patients with ulcerative skin lesions especially with ipsilateral ascending lymphatic nodules unresponsive to antibacterial treatment. Arthritis and bone infections occur after local spread from lymphocutaneous infections or rarely after hematogenous spread in immunocompromised subjects such as AIDS patients.

Extra-cutaneous infections are usually limited to a single site. Pulmonary infections occur after inhalation of spores by patients with underlying illnesses including COPD and alcoholism. The subacute to chronic infections may resemble reactivated tuberculosis.

8.9.2 Disseminated Disease

Hematogenous spread has been described in individuals with AIDS or hematologic malignancy. It may represent as widespread ulcerative cutaneous lesions with or without involvement of bones, joints, and the CNS. Ocular infections including chorioretinitis and endophthalmitis are rare manifestations presenting as visual disturbances.

8.9.3 Diagnosis and Differential Diagnosis

The fungi may be visualized in pus or tissue with GMS or PAS staining as small, round-, oval- to cigar-shaped cells. The definitive diagnosis is based on the cultivation of the fungus on fungal media at 25–30° for 3–5 days where *Sporothrix* grows as a mold. Identification relies on the micromorphology and demonstration of thermal dimorphism after incubation on blood or BHI agar at 37 °C which may not be possible for all isolates. Sporotrichosis needs to be differentiated from bacterial infections including nocardiosis, atypical mycobacterial infections, and fungal infections including blastomycosis, paracoccidioidomycosis, and cryptococcosis.

8.9.4 Management

Lymphocutaneous infections are not life-threatening but do not usually resolve without antifungal therapy. Potential complications include deep infections, scarring, and bacterial superinfections. Oral itraconazole is the treatment of choice (200 mg/day) for 3–6 months. Recalcitrant infections may be treated with higher dosage (2 × 200 mg/day), terbinafine (2 × 500 mg), or combinations. Fluconazole and voriconazole are less active. Experience with posaconazole is limited. Extra-cutaneous infections are treated with itraconazole (2 × 200 mg for 12 months) with therapeutic drug monitoring. Acutely ill patients with respiratory or CNS infections may need therapy with conventional (0.7 mg/kg/day) or liposomal amphotericin B (3–5 mg/kg/day).

8.10 Chromoblastomycosis

Chromoblastomycosis is a chronic fungal infection of the skin and subcutaneous tissues. The initial lesion is a small painless subcutaneous papule that occurs mostly on the lower extremities after minor trauma. A diagnostic hallmark of the infection is the microscopic detection of small, round, thick-walled brown cells (termed muriform cells) that differentiate chromoblastomycosis from subcutaneous phaeohyphomycosis and other infections. The fungi are associated with a granulomatous, purulent fibrotic inflammation. If left untreated, the lesions will enlarge to form multiple verrucous lesions. The lesions usually are painless except in the case of bacterial superinfection but may be pruritic. Scratching can result in satellite lesions by autoinoculation. In rare cases, metastatic lesions develop in the lymph nodes, brain, liver, bones, or elsewhere. Carcinomatous transformation may occur in long-standing skin lesions. A specific group of dematiaceous fungi present in the environment in soil, rotting wood, and decomposing plants is responsible for these slowly progressive infections that mostly occur in tropical countries including Brazil, Costa Rica, Southern Africa, Asia, and Australia but rarely also elsewhere.

8.10.1 Diagnosis

When verrucous lesions suggest the diagnosis, microscopic presentation of the typical muriform cells is needed to establish the diagnosis. They may be visualized in skin scrapings or histologic sections together with a granulomatous tissue reaction, microabscesses, and hyperkeratosis. In addition, cultures should be performed to isolate the causative agents. Cultivation should be performed for 4–6 weeks at 25–30 °C. Typically dark brown to tan molds will often grow within 1–2 weeks.

Differential diagnosis includes other fungal infections including blastomycosis, paracoccidioidomycosis, eumycetoma, phaeohyphomycosis, lobomycosis, or sporotrichosis, leishmaniosis, tuberculosis, leprosy, and syphilis.

8.10.2 Management

Chromoblastomycosis is difficult to treat with low cure rates and high risk of relapse. Scarring and bacterial superinfections are common complications. Complete surgical resection is indicated for small lesions. Alternatives may include local physical therapies including cryotherapy. Antifungal therapy should be prescribed before and after surgery to prevent local spread. In those with extensive lesions, antifungal therapy with itraconazole (200–400 mg/day) or terbinafine (500–1000 mg/day) for 6–12 months is used. Therapy should be continued for several months after clinical cure to prevent relapse. Posaconazole or amphotericin B in association with 5-flucytosine and the combination of itraconazole and terbinafine are alternative treatment options.

8.11 Eumycetoma

Eumycetoma is defined as a slowly progressive infection of the skin characterized by indurated swelling and the production of so-called grains, compact masses of fungal filaments, which are discharged through sinus tracts. The infection occurs after traumatic inoculation of diverse fungi into subcutaneous tissues mostly of the feet and hands. Local progression to underlying tissues including bones is possible, but spread through lymphatics or the blood is rare. Mycetomas are most common in arid tropical and subtropical regions, particularly in Senegal,

Sudan, Somalia, India, and South and Central America. Sporadic cases occur in many other parts of the world affecting mostly middle-aged men walking barefoot or having outdoor occupations. Besides *Madurella mycetomatis* and *Scedosporium apiospermum*, diverse melanized and non-melanized molds have been implicated as causative agents.

8.11.1 Diagnosis

Initial lesions (small subcutaneous nodules) appear several months after minor trauma afflicted by thorns or wood splinters. The infections evolve slowly to form abscesses with multiple sinuses containing characteristic grains. The lesions are mostly painless. Pain heralds the impeding rupture of a sinus onto the skin surface. Radiologic examination is useful in determining the extent of bone involvement. Bacterial superinfections may aggravate symptoms. The mycological diagnosis of mycetoma depends on the demonstration of grains. If possible, they should be obtained from an unruptured pustule (sinus) with a sterile needle by puncturing the lesion and squeezing its content onto a glass slide. If this is not possible, deep surgical biopsies are necessary. Superficial biopsies are seldom helpful. Cultivation of fungi or amplification of fungal DNA may identify causative agents.

8.11.2 Differential Diagnosis

Actinomycetoma is suggested by grains with small filaments, cultivation of aerobic actinomycetes, and response to antibacterial agents. Actinomycotic grains contain fine filaments (1 μm in diameter), while fungal etiology is suggested by grains containing masses of short fungal hyphae (2–4 μm in diameter). Histology shows the same picture including granulomatous inflammation. Cultures are incubated to grow actinomycetes and fungi at 25–30 and 37 °C for up to 6 weeks. Differentiation from chromoblastomycosis or cutaneous tuberculosis is usually possible by the clinical appearance with documentation of grains.

8.11.3 Management

Medical management is possible in patients without bone lesions and when supervision of the treatment over a number of months is possible. The most effective drugs include itraconazole (200–400 mg/day) and terbinafine (500–1000 mg/day) for up to 24 months. Posaconazole (2 × 400 mg/day) and voriconazole (2 × 200 mg) are alternatives. Surgical management is indicated for limited disease that can be completely removed and for patients with advanced disease for debulking during medical treatment.

8.12 Other Implantation Mycoses

Entomophthoramycosis is caused by molds belonging to the order Entomophthorales previously assigned to the Zygomycota. These fungi are characterized by broad, irregular-shaped, pauciseptate hyphae. In contrast to the Mucorales, these fungi are not angioinvasive. The fungi are found in soil, decaying wood, and decomposing vegetation in tropical regions. Two clinical forms are distinguished, basidiobolomycosis and conidiobolomycosis. *Basidiobolomycosis* manifests as a slowly progressive subcutaneous infection occurring after traumatic implantation of plant debris in tropical environments. The disease is caused by fungi of the genus *Basidiobolus*. Underlying bones are usually not affected. Lymphatic obstruction may occur and result in elephantiasis. Gastrointestinal infection may be caused by oral ingestion of soil, animal feces, or contaminated food. It presents with abdominal pain of subacute onset and fever, constipation, or diarrhea. Disseminated infections resemble mucormycosis. The diagnosis may be established by microscopy, histopathology, or culture from endoscopic biopsy specimens showing typical hyphae. Cultures may grow the organism in less than a week at 25–37 °C. The treatment of choice appears to be itraconazole which must be given for several months. Patients with gastrointestinal infection may need resection of the affected bowel followed by itraconazole for 3 months or more. *Conidiobolomycosis* is a chronic subcutaneous fungal infection, caused by *Conidiobolus corona-*

tus, originating in the nasal mucosa that invades adjacent facial tissue with the potential to cause severe disfigurement. Dissemination is uncommon. The disease has been reported in West Africa (Nigeria, Cameroon) and other tropical regions (Madagascar, India, China, South and Central America). The infection may present with nasal obstruction and later painless facial swelling and nasal discharge. Underlying bones are not affected. Disseminated infections resemble those of mucormycosis. The diagnosis may be established by smears or histopathological samples of nasal mucosa demonstrating typical hyphae. *Conidiobolus* grows rapidly, but cultivation frequently fails to grow the fungus. Antifungal therapy with itraconazole for at least 4 weeks after lesions have been cleared seems to be an acceptable treatment strategy. Surgery is usually not successful due to local spread.

8.12.1 Lacaziosis (Lobomycosis)

Lacaziosis refers to a rare, localized granulomatous skin and soft-tissue infection caused by *Lacazia loboi*. Infections are reported in Central and northern South America. The fungus has not been cultivated. Molecular tests suggest it to be a close relative of *Paracoccidioides*. The habitat is unknown. Besides humans, the infection has been diagnosed in dolphins suggesting an aqueous habitat. The disease presents as slowly progressing cutaneous lesions starting as a papule, evolving to a keloidal, verrucous, or ulcerating lesion. Autoinoculation may lead to additional lesions that may involve an entire limb. While regional lymph nodes may be affected, hematogenous spread is unusual. Long-standing lesions may undergo carcinomatous transformation. Diagnosis is established by histopathology. Grocott or PAS stains will reveal round to oval, thick-walled cells of *L. loboi* (>10 μm) in long unbranched chains joined by small tubules. Multiple buds may be present as in paracoccidioidomycosis. Differential diagnosis includes chromoblastomycosis, paracoccidioidomycosis, leishmaniosis, mycobacterial infections, keloids, and neoplasia. Effective medical treatment has not been evaluated. Promising results have been described in some patients receiving oral clofazimine (300 mg/kg). Localized lesions may be treated by surgery or cryotherapy.

8.13 Phaeohyphomycosis

The term phaeohyphomycosis refers to infections defined by the presence of melanized dark-colored fungal elements, consisting of hyphae, but also yeast-like cells or a combination of both in tissue samples. Phaeohyphomycosis is caused by melanized, dematiaceous fungi. This diverse group of fungi consists of more than 100 species that have been reported as rare human fungal pathogens. While dematiaceous fungi are found worldwide in soil in association with plants and in polluted water, individual fungal species may have a restricted distribution. While most encounters between humans and these fungi do not cause symptomatic illness, a broad spectrum of diseases, ranging from allergic disorders of the lungs and sinuses to localized cutaneous, subcutaneous, or deep infections, has been described. Localized subcutaneous infections are mostly seen in tropical and subtropical regions. Chronic sinusitis occurs worldwide. Both are mostly diagnosed in otherwise healthy persons. Life-threatening disseminated infections have been diagnosed in both immunocompromised and otherwise healthy subjects. The diagnostic workup relies on the pathologic examination of clinical specimens demonstrating melanized hyphae in tissue. The identification of cultivated fungi may require a reference laboratory as these agents may produce different culture morphologies under different culture conditions making identification without molecular tests sometimes difficult.

Localized phaeohyphomycosis may be cured by surgical resection. Published experience with antifungal therapy of these infections is limited to case reports and case series without evidence of randomized treatment trials.

Subcutaneous infections are the most frequently reported form of phaeohyphomycosis. Infections occur after inoculation by minor trauma and manifest as a nodule at the site of inoculation, often on the feet, hands, or head. In immunocompromised subjects the infection may present with pustules, ulcers, or eschars of the limbs. Rarely, subcutaneous lesions occur in immunocompromised hosts as part of a hematogenous disseminated infection. Typical agents include *Bipolaris*, *Exophiala*, and *Phialophora*, but many others have been described. Differential diagnosis includes other implantation mycoses and the endemic fungal infections. Resection of small lesions is curative. Itraconazole and terbinafine alone or in combination given for several months may be successful in some cases.

Keratitis, infections of the cornea, can cause severe visual impairment and blindness. Fungal keratitis is mainly caused by yeasts, hyaline molds, but also dematiaceous fungi including *Curvularia* and *Bipolaris*. Human infections follow traumatic inoculation of spores or by surgical procedures. The inoculation may involve plant material harboring fungal spores. The onset of infections is often insidious and a particular trauma may not be recognized by the patients. Symptoms include ocular pain, redness, diminished vision, and ocular discharge. Infections caused by dematiaceous molds progress more slowly than infections caused by bacteria, yeasts, *Aspergillus*, or *Fusarium*. The fungal elements may be seen by confocal microscopy. Identification of the causative agents requires cultivation or molecular tests such as PCR.

Rhinosinusitis caused by dematiaceous molds occurs in different clinical forms, mostly allergic fungal rhinosinusitis or chronic invasive rhinosinusitis. Allergic fungal rhinosinusitis is a noninvasive disease that may develop after inhalation of spores of fungi including *Alternaria*, *Bipolaris*, and *Curvularia*. Patients present with nasal polyposis and thick nasal or sinus mucus. The polyposis may form an expansive mass leading to a thinning of sinus walls. The diagnosis is favored by the presence of noninvasive fungi, eosinophilic mucin at the time of surgical debridement, eosinophilia, elevated serum IgE, and specific IgE against cultivated fungal pathogens. Chronic invasive rhinosinusitis is a slowly progressive destructive condition that may remain confined to the sinuses or spread to the orbit and the brain. This condition affects non-immunocompromised subjects presenting with long-lasting nasal discharge and obstruction, nasal polyposis, and headache.

Pulmonary infection is usually diagnosed in immunocompromised patients where it resembles invasive pulmonary aspergillosis with cough, fever, and presentation of nodular lung lesions with or without halo that may evolve to cavitation. In patients with asthma, colonization with fungi including *Bipolaris* and *Curvularia* may cause a clinical syndrome similar to allergic bronchopulmonary aspergillosis.

Cerebral phaeohyphomycosis is a rare but often fatal disease caused by neurotropic molds including *Cladophialophora bantiana*, *Ramichloridium mackenziei*, and agents of the genera *Bipolaris* and *Exophiala*. It occurs after inhalation of fungal spores and hematogenous dissemination. These infections have been diagnosed even in young healthy adults without obvious predisposition and are associated with case fatality rates exceeding 70%. Individuals manifest with headache, fever, and neurologic deficits due to brain abscess. The CSF is often unremarkable but may show signs of inflammation. Elevated opening pressure is a possible complication. As CSF cultures are often sterile, etiologic diagnosis is often possible after surgical resection only. Meningitis, encephalitis, and myelitis are other potential manifestations. The differential diagnosis includes bacterial CNS infections, toxoplasmosis, cryptococcosis, and the endemic fungal infections. Long-term survival is being reported when surgical resection of solitary nodules was performed. Antifungal treatment with agents showing good CNS levels such as voriconazole, posaconazole, or liposomal amphotericin B is frequently used.

Disseminated phaeohyphomycosis is an uncommon form of phaeohyphomycosis occurring in immunocompromised patients with hematological malignancies often during antifungal prophylaxis and is caused by the multidrug-resistant *Lomentospora (Scedosporium) prolificans* as a frequent pathogen. Patients may present with fever, lung-, and cutaneous lesions. These infections may be associated with a sepsis syndrome and the fungi are often cultivated from blood cultures late in the course of infection. As *L. prolificans* is usually resistant against many antifungals including amphotericin B, combinations of voriconazole with terbinafine and echinocandins may provide the most active antifungal approach. New antifungals with in vitro activity are entering clinical trials.

8.13.1 Diagnosis

As melanized fungi are widespread in the environment, they may be cultivated from the respiratory tract without clinical infection. Therefore, the diagnosis of phaeohyphomycosis often relies on the demonstration of hyphae in tissue. Microscopy reveals pleomorphic fungal elements consisting of yeast-like cells, pseudohyphae, and short, thin, and septate hyphal fragments. These elements can show pigmentation in wet mounts or HE-stained slides. The pigmentation may be easier to detect by the Fontana-Masson stain, and is not usually identified with Grocott's stain. Identification of the causative agents is necessary for correct management and can be established by cultivation on standard mycological culture media that will grow brown to black mold colonies. The identification of cultivated dematiaceous fungi by morphology is difficult due to variable morphology and may need to involve a reference laboratory.

8.13.2 Management

Evidence for the usefulness of antifungal agents is limited to case reports and small case series. Amphotericin B is active against most etiologic agents except for *S. prolificans*, some *Exophiala*, and *Rhinocladiella mackenziei* isolates. Itraconazole and terbinafine are options for subcutaneous infections. Eye infections may respond to topical natamycin and voriconazole. Respiratory tract infections may be treated with voriconazole or amphotericin B. Disseminated and central nervous system infections may respond to combination therapies including liposomal amphotericin B with voriconazole and echinocandins, but the best approach has not been validated.

8.14 Hyalohyphomycosis

Hyalohyphomycosis refers to mold infections characterized by non-melanized septated hyphae documented in tissue specimens. Etiologic agents include predominantly ascomycetous molds including *Fusarium* and *Scedosporium*. However, a growing list of other fungi is being reported as agents of hyalohyphomycosis. As the etiologic fungi often cannot be differentiated by tissue morphology but may differ in susceptibility against antifungals, identification of the causative agents by culture or molecular techniques guides treatment decisions. If the identification of the causative agents was established, specific names such as fusariosis or scedosporiosis are used. In immunocompetent patients, hyalohyphomycosis often presents as a localized infection after penetrating trauma. Inhalation of spores may lead to respiratory tract infections including pneumonia or sinusitis. Disseminated infections are possible and usually occur in immunocompromised patients. Predisposing conditions include hematologic malignancy and especially prolonged and profound neutropenia in leukemia. As these infections are rare, optimal antifungal therapies have not been defined. Treatment decisions are based on the in vitro susceptibility of the causative agents and may include surgery, as many agents show in vitro resistance against antifungals. In patients with underlying conditions, their reversal might be needed for successful outcomes.

8.15 Fusariosis

Fusarium is a diverse, globally distributed fungal genus encompassing plant and human pathogens. They also produce toxic metabolites which may contaminate food. The fungi can be cultivated from soil, water, fruits, and decomposing organic materials. Most of the human pathogenic species belong to the *Fusarium solani, Fusarium oxysporum*, and *Fusarium fujikuroi* species complexes. As identification at the species level by conventional morphology is unreliable, molecular approaches are needed for correct identification of these fungi. Clinical presentations of fusariosis may include nail, superficial, and deep skin infections or organ infections such as sinusitis, pneumonia, endophthalmitis, osteomyelitis, arthritis, and brain abscess that cannot be differentiated from other mold infections including aspergillosis and mucormycosis. *Fusarium* has a predilection for vascular invasion resulting in thrombosis, infarction, and necrosis. Dissemination occurs mostly in immunocompromised patients predominantly neutropenic patients and may present with sepsis syndrome and skin lesions. The diagnosis of fusariosis depends on the cultivation of the fungi from sterile specimens including blood cultures. In tissue samples, fusariosis is characterized by thin, septated mold hyphae with acute angle branching. However, differentiation from other agents of hyalohyphomycosis and even aspergillosis may be difficult. As *Fusarium* frequently shows in vitro resistance against many antifungals, these infections may manifest as breakthrough infections in patients receiving prophylactic or empiric antifungals.

8.15.1 Eye Infections

Keratitis is the most common infection caused by *Fusarium* and among the most common implantation mycosis of the eye. It has been mostly described in contact lens users, after eye surgery, or ocular trauma. Patients manifest with blurred vision, pain, photophobia, and local inflammation. Infections may progress to endophthalmitis with potential for loss of vision.

8.15.2 Skin and Nail Infections

Fusarium is a rare cause of onychomycosis. In addition to infected nails, cellulitis of adjacent tissues may represent as intertrigo, tinea pedis, and hyperkeratotic plantar lesions. Soft-tissue infections occur after penetrating trauma and may present with necrotic skin lesions.

Respiratory tract infections occur after inhalation of spores. They can present as sinusitis or pneumonia. Clinical differentiation from other mold infections is not usually possible. However dissemination with skin lesions is more prevalent in fusariosis.

Disseminated infection is frequent in immunocompromised patients, who present with fever unresponsive to antibacterial and antifungal therapy as *Fusarium* may be in vitro resistant to several antifungals. Ports of entry, including onychomycosis, may be visible as well as metastatic skin lesions. There are classically three different types of cutaneous lesions which are described: necrotic lesions, target lesions, and subcutaneous lesions. *Fusarium* may be cultivated from blood cultures in disseminated infections.

8.15.3 Diagnosis and Differential Diagnosis

A clinical differentiation from *Aspergillus* and other agents of hyalohyphomycosis is not possible in most cases. Therefore cultivation of *Fusarium* from skin, nail, and corneal scrapings, respiratory tract specimens, or blood cultures is needed to establish the diagnosis. Reference laboratories may be needed for correct identification to the species level and for in vitro resistance testing to guide therapeutic decisions. Specific PCR assays may provide a sensitive identification of *Fusarium* from clinical samples. There are no specific serologic tests available for *Fusarium*, but patients may have a positive beta-D-glucan or *Aspergillus* galactomannan antigen test.

8.15.4 Management

The treatment of keratitis includes the use of topical antifungals such as natamycin 5% (50 mg/ml eye drops) or voriconazole 1% (10 mg/ml eye drops). Voriconazole has been used in regimes combining topical and oral (400 mg/day) administration when deeper tissues are involved. Posaconazole (oral: 200 mg 4×/day) has been rarely used as salvage therapy, but results are encouraging. Liposomal amphotericin B has been used as systemic (5 mg/kg/day) or intravitreal therapy in the treatment of endophthalmitis often together with surgery. Onychomycosis may be treated with terbinafine (250–500 mg/day) or oral azoles including voriconazole and itraconazole (200–400 mg/day). The optimal treatment strategy of patients with severe *Fusarium* infection remains unclear. Localized disease may be cured by surgical debridement. Voriconazole (6 mg/kg/12 h as loading dose, 24 h, followed by 4 mg/kg/12 h) is the most active antifungal. Lipid-based amphotericin B formulations are often used at the highest tolerable dosage (>5 mg/kg/day). Combination therapies are frequently used for immunocompromised patients with disseminated, life-threatening infections. Most drug combinations of amphotericin, voriconazole, echinocandins, and terbinafine do not show antagonism in in vitro testing. Reversal of underlying conditions and surgical interventions are important for successful treatment strategies.

8.16 Scedosporiosis

Scedosporiosis refers to infections caused by the fungi of the genus *Scedosporium*. This mold can be isolated from soils, polluted waters, and decaying plants worldwide. Human infections are mainly caused by *Scedosporium apiospermum*, *Scedosporium boydii* (*previously Pseudallescheria boydii*), and *Scedosporium aurantiacum*. Infections caused by *Lomentospora prolificans* (previously *Scedosporium prolificans*) are described under disseminated phaeohyphomycosis. Spores of *Scedosporium* may be inhaled potentially leading to temporary or chronic colonization of the respiratory tract of patients with cystic fibrosis and rarely other chronic lung diseases. In addition, soft-tissue infections may follow traumatic implantation. *Scedosporium* can be cultivated from clinical specimens including respiratory and soft-tissue samples. The use of selective media containing benomyl improves their detection in the presence of bacteria or faster-growing fungi such as *Candida* and *Aspergillus*. There are no commercial-specific serologic assays available for scedosporiosis. In tissue samples, *Scedosporium* cannot be differentiated from other agents of hyalohyphomycosis, although detection of conidia in tissue may point to *Scedosporium*. *Scedosporium* is intrinsically resistant to antifungals including amphotericin B. Voriconazole is the most active antifungal. The optimal treatment approach has not been validated in clinical trials. Surgical interventions are an important part of the management of localized infections.

8.16.1 Soft-Tissue Infections

Subcutaneous infections have been described after penetrating trauma in previously healthy individuals. *Scedosporium* is a common cause of fungal mycetoma. Local dissemination to joints and bones and hematogenous spread to distant organs including bones and the central nervous system have been described even in non-immunocompromised hosts. *Scedosporium* is also found in ocular infections including keratitis and endophthalmitis and otitis externa.

Pulmonary infection may follow colonization of the respiratory tract in patients with chronic lung disease such as cystic fibrosis. Invasive infection is difficult to diagnose in the absence of a tissue biopsy. Manifestations may include fungus ball formation, pneumonia resembling invasive aspergillosis, and allergic bronchopulmonary aspergillosis. Pneumonia has also been described in immunocompromised hosts without preexisting lung conditions. A typical presentation is pneumonia and brain abscess after near drowning in waters containing the fungi.

Disseminated infections are predominantly diagnosed in immunocompromised patients including neutropenic cancer patients and allogeneic bone marrow and solid organ transplant recipients. However, dissemination to distant sites such as bones, joints, and the CNS is also diagnosed in previously healthy subjects.

Brain abscess may result from local spread in patients with sinusitis, after penetrating trauma or near drowning in polluted water after hematogenous dissemination from respiratory tract infections.

Clinical presentation and radiographic findings of *Scedosporium* infections are nonspecific. Therefore, the diagnosis relies on the cultivation of these slow-growing molds. Identification of *Scedosporium* as a causative agent offers important therapeutic clues as these fungi are resistant to amphotericin B and other antifungals. Identification to the species level and in vitro resistance testing is necessary for optimal patient management. When tissue biopsies show hyphae suggestive for hyalohyphomycosis in the absence of positive cultures, PCR may reveal the fungal etiology.

8.16.2 Management

Optimal treatment strategies have not been evaluated in clinical trials. In localized infections, surgical debridement should be considered. Voriconazole is the most active antifungal, while amphotericin B is intrinsically resistant. Combinations with antifungals including echinocandins and terbinafine are usually not antagonistic in vitro. Combination therapy has often been used in successfully treated patients with disseminated infections published in case reports. The reversal of underlying conditions is an integral part of the management of these infections.

8.17 Rare Yeast Infections

A number of yeasts that had been previously thought to represent harmless colonizers of the skin or to cause superficial skin disorders only are now recognized as significant pathogens causing systemic infections mostly in immunocompromised patients. Clinical presentation of these infections usually is fever unresponsive to antibacterials as in deep candidiasis due to bloodstream or pulmonary infections. Diagnosis relies on the cultivation from sterile sites such as blood cultures. Identification of these fungi can be accurately done by DNA sequencing or MALDI-TOF-MS with the use of high-quality databases. Some have been renamed repeatedly impairing the retrieval of information from the literature. Several of these yeasts show reduced in vitro susceptibility against antifungal agents used to prevent or treat candidemia including fluconazole and the echinocandins. Therefore, they may present as breakthrough infections in patients receiving prophylactic or empiric antifungal therapy. Management of these infections is based on antifungal treatment guided by in vitro resistance testing and reversal of underlying conditions such as removal of infected catheters. Due to the small numbers of infections reported, published experience is restricted to case reports and small case series, and the best management strategies are unknown.

Geotrichum candidum are filamentous ascomycetous yeasts. They have been described as agents of bloodstream infections mostly in cancer patients. As fluconazole and echinocandins are not active, as suggested by high MICs and breakthrough infections, newer azoles such as voriconazole or amphotericin B with or without flucytosine are therapeutic options.

Magnusiomyces capitatus previously named *Saprochaete capitata*, *Geotrichum capitatum*, *Trichosporum capitatum*, and *Blastoschizomyces capitatus* are ascomycetous yeasts found in environmental sources including soil, in dishwashers, and as part of the normal microbiota of humans. These fungi have been described as agents of bloodstream infections in neutropenic cancer patients. Infections are mostly diagnosed by cultivation from blood culture bottles. In vitro resistance testing suggests that fluconazole and echinocandins are not active. Voriconazole and posaconazole show good activity as flucytosine that may be used as a combination partner with amphotericin B.

Saprochaete clavata previously known as *Geotrichum clavatum* are ascomycetous yeasts causing infections typically diagnosed in patients with hematologic malignancy and neutropenia. Infections may present as fever of unknown origin, but deep organ involvement of the lung, spleen, liver, or kidneys is frequently identified.

Diagnosis is established by cultivation from blood cultures. Isolates may show in vitro resistance for echinocandins and reduced susceptibility for fluconazole, but newer triazoles are usually susceptible.

Malassezia are basidiomycetous yeasts and part of the normal skin flora. They can cause various skin conditions including pityriasis versicolor, seborrheic dermatitis, dandruff, or onychomycosis. Invasive infections have been described in patients receiving lipid containing parenteral nutrition, in cancer patients, and in the presence of central venous catheters. *Malassezia* infections may be difficult to diagnose as they may not be cultivated using standard laboratory methods. Amphotericin B and azoles including fluconazole and voriconazole have been suggested as therapeutic options, while the echinocandins and flucytosine appear to be in vitro resistant.

Rhodotorula are basidiomycetous yeasts commonly found in environments and as colonizers of the skin and the respiratory and gastrointestinal tract. Invasive infections have been reported in the presence of intravenous catheters and underlying hematologic malignancy. They are usually diagnosed by cultivation of these yeasts in blood culture bottles. *Rhodotorula* are regarded as intrinsically resistant to azoles and echinocandins but susceptible to amphotericin B and flucytosine.

Trichosporon are basidiomycetous yeasts widely distributed in the environment and regularly found as part of the human microbiota. The genus has undergone major taxonomic revisions. Therefore the existing literature may not provide correct species identification precluding the extraction of evidence for species-specific information. Most cases have been ascribed to *Trichosporon asahii* and *T. dermatis*. Invasive infections including fungemia, endocarditis, meningitis, and peritonitis have been described. In addition *Trichosporon mycotoxinivorans* may be an emerging pulmonary pathogen in the context of cystic fibrosis. Voriconazole seems to be the most active antifungal, while amphotericin B, echinocandins, and flucytosine are not active in vitro.

8.18 Yeast-Like Infections

Protothecosis refers to infections caused by achlorophyllic algae of the genus *Prototheca*. These algae are widespread in the environment in soils and water. They are thought to be less virulent than typical fungal pathogens. Human infections are reported rarely. They predominantly cause superficial infections in immunocompromised patients. Vesiculobullous skin lesions may progress to ulcerative lesions with purulent discharge and crusts after minor trauma with an incubation time of weeks to months. Deep systemic infections have been described with and without association with contaminated catheters. Diagnosis can be established when the algae are cultivated after 72 h on fungal media at 25–37 °C from sterile sites. They resemble yeast colonies. Microscopy demonstrates non-budding spherical unicellular organisms ranging from 3 to 30 μm with endospores. Therapy includes surgical intervention, drainage and excision, removal of contaminated catheters, and systemic antifungals especially in deep infections. Amphotericin B appears to be the most active antifungal in vitro. Azoles such as fluconazole, itraconazole, and voriconazole also show in vitro activity as do some antibacterials including gentamicin and polymyxin B.

Pythiosis is a term used for infections caused by *Pythium insidiosum*, which belongs to the order Oomycota of the kingdom Stramenopila. In contrast to true fungi, cell wall of these microbes contains cellulose instead of glucan, chitin, and mannan. They are found in aquatic environments where they form biflagellate, motile zoospores. Infections in the absence of water suggest additional niches. Infections occur in tropical as well as tempered regions. After traumatic implantation, clinical manifestations begin with a small itching papule that rapidly progresses to large, painful, ulcerating lesions and spreads to subcutaneous tissues. Ocular infections may manifest as keratitis or periorbital cellulitis. The vascular (arterial) form is characterized by invasion of blood vessels with thrombosis, infarction, and necrosis manifesting as claudication and later necrosis and hemorrhage. Diagnosis of pythiosis is based on the demonstration of broad, irregular septate hyphae with nonparallel walls resembling mucormycosis. They are very hard to detect in HE stains. They grow rapidly on Sabouraud dextrose agar at 37 °C as white submerged colonies. Despite lacking ergosterol in the cell wall, infections have been responded to antifungals such as amphotericin B, itraconazole, and terbinafine. Corneal infection may need surgical intervention. The vascular form requires prompt start of antifungals and surgical debridement.

Rhinosporidiosis is an infection of the nasal and other mucosal surfaces and the ocular conjunctiva by the protozoon *Rhinosporidium seeberi*. The pathogen has not been cultivated. It may have aquatic as well as terrestrial niches. The diagnosis relies on the demonstration of large, thick-walled structures of oval to spherical sporangiospores, containing endospores. Endospores are released from mature sporangiospores that develop into new sporangiospores. The disease occurs in tropical and subtropical regions worldwide, except for Australia, but is most often reported from India and Sri Lanka in rural areas among persons bathing in public ponds or working in stagnant water such as rice fields. The infection presents as nasal infections with nasal obstruction by large painless sessile or pedunculated papillomatous lesions containing the sporangiospores. In some cases, lesions develop on the conjunctiva or the ears. Diagnosis relies on microscopic examination of biopsy specimens demonstrating sporangia of different stages and sizes. Mature sporangia resemble spherules of *Coccidioides* and can be differentiated from those of *Emmonsia* by the zonation of the internal sporangiospores. The treatment of choice is surgical resection.

Clinical Syndromes: Pneumocystis 9

Peter-Michael Rath

9.1 Introduction

Pneumocystis spp. are typically opportunistic pathogens, causing an asymptomatic or mild pneumonia in immunocompetent humans and fulminant infections (*Pneumocystis* pneumonia, PCP) in immunocompromised patients. It has been estimated that PCP is the third most common invasive fungal infection worldwide with more than 400,000 life-threatening infections per year and a mortality rate of 20–80% [1] .

Pneumocystis spp. colonize the lungs of mammalian hosts. The long co-evolution of millions of years results in a high host specificity. For example, the human-relevant species, now named *P. jirovecii*, is not pathogenic in mice [2]. Up to now, five species have been identified: *P. carinii* and *P. wakefieldiae* in rats, *P. murina* in mice, *P. oryctolagi* in rabbits, and *P. jirovecii* in humans [3].

9.2 *Pneumocystis jirovecii*

The taxonomic classification of *Pneumocystis* changed over time. Initially described as a form of *Trypanosoma cruzi* in guinea pigs by Chagas in 1909, Delanoe and Delanoe recognized that it is a new species in a new genus and purposed the name *Pneumocystis carinii* in 1912 in honour of Dr. Carini (reviewed in [4]). It was believed for a long time that the organism is a parasite; however morphological and molecular data from the 1970s and 1980s clearly indicate that *Pneumocystis* is a fungus belonging to a deep basal branch of *Ascomycota* [4] in close association with *Taphrina*, *Saitoella*, and *Schizosaccharomyces* [5]. However, *Pneumocystis* is an unusual fungus in that the organism lacks ergosterol in its plasma membrane, resulting in insensitivity to classical antifungals as polyenes or azoles. The now generally accepted name of the human-relevant species is *P. jirovecii* [6]. Otto Jirovec was a Czech parasitologist describing *Pneumocystis* as the agent of plasma cell pneumonia in children in 1951.

Pneumocystis has a complex life cycle consisting of small (1–4 μm), ameboid trophozoites which bind to the alveolar type 1 cells and sporocysts which evolve to cysts (5–8 μm) with eight haploid nuclei. The life cycle has been extensively reviewed by Chabé et al. [7]. The cysts induce a strong immune response mainly due to ß-glucans in the cell wall. Both the immune response and the uncontrolled, excessive proliferation of trophic forms in a foamy matrix are responsible for the typical clinical picture with plasma cell pneumonia and disturbed oxygenation, hypercapnia, and elevated lactate dehydrogenase (LDH) in serum as a sign of lung injury.

P.-M. Rath
Institute of Medical Microbiology, University Hospital of Essen, Essen, Germany
e-mail: pm.rath@uni-due.de

E. Presterl (ed.), *Clinically Relevant Mycoses*, https://doi.org/10.1007/978-3-319-92300-0_9

As reviewed by Kelly and Shellito [8], macrophages represent the first line of defence. The innate immunity, combined with both T and B lymphocytes, results not only in resolution of infection but also in long-term protection from clinically relevant infections. An impaired local or systemic immune system allows the organism to proliferate in the alveoli and to induce clinically relevant symptoms. Whereas earlier predominantly described in immunocompromised children and as an AIDS-defining disease in HIV-infected patients, the focus shifted to patients with haemato-oncological diseases and autoimmune diseases as well as to organ transplant recipients in the past two decades.

9.3 Epidemiology

The source of infection and the route of transmission are not clear. A number of data suggest primarily an airborne transmission with humans as the sole source of *P. jirovecii*.

Animal experiments indicate that the cysts are more relevant in transmission than the trophic forms [9, 10]. Serological data indicates that the initial contact occurs within the first 5–10 years of life (reviewed in [11]). A seroconversion rate of 85% was found up to an age of 10 years. The first contact seems to result in an asymptomatic or mild infection in immunocompetent children. In immunosuppression due to infections or immunosuppressive treatment or in severe malnutrition, clinically relevant symptoms occur. Whereas first reported in children with malnutrition in the 1950s, the incidence increased dramatically with the emergence of the HIV pandemia later in the 1980s. During the following years, the frequency of infections in these patients decreased due to the advances in the treatment of HIV in the developed countries. However, other patients are also at risk for PCP, especially patients with solid cancers, with hematologic malignancies, and after organ transplantation. Many immunosuppressive drugs are associated with a risk for clinically relevant infection, for example, monoclonal antibodies (Aletuzumab and other), TNF-alpha-inhibitors, purine analogous like azathioprine, antimetabolites like methotrexate, anticalcineurins like cyclosporine, or alkylating agents like cyclophosphamide [12]. Some data indicate that the infection rate is increasing in these patients [13].

It seems that *Pneumocystis* colonizes permanently or intermittently the healthy lung. *Pneumocystis*-DNA was found in up to 70% of healthy individuals by using sensitive methods [14]. As reviewed by Calderón [11], a high rate of colonized but not ill HIV patients (10–69%) was found. *P. jirovecii* can also be detected in children with bronchiolitis (24%) or respiratory infections (15–32%), or because of various other causes (17–100%) [15]. In one study from Chile *Pneumocystis* was detected in the lung of 82% of children with sudden unexpected death by PCR (of which 94% were also positive by microscopy) [16]. In adults, *P. jirovecii* was found in respiratory samples in 15–58% of immunosuppressed patients and in up to 30–55% in adults with pulmonary non-PCP diseases. In haemodialysis patients [17] and renal transplant recipients, 21% and 19%, respectively, were colonized, detected by PCR from induced sputa [18].

A reinforced colonization may play a role in the clinical course of chronic lung diseases like COPD [19] or cystic fibrosis [20], due to a pro-inflammatory effect.

Nosocomial outbreaks have been described, especially in renal transplant units but also in other settings [21]. In face of these data, some guidelines recommend to separate infected patients and patients at risk for pneumocystosis [22]. Indeed, *Pneumocystis*-DNA can be detected not only in the ambient air but also in higher concentrations in the air of rooms with infected as well as colonized patients [23]. Some data indicates that health-care workers also may play a role in nosocomial infections. Those with contact to patients with pneumocystosis have higher antibody titers than workers without contact to such patients [24]. In one study a colonization rate of 9% was found in ICU health-care workers with contact to patients with PCP [25]. Therefore, health-care workers may be an in-hospital reservoir for *Pneumocystis*.

9.4 Clinical Picture

Pneumocystis pneumonia should be considered in any immunosuppressed patient who shows fever, respiratory symptoms, and an abnormal X-ray. The detection by microscopic methods and/or PCR is essential for a definitive diagnosis, because symptoms are nonspecific and may be caused by a number of infectious and non-infectious agents. Clinical presentation differs between HIV-infected and non-infected patients. Patients with a severely suppressed immune system like AIDS with a T-cell count <200/µl show a high fungal load in their lung but only minor inflammation, while other patients with a partially suppressed immune system, for example, organ transplant recipients, show a low number of fungal cells but a severe clinical picture due to a strong inflammatory reaction.

The clinical signs in HIV-positive patients are subacute with fever, progressive dyspnoea, and dry cough [12]. In non-HIV-infected patients, the clinical picture is more acute, and the prognosis is significantly poorer. The poorer prognosis may be linked to a delay in diagnosis and initiation of treatment in those patients [26, 27]. Diffuse bilateral interstitial infiltrates are the typical signs on X-ray. In CT scan bilateral ground glass opacities are characteristic (Fig. 9.1). Seldom lobar infiltrates, nodules, or cavities are seen. Extrapulmonary manifestations seem to be rare [28], although systematic investigations are missing.

9.5 Laboratory Diagnosis

The detection of the pathogen is essential for the diagnosis of pneumocystosis, because clinical and radiological signs are unspecific, as mentioned above. The laboratory methods have been reviewed recently in more detail by Rath and Steinmann [29].

9.6 Microscopy

The traditional laboratory diagnosis of pneumocystosis is based on the microscopic detection of cysts or trophozoites in deep respiratory materials, i.e. in bronchoalveolar lavage fluid. Other materials, for example, induced sputum, show a reduced sensitivity.

Most commonly used stains are the Papanicolaou, Wright-Giemsa, Grocott-Gomori silver, and toluidine blue *O* stains. Using Papanicolaou or Giemsa stain, simultaneous detection of trophic forms and cysts is possible (Fig. 9.2), while with all other stains, only cysts are detectable. Examples are shown in Fig. 9.3. Which stain is used in a laboratory depends on the specific circumstances in the lab, i.e. which stain is established and which experience exists. In a large study with more than 300 respiratory samples investigated by four staining methods (Calcofluor white, Grocott-Gomori silver, Diff-Quik, and an immunofluorescence assay), it was shown that only Calcofluor white and the sil-

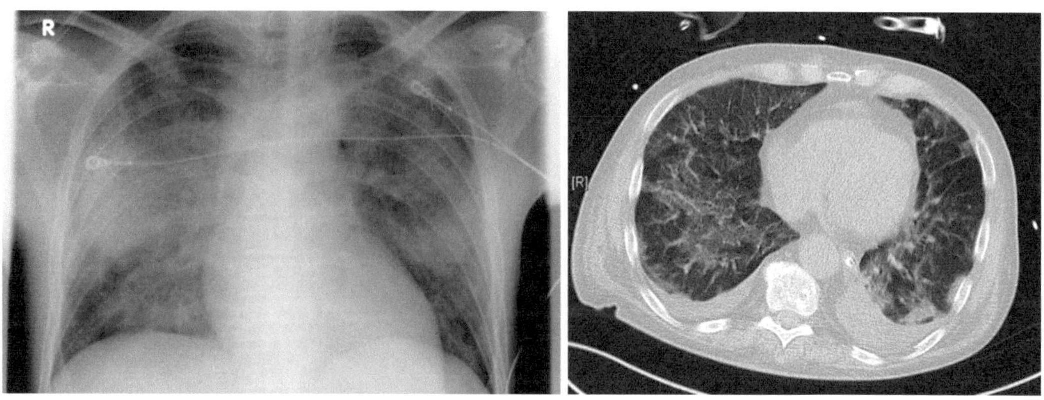

Fig. 9.1 X-ray and CT scan of an immunosuppressed child (*left*) and an adult (*right*) with pneumocystosis

ver stain had a positive and negative predictive value of >90% [30]. In HIV patients immunofluorescence assays showed a higher sensitivity of 67% than cytochemical stains (43%) when using induced sputum samples and compared with BAL [31]. Therefore, such assays should be preferred.

Although a permanent cell culture model has been described recently [32], such systems are not established for routine diagnosis.

9.7 Molecular Detection

Since some years PCR systems are commercially available, and these systems more and more replace the microscopic detection due to the higher sensitivity and specificity. In addition, other than deep respiratory samples can be used without loss of sensitivity. For example, in one study a high sensitivity was found when using nasopharyngeal aspirates for detection [33]. However, many systems are not validated systematically in different patient populations and seem to have varying sensitivities resulting in different cut-offs. Furthermore, based on a qualitative positive result, no discrimination is possible between (asymptomatic) colonization and disease. Recent data indicate that this is possible using quantitative assays [34]. In addition, it was purposed that different cut-offs should be used depending on the HIV status to differentiate between infection and colonization [35]. Currently, we recommend to use both an immunofluorescence assay and a quantitative PCR for the diagnosis of PCP. A positive immunofluorescence result correlates well with a clinically significant infection. If a lab decides to use PCR only, a quantitative assay is recommended, and individual cut-offs should be established for the different patient groups considering clinical and radiological findings.

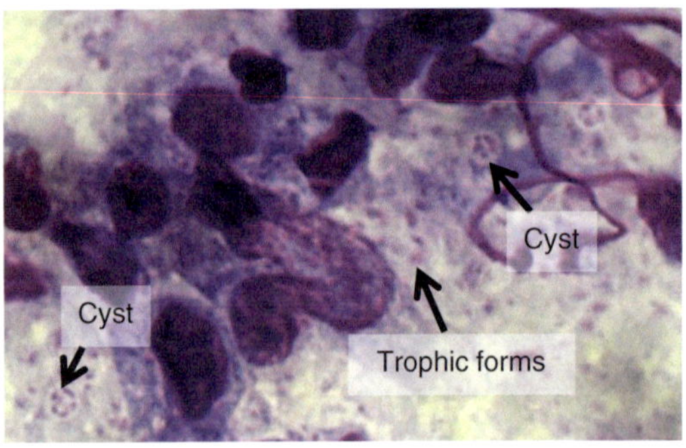

Fig. 9.2 Giemsa stain of *Pneumocystis* trophozoites and cysts in bronchoalveolar lavage fluid (magnification ×1000)

9.8 Serology

Because of the high seroprevalence on the one hand and the high proportion of immunosuppressed patients on the other hand, serological investigations for diagnosis of PCP are not applicable. Therefore, no commercial test is available.

However, some biomarkers are currently under investigation [36] from which (1-3)-ß-D-Glucan

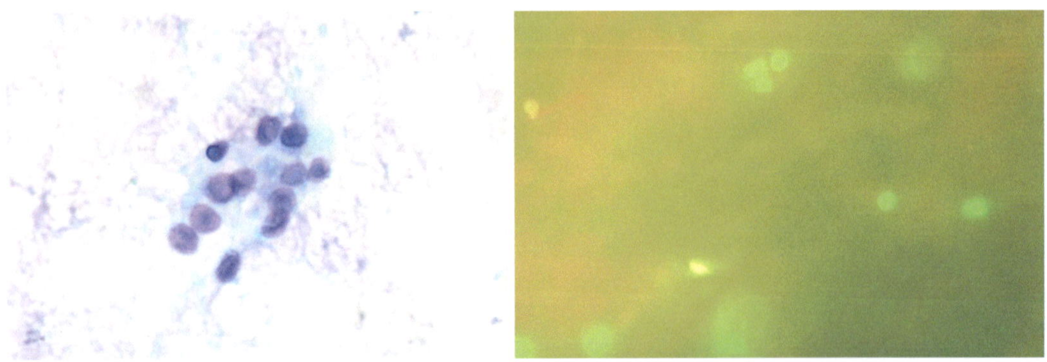

Fig. 9.3 Toluidine blue *O* (*left*) and a immunofluorescence stain of *Pneumocystis* cysts in bronchoalveolar lavage fluid (magnification ×1000)

(BDG) is the most extensively investigated one. BDG is elevated in patients with clinically relevant pneumocystosis [37], but many other fungal infections as well as the administration of blood products and antibiotics, the use of gauze, and even dialysis resulted in elevated serum BDG levels [38].

In pneumocystosis a meta-analysis showed a sensitivity of 95% and a specificity of 85% [39]. In a more recent analysis, a sensitivity of 91% and a specificity of 75% were found [40]. Sensitivity was significantly higher in HIV-positive patients (92%) than in HIV-negative patients (85%), whereas the specificity was similar (78% vs. 73%). The authors concluded that a negative BDG is useful to rule out PCP only in HIV patients. Combining PCR and BDG results seems to be useful in the discrimination between clinically relevant infection and colonization [41]. Some recent data indicates that the determination of BDG in bronchoalveolar lavage fluid may also be helpful to discriminate patients with clinical relevant infection and those with (asymptomatic) colonization [42].

9.9 Prophylaxis of Pneumocystosis

Given the high incidence of pneumocystosis in immunosuppressed patients, prophylaxis is recommended in high-risk patients. For a detailed discussion of *Pneumocystis* prophylaxis and treatment, the reader is referred to current recommendations. In short a CD4 cell count <200 cells/µl is a useful marker to identify patients at risk in HIV and non-HIV patients [43]. In these patients trimethoprim/sulfamethoxazole (either 80/400 mg daily or 160/800 mg three times weekly) should be given during the period of risk as first-line treatment. Second-line alternatives are pentamidine, atovaquone, or dapsone (Table 9.1). Prophylaxis should be continued in HIV patients until the CD4+ cell count increases to >200 cells/µl for more than 3 months [45], or for allogenic HSCT patients until 6 months after engraftment, or longer in patients having chronic GvHD or in patients under immunosuppressive treatment [44].

9.10 Treatment

High-dose trimethoprim/sulfamethoxazole (15–20 mg/kg trimethoprim and 75–100 mg/kg sulfamethoxazole, TMP-SMX) for 2–3 weeks is the treatment of choice in HIV- and non-HIV-infected patients [45, 46]. TMP-SMX is well-tolerated by non-HIV-infected patients, but many HIV-infected patients suffer adverse reactions, including rash, cytopenia, hepatitis, nephritis, and others. Alternative regimes consist of clindamycin plus primaquine (the preferred combination in patients who do not tolerate TMP-SMX), pentamidine, TMP plus dapsone, or atovaquone (Table 9.2). Secondary prophy-

Table 9.1 Prophylaxis for PCP (Adapted from [44, 45])

Substance	Dose
Trimethoprim/sulfamethoxazole	80/400 mg daily or 160/800 mg/day or thrice a week
Dapsone	2 × 50 mg/day
Atovaquone	1500 mg/day
Pentamidine inhalation	300 mg once/month

Table 9.2 Treatment of PCP (Adapted from [44, 45])

Substance	Dose
TMP/SMX	15–20 mg/kg/75–100 mg/kg
Pentamidine iv	4 mg/kg/day
Primaquine+clindamycin	15–30 mg/day + 3 × 600 mg/day
Atovaquone	2–3 × 750 mg/day

laxis can be stopped when the CD4 cell count has increased to >200 cells/µl for a period of more than 3 months in HIV patients [45].

In the first few days of treatment, an aggravation of symptoms is characteristic, probably due to an increased release of glucans through the lysis of cysts. Therefore, the administration of corticosteroids is recommended starting within the first 3 days of treatment in HIV patients with moderate to severe PCP, resulting in a 0.55 times reduction in the mortality [47]. However, patients should be carefully monitored for other opportunistic infections and complications of steroid treatment. The recommended dosing is 40 mg prednisolone bid on days 1–5, than 40 mg once per day on days 6–10, thereafter 20 mg per day on days 11–21 [45]. The role of corticosteroid treatment in non-HIV patients is less clear. In a recently published meta-analysis, no benefit of adjunctive corticosteroid treatment in such patients was found [48].

The role of echinocandins in the treatment of PCP is not cleared up to now. This class of antifungals inhibits the synthesis of (1-3)-ß-D-glucan which is a component of the cell wall of many fungi (except *Cryptococcus* and *Zygomycetes*) as well as in the cysts of *Pneumocystis*. In animal experiments echinocandin treatment resulted in a depletion of *Pneumocystis* cysts, but not the trophozoites [9]. A number of case reports, in which caspofungin has been used as salvage therapy or in combination with other agents, have been published with conflicting results. Furthermore, breakthrough infections have been reported in patients treated with an echinocandin for other reasons [49]. Consequently, the most recent ECIL guideline for the treatment of pneumocystosis in haematological patients did not recommend an echinocandin monotherapy [46].

Conflict of Interests None

References

1. Brown GD, Denning DW, Gow NAR, Levitz SM, Netea MG, White TC (2012) Hidden killers: human fungal infections. Sci Transl Med 4:165rv13
2. Durand-Joly I, Aliouat EM, Recourt C, Guyot K, François N, Wauquier M, Camus D, Dei-Cas E (2002) *Pneumocystis carinii* f. sp. *hominis* is not infectious for SCID mice. J Clin Microbiol 40:1862–1865
3. Aliouat-Denis C-M, Chabé M, Demanche C, Aliouat EM, Viscogliosi E, Guillot J, Delhaes L, Dei-Cas E (2008) *Pneumocystis* species, coevolution and pathogenic power. Infect Genet Evol 8:708–726
4. Aliouat-Denis C-M, Martinez A, Aliouat EM, Pottier M, Gantois N, Dei-Cas E (2009) The *Pneumocystis* life cycle. Mem Inst Oswaldo Cruz 104:419–426
5. Ma L, Huang D-W, Cuomo CA, Sykes S, Fantoni G, Das B, Sherman BT, Yang J, Huber C, Xia J, Davey E, Kutty G, Bishop L, Sassi M, Lempicki RA, Kovacs JA (2013) Sequencing and characterization of the complete mitochondrial genomes of three *Pneumocystis* species provide new insights into divergence between human and rodent *Pneumocystis*. FASEB J 27:1962–1972
6. Stringer JR, Beard CB, Miller RF (2009) Spelling *Pneumocystis jirovecii*. Emerg Infect Dis 15:506
7. Chabé M, Aliouat-Denis C-M, Delhaes L, Aliouat EM, Viscogiosi E, Dei-Cas E (2011) *Pneumocystis*: from a doubtful unique entity to a group of highly diversified fungal species. FEMS Yeast Res 11:2–17
8. Kelly MN, Shellito JD (2010) Current understanding of *Pneumocystis* immunology. Future Microbiol 5:43–65
9. Cushion MT, Linke MJ, Ashbaugh A, Sesterhenn T, Collins MS, Lynch K, Brubaker R, Walzer PD (2010) Echinocandin treatment of *Pneumocystis* pneumonia in rodent models depletes cysts leaving trophic burdens that cannot transmit the infection. PLoS ONE 5:e8524
10. Martinez A, Halliez MCM, Aliouat EM, Chabé M, Standaert-Vitse A, Fréalle E, Gantois N, Pottier M, Pinon A, Dei-Cas E, Aliouat-Denis C-M (2013) Growth and airborne transmission of cell-sorted life cycle stages of *Pneumocystis carinii*. PLoS ONE 8:e79958
11. Calderón EJ (2009) Epidemiology of *Pneumocystis* infection in humans. J Mycol Méd 19:270–275
12. Roux A, Gonzales F, Roux M, Mehrad M, Menotti J, Zahar J-R, Tadros V-X, Azoulay E, Brillet P-Y, Vincent F (2014) Update on pulmonary *Pneumocystis jirovecii* infection in non-HIV patients. Méd Mal Infect 44:185–198
13. Maini R, Henderson KL, Sheridan EA, Lamagni T, Nichols G, Delpech V, Phin N (2013) Increasing *Pneumocystis* pneumonia, England, UK, 2000–2010. Emerg Infect Dis 19:386–392
14. Ponce CA, Gallo M, Bustamante R, Vargas SL (2010) *Pneumocystis* colonization is highly prevalent in the autopsied lungs of the general population. Clin Infect Dis 50:347–353
15. Morris A, Wei K, Afshar K, Huang L (2008) Epidemiology and clinical significance of *Pneumocystis* colonization. J Infect Dis 197:10–17
16. Vargas SL, Ponce CA, Gallo M, Pérez F, Astorga J-F, Bustamante R, Chabé M, Durand-Joly I, Iturra P, Miller RF, Aliouat EL, Dei-Cas E (2013) Near-universal prevalence of *Pneumocystis* and asso-

ciated Increase in mucus in the lungs of infants with sudden unexpected death. Clin Infect Dis 56:171–179

17. Fritsche C, Ghanem H, Koball S, Mueller-Hilke B, Reisinger EC (2017) High *Pneumocystis jirovecii* colonization rate among haemodialysis patients. Infect Dis 49:132–136
18. Fritzsche C, Riebold D, Fuehrer A, Mitzner A, Klammt S, Mueller-Hilke B, Reisinger EC (2013) *Pneumocystis jirovecii* colonization among renal transplant recipients. Nephrology 18:382–387
19. Morris A, Netravali M, Kling HM, Shipley T, Ross T, Sciurba FC, Norris KA (2008) Relationship of *Pneumocystis* antibody response to severity of chronic obstructive pulmonary disease. Clin Infect Dis 47:e64–e68
20. Green HD, Bright-Thomas RJ, Mutton KJ, Guiver M, Jones AM (2016) Increased prevalence of *Pneumocystis jirovecii* colonization in acute pulmonary exacerbations of cystic fibrosis. J Infect 73:1–7
21. Yiannakis EP, Boswell TC (2016) Systematic review of outbreaks of *Pneumocystis jirovecii* pneumonia: evidence that *P. jirovecii* is a transmissible organism and the implications for healthcare infection control. J Hosp Infect 93:1–8
22. Siegel JD, Rhinehart E, Jackson M, Chiarello L; The Healthcare Infection Control Practices Advisory Committee (2007) Guideline for isolation precautions: preventing transmission of infectious agents in healthcare settings. http://www.cdc.gov/ncidod/dhqp/pdf/isolation2007.pdf
23. LeGal S, Pougnet L, Damiani C, Fréalle E, Guéguen P, Virmaux M, Ansart S, Jaffuel S, Couturaud F, Delluc A, Tonnelier J-M, Castellant P, Le Meur Y, Le Floch G, Todet A, Menotti J, Nevez G (2015) *Pneumocystis jirovecii* in the air surrounding patients with *Pneumocystis* pulmonary colonization. Diagn Microbiol Infect Dis 82:137–142
24. Fong S, Daly KR, Tipirneni R, Jarlsberg LG, Djawe K, Koch JV, Swartzman A, Roth B, Walzer PD, Huang L (2013) Antibody responses against *Pneumocystis jirovecii* in health care workers over time. Emerg Infect Dis 19:1612–1619
25. Valade S, Azoulay E, Damiani C, Derouin F, Totet A, Menotti J (2015) *Pneumocystis jirovecii* airborne transmission between critically ill patients and health care workers. Intensive Care Med 41:1716–1718
26. Kovacs JA, Hiemenz JW, Macher AM, Stover D, Murray HW, Shelhamer J et al (1984) *Pneumocystis carinii* pneumonia: a comparison between patients with the acquired immunodeficiency syndrome and patients with other immunodeficiencies. Ann Intern Med 100:663–671
27. Bienvenu AL, Traore K, Plekhanova I, Bouchrik M, Bossard C, Picot S (2016) *Pneumocystis* pneumonia suspected in 604 non-HIV and HIV patients. Int J Infect Dis 46:11–17
28. Ng VL, Yajko DM, Hadley WK (1997) Extrapulmonary pneumocystosis. Clin Microbiol Rev 10:401–418
29. Rath P-M, Steinmann J (2014) Update on diagnosis of Pneumocystis pulmonary infections. Curr Fungal Infect Rep 8:227–234
30. Procop GW, Haddad S, Quinn J, Wilson ML, Henshaw NG, Reller LB, Artymyshyn RL, Katanik MT, Weinstein MP (2004) Detection of *Pneumocystis jiroveci* in respiratory specimens by four staining methods. J Clin Microbiol 42:3333–3335
31. Cruciani M, Marcati P, Malena M, Bosco O, Serpelloni G, Mengoli C (2002) Meta-analysis of diagnostic procedures for *Pneumocystis carinii* pneumonia in HIV-1-infected patients. Eur Respir J 20:982–989
32. Schildgen V, Mai S, Khalfaouri S, Lüsebrink J, Pieper M, Tillmann RL, Brockmann M, Schildgen O (2014) Pneumocystis jirovecii can be productively cultured in differentiated CuFi-8 air was cells. MBio 5:e01186–e01114
33. To KKW, Wong SCY, Xu T, Poon RWS, Mok K-Y, Chan JFW, Cheng VCC, Chan K-H, Hung IFN, Yuen K-Y (2013) Use of nasopharyngeal aspirate for diagnosis of *Pneumocystis* pneumonia. J Clin Microbiol 51:1570–1574
34. Sasso M, Chastang-Dumas E, Bastide S, Alonso S, Lechiche C, Bourgeois N, Lachauda L (2016) Performances of four real-time PCR assays for diagnosis of *Pneumocystis jirovecii* pneumonia. J Clin Microbiol 54:625–630
35. Louis M, Guitard J, Jodar M, Ancelle T, Magne D, Lascols O, Hennequin C (2015) Impact of HIV infection status on interpretation of quantitative PCR for detection of *Pneumocystis jirovecii*. J Clin Microbiol 53:3870–3875
36. Esteves F, Calé SS, Badura R, de Boer MG, Maltez F, Calderón EJ, van der Reijden TJ, Márquez-Martín E, Antunes F, Matos O (2015) Diagnosis of *Pneumocystis* pneumonia: evaluation of four serologic biomarkers. Clin Microbiol Infect 21:379.e1–379.e10
37. Finkelman MA (2010) *Pneumocystis jirovecii* infection: cell wall(1→3)-β-D-glucan biology and diagnostic utility. Crit Rev Microbiol 36:271–281
38. Theel ES, Doern CD (2013) ß-D-glucan testing is important for diagnosis of invasive fungal infections. J Clin Microbiol 51:3478–3483
39. Karageorgopoulos DE, Qu J-M, Korbila IP, Zhu J-G, Vasileiou VA, Falagas ME (2013) Accuracy of ß-D-glucan for the diagnosis of *Pneumocystis jirovecii* pneumonia: a meta-analysis. Clin Microbiol Infect 19:39–49
40. Li W-J, Guo Y-L, Liu T-J, Wang K, Kong J-L (2015) Diagnosis of pneumocystis pneumonia using serum (1-3)-β-D-glucan: a bivariate meta-analysis and systematic review. J Thorac Dis 7:2214–2225
41. Damiani C, Le Gal S, Da Costa C, Virmaux M, Nevez G, Totet A (2013) Combined quantification of pulmonary pneumocystis jirovecii DNA and serum (1-3)-D-glucan for differential diagnosis of *Pneumocystis* pneumonia and *Pneumocystis* colonization. J Clin Microbiol 51:3380–3388
42. Damiani C, Le Gal S, Goin N, Di Pizio P, Da Costa C, Virmaux M, Bach V, Stéphan-Blanchard E, Nevez G, Totet A (2015) Usefulness of (1,3) ß-D-glucan detection in bronchoalveolar lavage samples in

Pneumocystis pneumonia and *Pneumocystis* pulmonary colonization. J Mycol Méd 25:36–43
43. Messiaen PE, Cuyx S, Dejagere T, van der Hilst JC (2017) The role of CD4 cell count as discriminatory measure to guide chemoprophylaxis against *Pneumocystis jirovecii* pneumonia in human immunodeficiency virus-negative immunocompromised patients: a systematic review. Transpl Infect Dis 19:e12651
44. Maertens J, Cesaro S, Maschmeyer G, Einsele H, Donnelly JP, Alanio A, Hauser PM, Lagrou K, Melchers WJG, Helweg-Larsen J, Matos O, Bretagne S, Cordonnier C (2016) ECIL guidelines for preventing *Pneumocystis jirovecii* pneumonia in patients with haematological malignancies and stem cell transplant recipients. J Antimicrob Chemother 71:2397–2404
45. Kaplan JE, Benson C, Holmes KK, Brooks JT, Pau A, Masur H (2009) Guideline for prevention and treatment of opportunistic infections in HIV-infected adults and adolescents. MMWR 58(RR04):1–198
46. Maschmeyer G, Helweg-Larsen J, Pagano L, Robin C, Cordonnier C, Schellongowski P (2016) ECIL guidelines for treatment of *Pneumocystis jirovecii* pneumonia in non-HIV-infected haematology patients. J Antimicrob Chemother 71:2405–2413
47. Wang L, Liang H, Ye L, Jiang J, Liang B, Hunag J (2016) Adjunctive corticosteroids for the treatment of *Pneumocystis jiroveci* pneumonia in patients with HIV: A meta-analysis. Exp Ther Med 11:683–687
48. Fujikura Y, Manabe T, Kawana A, Kohno S (2017) Adjunctive corticosteroids for *Pneumocystis jirovecii* pneumonia in non-HIV-infected patients: A systematic review and meta-analysis of observational studies. Arch Bronconeumol 53:55–61
49. Kamboj M, Weinstock D, Sepkowitz KA (2006) Progression of *Pneumocystis jiroveci* pneumonia in patients receiving echinocandin therapy. Clin Infect Dis 43:e92–e94

Clinically Relevant Mycoses Dermatomycoses

10

Gabriele Ginter-Hanselmayer and Pietro Nenoff

10.1 Definition of Dermatomycoses

The term dermatomycoses comprises superficial fungal infections of the skin and their appendages like the hair follicles and the nail apparatus. These superficial mycoses may be caused by dermatophytes or yeasts and, to a less extend, by moulds. These infections are of high importance in medical disciplines not only for the dermatologist but also for physician and the paediatrician and of course for the patients affected. With regard to the treatment of these fungal infections, the costs of topical antifungals will surpass topical corticosteroids in the healthcare system.

10.2 Superficial Mycoses Caused by Dermatophytes (Dermatophytoses, Ringworm Infection)

Dermatophytoses are caused by different classes of dermatophytes with potency to invade the stratum corneum as well as the hair follicle and the nail apparatus. If caused by anthropophilic species, they produce little to no inflammatory host-mediated immune response resulting in chronic course of infection and missing self resolution. Zoophilic or geophilic species may cause acute, inflammatory mycoses.

Dermatophytoses are of worldwide distribution. Their epidemiology depends from many circumstances, i.e. geographical regions, occupational and social aspects, travel, migration, preventive education and modern conveniences such as antifungal therapy. Awareness given to these infections is of crucial importance reflecting the states of civilization and medical systems. In general the distribution of different dermatophyte species varies in the course of time in different regions.

10.2.1 Etiologic Agents

10.2.1.1 History and New Developments of Classification

The dermatophytes, a group of fungi that infect keratinous tissues, belong to the oldest groups of microorganisms that have been recognized as agents of human disease. The taxonomy of these fungi was initiated in 1841 with studies of Robert Remak and David Gruby [1].

Between 1840 and 1875, five of the main species known today, viz. *Microsporum audoui-*

G. Ginter-Hanselmayer (✉)
Department of Dermatology and Venereology Graz, Medical University of Graz, Graz, Austria
e-mail: gabriele.ginter@klinikum-graz.at

P. Nenoff
Labor für Medizinische Mikrobiologie, Partnerschaft Prof. Dr. med. Pietro Nenoff & Dr. med. Constanze Krüger, Rötha OT, Germany
e-mail: nenoff@mykologie-experten.de

E. Presterl (ed.), *Clinically Relevant Mycoses*, https://doi.org/10.1007/978-3-319-92300-0_10

nii, *Epidermophyton floccosum*, *Trichophyton schoenleinii*, *T. tonsurans* and *T. mentagrophytes*, had already been described. This was several decades before the discovery of Pasteur's invention of axenic culture [2].

The only ubiquitous modern dermatophyte missing from the list is *Trichophyton rubrum*, which has been hypothesized to have emerged in the twentieth century [3, 4].

After Pasteur's time, culturing of dermatophytes and description of new species have taken off enormously. Species were defined on the basis of combined clinical pictures and morphological characters in vitro. During the following decades, application of new methodological standard led to an explosion of new species and recombined names. Subsequently anamorph nomenclature stabilized by the wide acceptance of *Epidermophyton*, *Microsporum* and *Trichophyton* as the genera covering all dermatophytes.

In the last decades of the twentieth century, the conventional approach to dermatophyte taxonomy combined clinical appearance, cultural characteristics, microscopy and physiology. Because each of these morphologies had it limitations, a novel multilocus phylogenetic taxonomy for the dermatophytes was recently established by the working group of Sybren de Hoog et al. by sequencing for rDNA ITS and partial LSU, the ribosomal 60S protein and fragments of ß-tubulin and translation elongation factor 3 of type and reference strains of members of the onygenalean family *Arthrodermataceae*. The resulting phylogenetic trees reached an acceptable level of stability for dermatophytes and dermatophyte-like fungi. In the newly proposed taxonomy, 7 genera are categorized like the following: *Trichophyton* contains 16 species, *Epidermophyton* 1 species, *Nannizzia* 9 species, *Microsporum* 3 species, *Lophophyton* 1 species, *Arthroderma* 21 species and *Ctenomyces* 1 species. Of these seven genera only *Trichophyton*, *Epidermophyton*, *Microsporum* and *Nannizzia* are clinically relevant with the remaining three genera containing geophilic species (Table 10.1) [5].

10.2.1.2 Classification According to Their Natural Habitat (Ecology)

Reflecting the source of infection dermatophytes may be classified according to their ecology in anthropophilic, zoophilic and geophilic species. Anthropophilic species naturally colonize humans, are being transmitted between humans and usually cause chronic, mild, noninflammatory infections often reaching epidemic proportions. The zoophilic species primarily infect or colonize lower animals and can be transmitted to humans leading to severe inflammation in the host. Geophilic

Table 10.1 Clinical relevant genera of dermatophytes [5]

Trichophyton	*Epidermophyton*	*Microsporum*	*Nannizzia*
T. tonsurans	*E. floccosum*	*M. audouinii*	*N. aenygmaticum*
T. equinum		*M. canis*	*N. duboisii*
T. interdigitale		*M. ferrugineum*	*N. corniculata*
T. mentagrophytes			*N. fulva*
T. simii			*N. gypsea*
T. schoenleinii			*N. incurvata*
T. quinckeanum			*N. nana*
T. erinacei			*N. persicolor*
T. eriotrephon			*N. praecox*
T. benhamiae			
T. concentricum			
T. verrucosum			
T. bullosum			
T. rubrum			
T. soudanense			
T. violaceum			

Table 10.2 Classification of clinically relevant dermatophytes according to their natural habitat (ecology)

Anthropophilic	Zoophilic	Geophilic
Trichophyton rubrum	*Trichophyton mentagrophytes*	*Nannizzia fulva*
Trichophyton interdigitale	*Trichophyton equinum*	*Nannizzia gypsea*
Trichophyton schoenleinii	*Trichophyton erinacei*	*Nannizzia persicolor*
Trichophyton soudanense	*Trichophyton simii*	*Nannizzia praecox*
Trichophyton violaceum	*Trichophyton verrucosum*	
Trichophyton tonsurans	*Trichophyton benhamiae*	
Epidermophyton floccosum	*Trichophyton quinckeanum*	
Microsporum audouinii	*Microsporum canis*	
Microsporum ferrugineum		

species saprophyte in the soil and may have infectious potency in lower animals or humans causing acute, inflammatory mycoses that may quickly resolve (Table 10.2).

10.2.1.3 Sexual States (Anamorph, Teleomorph)

In most dermatophytes no sexual state (=anamorph) is known; therefore the term 'fungi imperfecti' was created in the past. Dermatophytes with known sexual phase (=teleomorph) were formerly categorized into two genera, *Nannizzia* and *Arthroderma*. In truly anthropophilic species, no sexual phases are known, while geophilic species show vigorous mating. Sexual states are generally not isolated from skin, hair or nail cultures, probably because only one mating type initiated the infection.

With regard to the change in the 'Botanical Code of Nomenclature', the dermatophytes are now classified by their phylogenetic relationship, which means in genomic sequencing, species names are not more referred to sexual states [5].

10.2.1.4 Clinically Relevant Species of Dermatophytes (Anthropophilic Source)

Trichophyton rubrum

Initially endemic in Southeast Asia and Africa, by soldiers and slaves brought to America:

- Worldwide distribution
- Main agent of tinea pedis and tinea unguium worldwide
- Causes tinea pedis, tinea cruris, tinea corporis, tinea manuum (infrequent tinea barbae, tinea capitis)
- Follicular granulomatous lesions: Majocchi's granuloma
- Chronic infections

Trichophyton interdigitale (formerly *Trichophyton mentagrophytes* var. *interdigitale*)

- Anthropophilic
- Worldwide distribution
- Tinea pedis (interdigital spaces of the feet)

Trichophyton tonsurans

Initially endemic in Central America and the Caribbean—by Spanish colonists brought to North America:

- North America, Europe (in particular in Great Britain), Africa, rarely in Asia
- Most common agent of tinea capitis in North America and Great Britain
- Causes tinea capitis, tinea corporis, tinea pedis and tinea unguium
- 'Black dot' tinea capitis or kerion formation

Trichophyton soudanense

- Endogenous distribution in West Africa and countries with West African immigration: Europe, Great Britain, the United States, Brazil
- Causes tinea capitis, tinea corporis, tinea unguium [6]

Trichophyton violaceum

- Endogenous distribution in Asia, Africa (East and North Africa), Russia, Europe and South and Central America
- Causes tinea capitis with kerion and favus formation
- Causes tinea corporis, tinea pedis and tinea unguium

Trichophyton schoenleinii

- Eurasia, North Africa, Western Hemisphere
- Causes tinea capitis, tinea corporis, noninflammatory tinea unguium
- Causes favus in humans

Epidermophyton floccosum

- Worldwide distribution
- May reach epidemiological proportions
- No hair invasion
- Noninflammatory tinea
- Causes tinea pedis, tinea cruris, tinea corporis, tinea unguium

Microsporum audouinii

- Endogenous distribution in Africa, more frequently in West African countries
- Sporadic occurrence in Europe (France, Italy, Spain, Portugal, Denmark), Australia
- Causes tinea capitis, tinea corporis and occasionally other dermatophytoses

10.2.1.5 Clinically Relevant Species of Dermatophytes (Zoophilic Source)

Trichophyton mentagrophytes (zoophilic, formerly *Trichophyton mentagrophytes* var. *mentagrophytes*)

- Worldwide distribution
- Infection in humans and lower animals (e.g. rodents)
- Inflammatory tineas with dermatophytid reaction
- Causes tinea corporis, tinea pedis, tinea barbae, tinea capitis, tinea unguium

Trichophyton verrucosum

- Worldwide distribution
- Infections in cattle and individuals in contact with cattle
- Possible occupational infection in farmers
- Highly inflammatory infections with kerion formation
- Causes tinea corporis, tinea faciei, tinea barbae, tinea capitis

Trichophyton benhamiae (formerly *Trichophyton* anamorph of *Arthroderma benhamiae*)

- Transmission mainly by colonized or infected guinea pigs
- First isolated in hedgehogs in Japan
- Steep increase in European countries, source of infection often pets, e.g. guinea pigs
- Highly inflammatory infections with kerion formation and lymph node enlargement and dermatophytid reaction
- Causes tinea corporis, tinea faciei, tinea capitis, tinea genitalis

Trichophyton quinckeanum [7]

- Zoophilic
- Cause of the so-called mice favus
- Causes tinea capitis and tinea corporis, both in children and more frequently in adults
- Middle East, Arab world, Egypt, Iran, Central Asia, European countries (recently increasingly isolated in Germany)
- Source of infection are camels and mice but in Europe more frequently cats

Microsporum canis

- Worldwide distribution
- Highly contagious organism
- Transmission mainly by colonized or infected kittens
- Childhood population mainly affected
- Tinea with kerion formation possible
- Causes tinea corporis, tinea faciei, tinea genitalis, tinea capitis

10.2.2 Dermatophytoses (Tinea of the Glabrous Skin, Ringworm Infection)

10.2.2.1 General Considerations

Diseases caused by dermatophytes—dermatophytoses—are named by the body part designation (in Latin) with the preface *tinea* or ringworm. Beside the glabrous skin appendages like scalp hair follicles and the nail apparatus can be infected. The clinical presentations reflect the

Table 10.3 Dermatophytes (tinea) with regard to the site of infection

Organism	Site of infection
Tinea faciei	Face
Tinea corporis	Glabrous skin (face, trunk, extremities)
Tinea cruris (inguinalis)	Groin
Tinea manus (*pl.* manuum)	Hand
Tinea pedis (*pl.* pedum)	Feet (plantar surface, interdigital spaces)
Tinea barbae	Beard
Tinea capitis	Scalp hair
Tinea unguium	Nail

etiologic agent as source of infection and interaction of the host immune system and may vary from erythematous scaly eruptions to highly inflammatory infections (Table 10.3).

Dematophytes have the ability to produce keratinases and digest keratin in vitro [8].

By this ability the dermatophytes are permitted to sustain itself on the skin, hair or nails. The host immune system plays a significant role limiting the scope of dermatophyte invasion. The cell-mediated immune system in conjunction with the antimicrobial activity of polymorphonuclear leukocytes and serum factors restricts dermatophyte fungi to the stratum corneum [9–11].

When defects in the immune system such as neutropenia occur, locally invasive dermatophyte abscesses may result. In contrast, defects in cell-mediated immunity, such as occurring in HIV infection, predispose to widespread cutaneous infection. In addition to limit the scope and extent of infection, the host immune system mediates the cutaneous eruption and explains the broad variety of clinical features from a given organism.

Another important feature especially of anthropophilic dermatophytes is to sustain chronic infections. Chronic infections are characterized by long-standing, extensive disease with little to no inflammatory response that often involves the palms and soles. In these infections, dermatophyte fungi grow on new-formed keratin as older skin cells are shed. Chronicity means dermatophytic skin invasion proceeds faster than the epidermal turnover. The clinical presentation in long-standing dermatophyte infections yields usually non-inflammatory lesions with only slight scaling and erythema. Several features like sweat, occlusion by tight-fitting shoes, high temperatures and other occupational circumstances are thought to be in close association with chronic dermatophytosis. With regard to additional predisposing circumstances, vascular diseases, metabolic disorders like diabetes, malignancies and genetic disorders like ichthyosis seem to be of possible importance [12].

Infections by zoophilic organisms like *Microsporum canis* or *Trichophyton verrucosum* present as highly inflammatory lesions and are generally short in duration with the possibility of spontaneous resolvement [12].

10.2.2.2 Site of Infection

The clinical presentation of dermatophytosis is beside the etiologic organism mediated by the anatomic site infected. Infections on palms and soles are of chronic course in view of the thickened hyperkeratotic skin. Chronic tinea pedis, tinea cruris and tinea manuum are generally associated with pedal onychomycosis.

Tinea Faciei (Syn. Ringworm of the Face, Tinea Faciale)

Tinea faciei is characterized by erythematous, centrifugally growing, discretely scaly lesions with prominent borders, frequently on the cheeks but also on the eyelids and sometimes in the submandibular region. Mild pruritic (or even non-pruritic), scaly facial lesions with accentuated borders should therefore always prompt a mycologic workup to rule out tinea faciei [13]. Among others, differential diagnostic considerations include impetigo, atopic dermatitis, contact dermatitis, discoid lupus erythematodes and herpes zoster. In children, zoophilic dermatophytes—zoophilic strains of *T. mentagrophytes* as well as *M. canis* and *Trichophyton benhamiae*—are the primary pathogens in tinea faciei. Steroid-modified tinea faciei so-called tinea incognita is possible [14].

- In facial dermatosis with recalcitrant course, a mycology workup should be ruled out (Figs. 10.1 and 10.2).

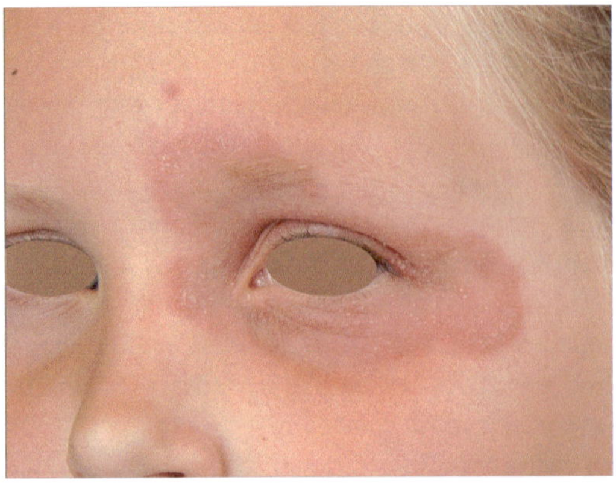

Fig. 10.1 Periorbital tinea due to *Trichophyton benhamiae*

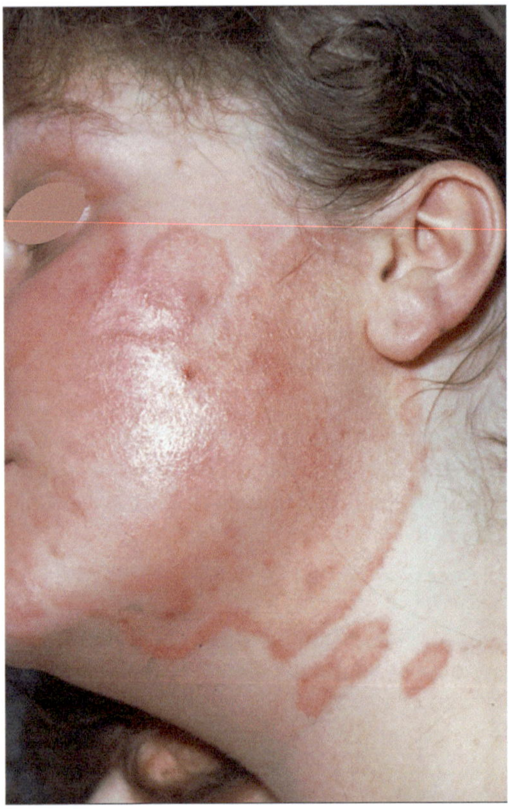

Fig. 10.2 Tinea faciei due to *Trichophyton mentagrophytes*

Tinea Corporis (Ringworm of the Body, Tinea Circinata)

Tinea corporis refers to dermatophytosis of the glabrous skin and may be found on the trunk and the extremities. All dermatophytes, anthropophilic and zoophilic species, are capable of causing tinea corporis with *Trichophyton rubrum* and *Trichophyton mentagrophytes* as main agents. In the USA, Latin America (Mexico) but also Great Britain, the anthropophilic species *T. tonsurans* is the second most common pathogen of tinea corporis after *T. rubrum*. In Africa, *T. violaceum* and *M. audouinii* play a crucial role [15].

In childhood population zoophilic dermatophytes like *Microsporum canis* and *Trichophyton benhamiae* are the most frequently isolated causative fungi. Source of infection are small, domesticated, furry animals that either suffer from dermatophytosis or simply represent asymptomatic carriers of zoophilic dermatophytes [13].

Tinea corporis may present as scaling erythematous lesions with annular figures and accentuated borders. In infections of zoophilic source, highly inflammatory eruptions like vesicular and bullous lesions may develop. The lesions may confluence and tend to centrifugal enlargement. With regard to the etiologic agent and the host immune response, itching and burning may be of subjective complaints. Cutaneous presentations of tinea corporis may mimic other scaling conditions like psoriasis vulgaris, impetigo, atopic dermatitis, contact dermatitis, granuloma annulare, erythema multiforme, pityriasis rosea and T cell lymphoma [12].

Generalized tinea corporis involving at least four different body sites excluding the groins are the criteria for the so-called *T. rubrum* syndrome. This extensive dermatomycosis develops after autoinoculation from a prior existing tinea pedis and tinea unguium. An immunosuppressive treatment—e.g. by glucocorticoids, leflunomide and fumaric acid esters—but also pre-existing immunocompromised diseases like rheumatoid arthritis represent disposing factors for the *T. rubrum* syndrome (Figs. 10.3 and 10.4) [16].

Tinea Inguinalis (Syn. Ringworm of the Groin, Eczema Marginatum, Tinea Cruris)

The term 'tinea cruris' (syn. tinea inguinalis) refers to dermatophytosis of the proximal medial aspects of the thighs, perineum and buttocks. Scrotum and penis are generally spared. Tinea cruris is common in males with pre-existing tinea

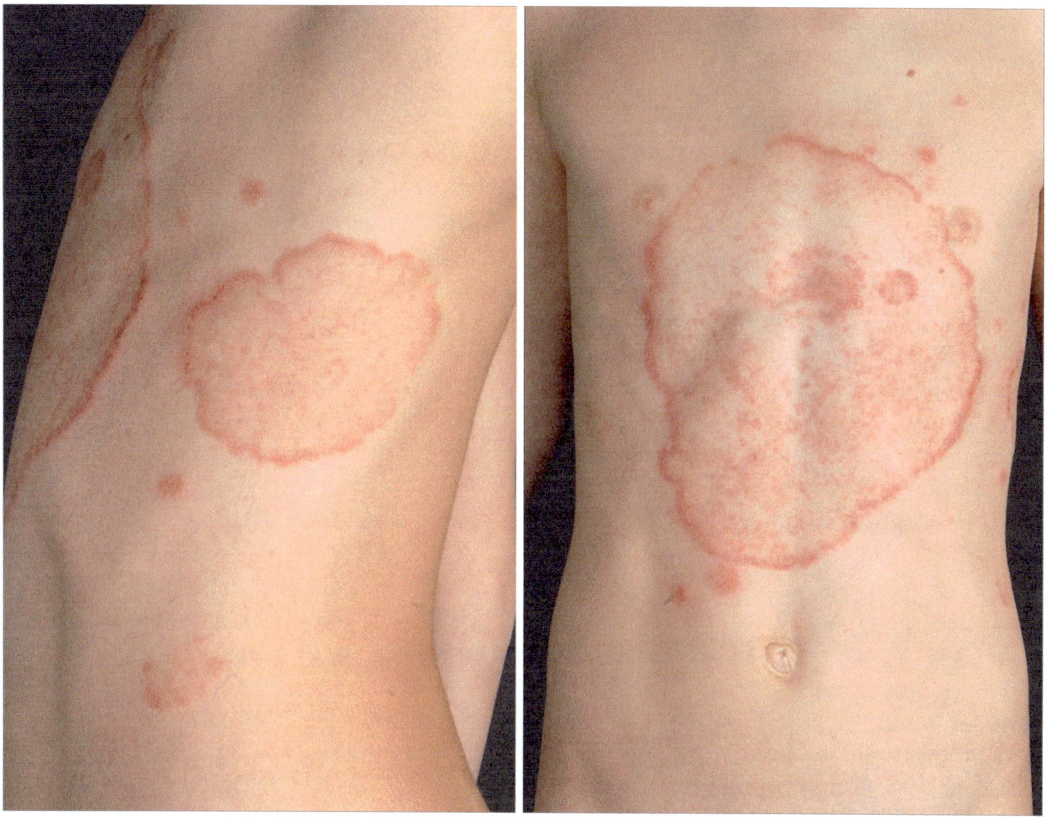

Fig. 10.3 Tinea corporis in a child simulating Lyme disease (migrating erythema)

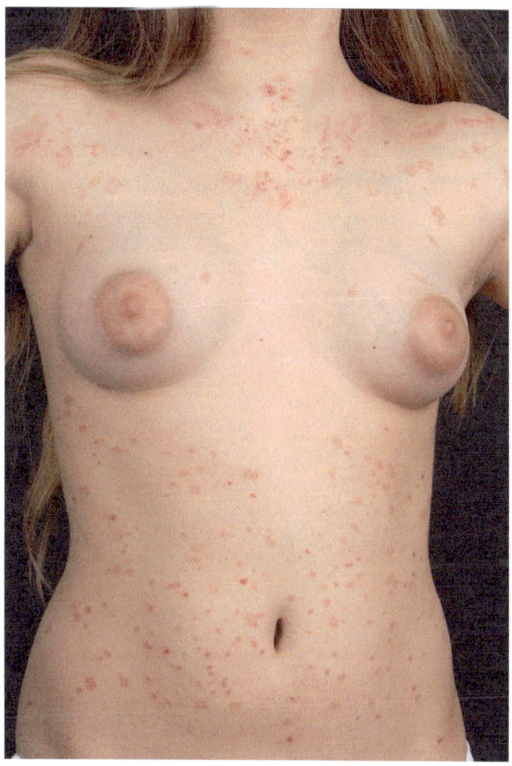

Fig. 10.4 Tinea corporis resembling exanthema due to *Microsporum canis*

pedis and pedal onychomycosis with autoinoculation as source of infection. Additional risk factors are heavy perspiration, tight-fitting clothing, contact sports and environmental factors like high temperatures and humidity [12, 13]. Although *T. rubrum* is a common pathogen, *T. interdigitale* and *E. floccosum* have also been isolated in the inguinal region.

Due to the accentuated borders of the macerated and scaly lesions in tinea inguinalis, the clinical picture corresponds to the so-called eczema marginatum (Hebra), first described in 1860 by Ferdinand Ritter von Hebra (1816–1880), founder of the Vienna School of Dermatology.

Differential diagnosis includes intertrigo, intertriginous candidiasis, erythrasma and inverse psoriasis.

- In infected persons both regions—genital area and feet—should be examined (Fig. 10.5).

Tinea Manus (pl. Manuum) (Syn. Ringworm of the Hand)

Tinea manus (pl. manuum) is referred to as dermatophyte infection of the hand. One or both hands can be infected, but unilateral involvement is most common. Tinea manus is mainly characterized by a dry, mild scaling, hyperkeratotic palm. In some cases the dorsum of the hand, the lateral aspects and the interdigital spaces may reveal scaling erythemas, sometimes with distinct scaling borders. Concurrent fingernail onychomycosis ensures the true diagnosis of fungal infection, whereas in most cases toenail onychomycosis may be the primary cause of this condition. The etiologic organisms of tinea manus are the same as in tinea pedis with *T. rubrum* as the most common agents, with *T. mentagrophytes* (*T. interdigitale*) and *Epidermophyton floccosum* being the others. Differential diagnosis includes eczema, psoriasis and cutaneous T cell lymphoma. Tinea manus yields generally an extremely chronic course and does not respond to topical antimycotic treatment.

Oral Treatment

Terbinafine 250 mg daily for 2–4 weeks
Itraconazole 200 mg daily for 4 weeks
Itraconazole 400 mg daily for 1 week (pulsing)—2 to 3 consecutive months

- In infected persons, feet and nails should be inspected.
- Oral antifungal agents are indicated for cure.
- Underlying fungal nail infection needs treatment (Figs. 10.6 and 10.7).

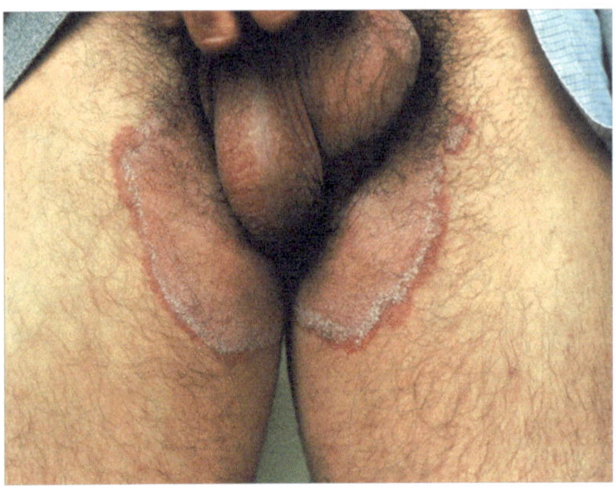

Fig. 10.5 Tinea inguinalis due to *Trichophyton rubrum*

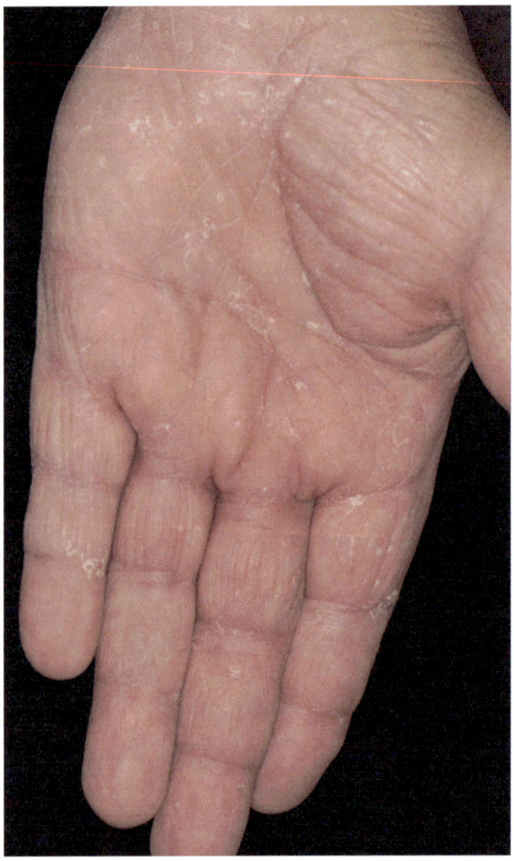

Fig. 10.6 Tinea manus with fine scaling in the creases on the palms

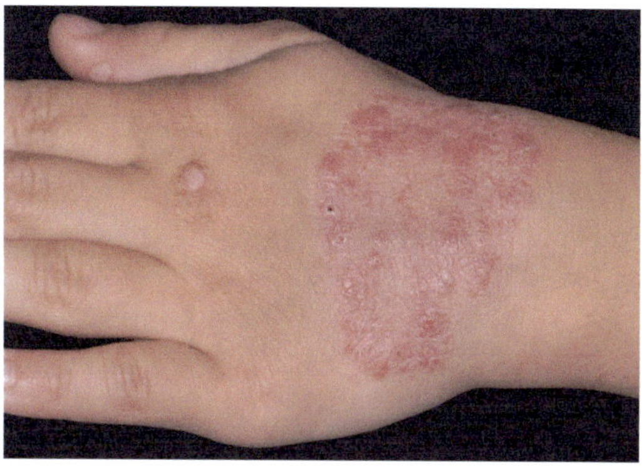

Fig. 10.7 Tinea manus on the dorsum of the hand in a child

Tinea Pedis (pl. Pedum) (Syn. Foot Ringworm, Athlete's Foot)

Tinea pedis is the most common fungal infection worldwide, affecting 30–70% of the population. It is a disease of civilized humans, with adults and predominately male patients most commonly affected [17].

Less frequently the childhood population can be affected, mainly starting at puberty. High humidity in warm climates, sporting, frictions by occlusive shoes, moisture and wet feet are predisposing factors. In addition, the practice of sharing baths, showers, swimming pools and even shoes facilitate the spread of infection.

There are three clinical presentations of tinea pedis. The most common form is the interdigital form with infection of the intertriginous webspace, mainly the fourth to the fifth interspace. The skin involved appears white and macerated; erosions may develop in the course of infection. The infection will extend to other toes and the soles. Hyperhidrosis, pruritus and odour may be accompanying features. Superinfection by bacteria may compete to the infection. The course of this infection usually is chronic and recalcitrant with a high recurrence rate.

In the second form, vesiculobullous lesions may develop from the webspace and extend to the soles and dorsum of the foot. Itch and secondary infection may result in cellulitis with lymphangitis.

The third form is referred to as 'moccasin type' of tinea pedis. In this type the infection involves the sole, heel and sides of the feet according to a moccasin with scaling erythema. The lesions may appear patchy and discrete and are often accompanied by onychomycoses. As symptoms may not be apparent, the chronic course of infection will not be recognized by the herewith affected person.

The 'two foot-one hand' syndrome describes a recalcitrant dermatophyte infection of the soles of both feet and the palm of one hand (mostly the left) with extensive chronic course and accompanying fungal nail infection.

10.2.2.3 Etiologic Agents

Etiologic agents of tinea pedis usually are of anthropophilic source. *Trichophyton rubrum* is the most common causative agent involved in tinea pedis, followed in order of decreasing frequency by *Trichophyton interdigitale* and *Epidermophyton floccosum*. Whereas *T. rubrum* produces noninflammatory tinea of the feet with extended chronic course, highly inflammatory features like vesicles and pustules and fissures may be caused by *T. interdigitale*/*T. mentagrophytes*. Infections can also be mixed and include *Candida* and bacteria, especially in the interdigital type [17].

Cultivation of dermatophytes from normal toe webs corresponds to colonization and may give rise to true infection in the case of stratum corneum barrier disruption.

10.2.2.4 Complications

Interdigital tinea pedis may be the site for secondary infection by gram-negative bacteria or staphylococci resulting in cellulitis. In inflammatory tinea pedis, ID reactions (autoeczematization) with vesiculation and eczematous eruptions on the fingers, palms and toes may develop.

Treatment

- Topical antifungal agents (azoles, allylamine, ciclopirox olamine).
- Oral antifungal agents in moccasin tinea pedis:
  - Terbinafine 250 mg daily for 2–4 weeks
  - Itraconazole 200 mg daily for 4 weeks

- Itraconazole 400 mg daily for 1 week (pulsing)—2 to 3 consecutive months
- Underlying pedal onychomycosis needs treatment.
- Disinfection of shoes (Figs. 10.8, 10.9 and 10.10).

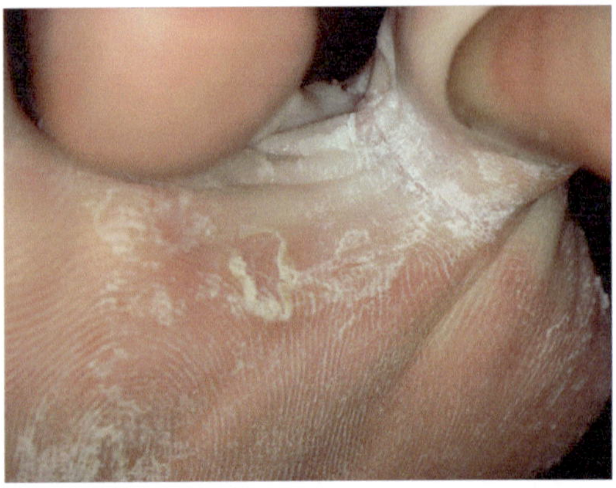

Fig. 10.8 Tinea pedis—interdigital form

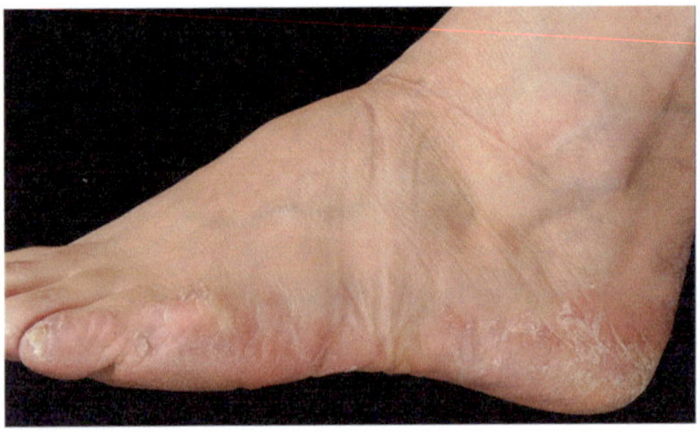

Fig. 10.9 Tinea pedis—moccasin type

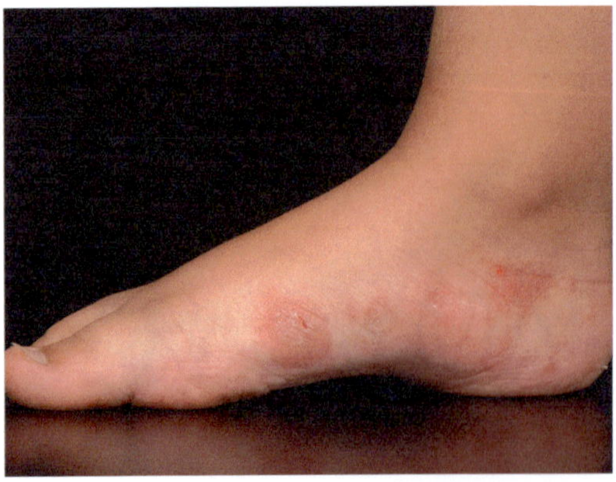

Fig. 10.10 Childhood tinea pedis

Two Feet-One Hand Syndrome

A fungal infection of the left hand and both feet, frequently involving fingernails and toenails, is referred to as 'two feet-one hand syndrome' (TFOHS). Usually *T. rubrum* is the causative pathogen, occasionally *T. mentagrophytes/T. interdigitale* [13, 18].

TFOHS more frequently affects men and is caused by dermatophyte transmission from pre-existing tinea pedis or fungal nail infection to the (left) hand, e.g. by scratching or by pedicure. The non-dominating hand (usually the left) is mostly affected, whereas the dominating or 'working' hand shows a better-developed protective stratum corneum. In general the course of this syndrome is recalcitrant with persistence of the infection over years and the need of long-duration systemic treatment regimen.

Trichophyton rubrum Syndrome

Trichophyton rubrum syndrome (syn. chronic dermatophytosis syndrome, generalized chronically persistent rubrophytia, tinea corporis generalisata, dry-type *T. rubrum* infection) represents a chronic and generalized dermatophytosis. According to the definition, at least four body sites are affected: feet (plantar), hands (palmar), nails as well as one other site. The inguinal region which is a common site of tinea is explicitly excluded. The second diagnostic criterion in *T. rubrum* syndrome includes microscopic fungal detection from all four sites. The third criterion should be the cultural detection of *T. rubrum* from at least three out of four sites.

It is still unclear whether *T. rubrum* syndrome represents a distinct nosologic entity. Treatment with corticosteroids seems to be a predisposing factor. The syndrome is of utmost course and may be refractory even to long-duration treatments [13].

10.2.3 Tinea of the Hair Follicle

10.2.3.1 Tinea Capitis (Syn. Ringworm of the Scalp, Tinea Tonsurans)

Fungal scalp infection (tinea capitis) is defined as infection of the hair follicle by dermatophytes and presents with a different amount of erythema, scaling and hair loss. Tinea capitis is the most common infection of the scalp in childhood [19].

Both genders may be affected: while in the past boys were thought to be more frequently affected, particularly with respect to *Microsporum canis* infections, this gender difference seems to have disappeared [20].

Currently, even in the USA, there is an even distribution between girls and boys [21].

Etiologic Agents in Europe

The causative organism in tinea capitis may be of zoophilic or anthrophilic source.

In European countries, mainly in Central and Southern Europe, *Microsporum canis* and *Trichophyton benhamiae* are the most common agents, followed by zoophilic strains of *T. mentagrophytes* and *T. verrucosum*. Due to the increase in immigration by people from Africa, the epidemiologic situation with causative agents of tinea capitis has changed dramatically in Europe with a steep swift from zoophilic to anthropophilic dermatophytes. In France (Paris) and Switzerland and in urban areas of Germany (f.e. Munich, Bonn, Würzburg), outbreaks with the anthropophilic fungus *M. audouinii* have been reported [22].

The same holds for the anthropophilic *T. violaceum* brought to Europe (Zürich, Göteburg) by immigrants from Eastern African countries (Eritrea, Ethiopia, Somalia, Kenya, Uganda), whereas *T. soudanense* mainly originates from the western parts of Africa (Nigeria, Mali, Senegal, Angola) [23].

In the USA and the UK, the majority of fungal scalp infections are caused by the anthropophilic *Trichophyton tonsurans*. The main problem with this epidemiological shift to anthropophilic causative agents is the possible transmission by inert items such as reaching epidemiological proportions.

Geophilic dermatophytes with *Nannizzia gypsea* being the clinically most relevant species rarely cause tinea capitis. Present in soil and dust, children may contract them, e.g. while playing outside, with subsequent infection of the skin and occasionally the scalp [13].

Pattern of Hair Involvement

Hair root involvement by dermatophytes may be endothrix, ectothrix or favic. In endothrix infections, seen in *T. tonsurans*, *T. violaceum*, *T. soudanense* and *T. verrucosum*, tinea capitis, arthrospores and mycelia are found inside the hair shaft, without any destruction of the cuticle. In ectothrix infections by *M. canis*, *M. audouinii* and *T. mentagrophytes* (zoophilic type), spores and hyphae aggregate in a cuff-like fashion outside the hair shaft. In favic pattern (mainly caused by *T. schoenleinii*), the infection presents with airspaces within the hair.

Classification According to Clinical Presentation

Tinea capitis can be differentiated according to the *genus* level into *Trichophyton* and *Microsporum* tinea capitis or with relation to the infectious mode of the hair shaft (endothrix vs. ectothrix mode vs. favic pattern). The most common classification describes the clinical picture of tinea capitis with special regard to the different amounts of inflammation varying from a noninflammatory to highly inflammatory state. In general zoophilic strains may cause highly inflammatory infections with purulent discharge and pains with exception to be drawn in attention.

Grey Patch Tinea Capitis

This type is characterized by disc-like alopecic lesions covered by whitish-grey scales. Hairs break off directly above the skin surface resulting in a typical picture of 'stubble field' appearance. In some cases, an inflammatory component with erythema may be completely missing responding to noninflammatory-type tinea capitis. Without treatment the lesions show centrifugally growing and recalcitrant chronic course over months. Grey patch tinea capitis is mainly seen in *M. canis*, *M. ferrugineum*, *Nannizzia incurvata* and *T. benhamiae* infections. Favus (caused by *T. schoenleinii*) with so-called scutulum formation may also simulate this type (Figs. 10.11 and 10.12).

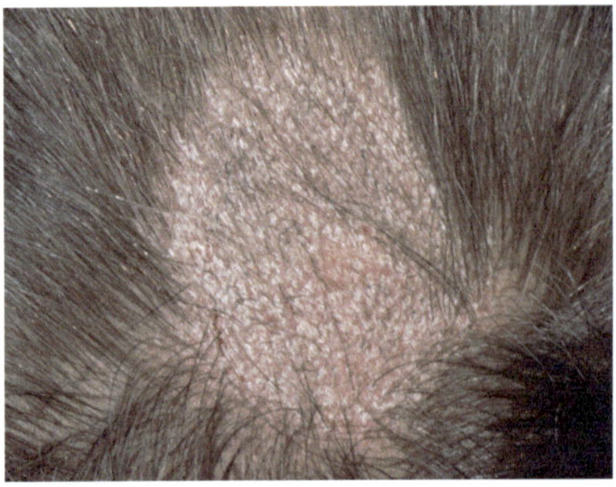

Fig. 10.11 Noninflammatory-type tinea capitis due to *Microsporum canis* ('grey patch' tinea capitis)

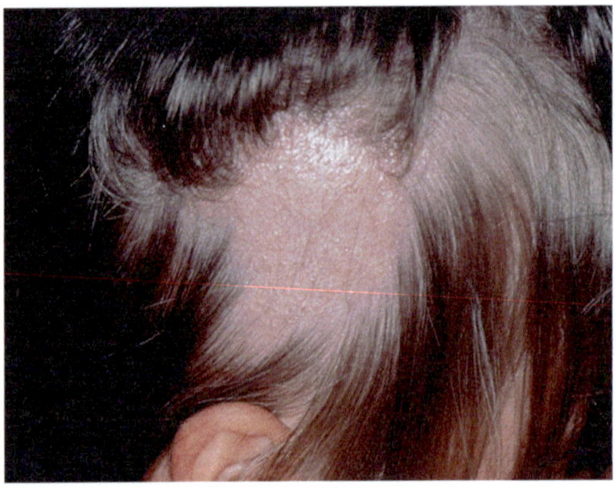

Fig. 10.12 Noninflammatory-type tinea capitis due to *Microsporum canis* resembling alopecia

Moth-Eaten Tinea Capitis

This type presents with distinct scaling small-sized alopecic lesion described as moth-eaten appearance. The clinical picture is the same as in alopecia syphilitica.

Black Dot Tinea Capitis

This clinical manifestation impresses as black (or white or yellow) dots at the scalp following hair shaft breakage representing a noninflammatory type of tinea capitis. This type of infection is mainly caused by dermatophytes of anthropophilic source like *T. tonsurans* (most commonly seen in the Afro-Caribbean population in the USA), *T. mentagrophytes*, *T. soudanense*, *T. violaceum* and *M. audouinii* and is most commonly seen in curling hair type (Fig. 10.13).

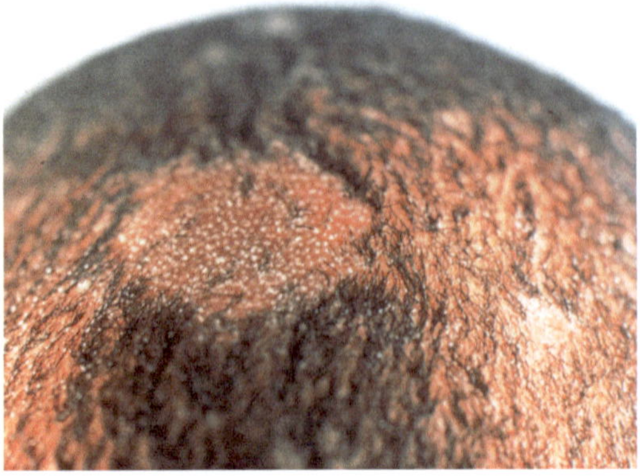

Fig. 10.13 Noninflammatory type tinea capitis due to *Trichophyton tonsurans* ('black dot' tinea capitis)

Pityriasis Capillitii-Type Tinea Capitis

This kind of tinea capitis presents with diffuse scaling of the scalp without signs of inflammation and is mainly caused by *T. tonsurans*, *T. violaceum*, *T. soudanense* and *M. audouinii* (Fig. 10.14).

Pustular Tinea Capitis

Fungal infections of the hair root may present as scattered pustules covering the scalp; in addition hair loss may be visible. *T. violaceum*, *T. soudanense* and *T. mentagrophytes* have to be considered as causative agents (Fig. 10.15).

Kerion (Tinea Capitis Profunda)

The most severe form of tinea capitis is characterized by an abscess-like deep infection of the scalp and accompanying nuchal or cervical lymphadenopathy. The hairs in the surrounding of the charging mass may be epilated without difficulty. This highly inflammatory condition may cause pain and febrile temperature. According to the course of infection, it will result in permanent scaling due to hair loss. This type of infection is mainly caused by zoophilic dermatophytes like *T. mentagrophytes*, *T. verrucosum* but also *T. benhamiae* (Fig. 10.16).

Favus

Tinea capitis of favus type has disappeared in Europe but may still be found in Turkey, Iran and Northern African countries. Causative agent is *T. schoenleinii*.

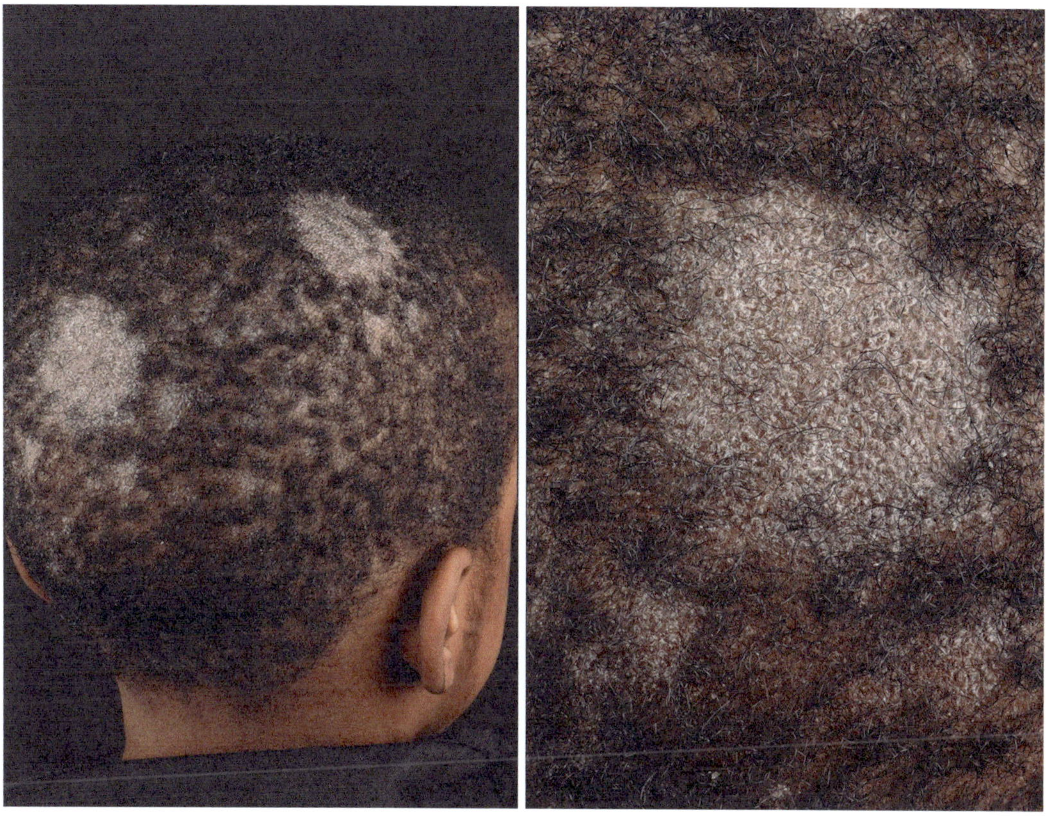

Fig. 10.14 Pityriasis capillitii-type tinea capitis due to *Trichophyton soudanense*

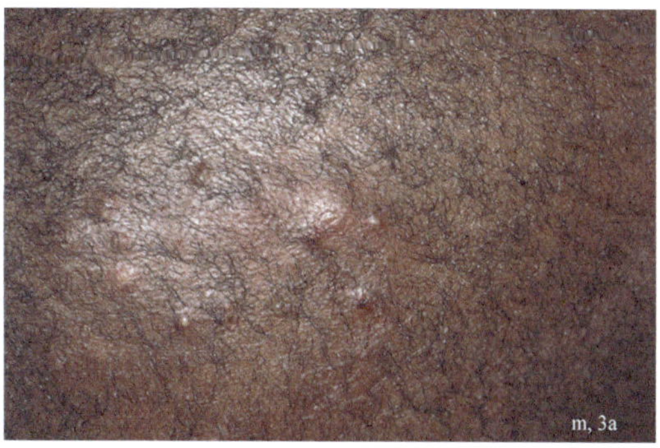

Fig. 10.15 Pustular tinea capitis due to *Trichophyton soudanense*

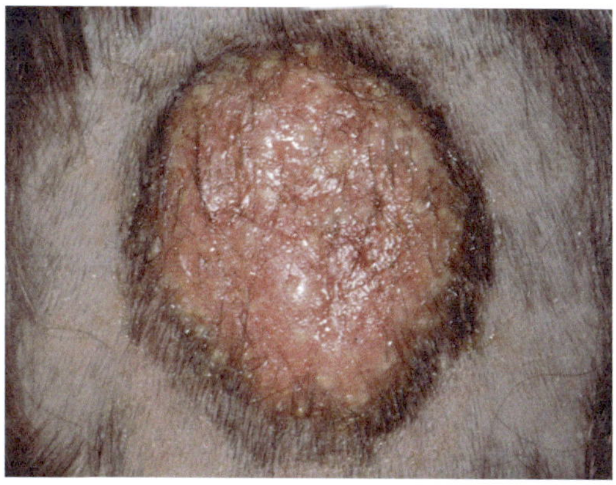

Fig. 10.16 Tinea capitis profunda (kerion-type) due to *Nannizzia gypsea*

Tinea Capitis in Adults

Even though childhood population is usually affected by tinea capitis, mycotic scalp infection may be seen in adults and elderly. The infection manifests as a different amount of erythema, scaling and hair loss and may simulate disorders like discoid lupus erythematosus, psoriasis or other forms of hair loss. The true nature of the condition may be proofed by histology. The infection may be caused by *M. canis*, *T. schoenleinii* or *M. audouinii* and even by *T. rubrum* as result of autoinoculation (Fig. 10.17) [13].

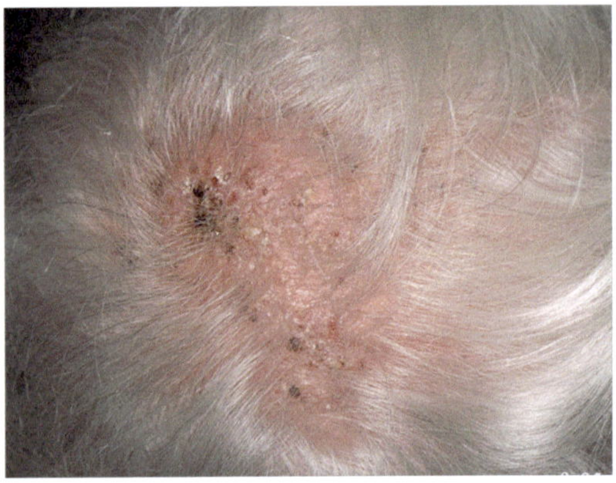

Fig. 10.17 Tinea capitis microsporica in an elderly

Differential Diagnoses of Tinea Capitis

There is a broad range of disorders of the scalp to be drawn in attention:

- Scaling disorders like psoriasis capitis, pityriasis capillitii, pityriasis amiantacea (formerly tinea amiantacea) and seborrheic dermatitis of the scalp
- Bacterial infections like bacterial abscesses, impetigo, pyodermas (furuncle, carbuncle)
- Different forms of hair loss like alopecia areata, scarring alopecia
- Autoimmune disorders like discoid lupus erythematosus, lichen planopilaris
- Other disorders like erosive pustular dermatitis of the scalp, sterile eosinophilic pustulosis (Ofuji), folliculitis decalvans, dissecting cellulitis, folliculitis et perifolliculitis capitis abscedens et suffodiens (Hoffmann), acne keloidalis nuchae
- Syphilis II (alopecia syphilitica)

The correct diagnosis is a challenge with regard to microbiological investigations and histology.

Carrier State (=Asymptomatic Tinea Capitis)

The cultural isolation of dermatophytes from a scalp without any signs of infection is termed carrier state. The situation with scalp contamination by dermatophytes, mainly *T. tonsurans* and *M. audouinii*, has been observed in children and adults. The causative role of pathogen carriers is of suggestive nature—given the fact that contamination by dermatophytes is an invisible source of transmission or gives rise for true infection [24, 25].

Treatment

General Considerations

Tinea capitis needs to be treated with an oral agent because the antifungal needs to penetrate into the hair follicle. Topical antifungal agents used as sole therapy are therefore ineffective [26].

Treatment needs to be continued until mycological cure is proved as microscopically documented by a fungus-free hair root and the inability of the causative organism to grow on culture. Treatment duration in general depends on the causative agent and the thereby administered oral antifungal and the clinical response of the patient. Fully hair regrowth is a matter of time and needs patience. Scarring alopecia may be a task for aesthetic/plastic surgery [27].

Systemic Treatment

Oral antifungal agents are the primary interventions for treating tinea capitis (e.g. griseofulvin, terbinafine, ketoconazole [not yet available in Europe, black box warning of the FDA due to hepatotoxicity and QT prolongation and drug interactions], fluconazole and itraconazole). Griseofulvin and terbinafine should be considered as first-line choice. Terbinafine is most effective for *Trichophyton* infections, whereas griseofulvin is the drug of choice in *Microsporum canis* infections. Itraconazole and fluconazole are alternative treatments [28]. Oral ketoconazole has been withdrawn from use in the UK and Europe since 2013 [29].

The problem with systemic treatment in childhood population is that not all medication for tinea capitis are available in paediatric formulation (f.e. suspension) and most agents are not licensed in this age group (Table 10.4).

The use of systemic antibiotics or corticosteroids has to be considered in special cases but seems to be of no advantage.

Topical Treatment

In addition to systemic treatment, topically antifungal agents like antifungal shampoos containing azoles (ketoconazole 2% shampoo) or 2.5% selenium disulphide at least twice weekly and

Table 10.4 Systemic treatment of tinea capitis in childhood

Griseofulvin Tablets, suspension	15–20–25 mg/kg BW daily (fatty meals) 6–8–12 weeks
Terbinafine (not licensed/ off-label use) Tablets (USA: oral granules for suspension)	62.5 mg daily (<20 kg BW) 125 mg daily (>20–40 kg BW) 250 mg daily (>40 kg BW) *Trichophyton* TC: 2–4 weeks (kerion 8–12 weeks) *Microsporum* TC: 6–12 weeks
Itraconazole (not licensed in tinea capitis/off-label use) Capsules (50 mg, 100 mg) Suspension (10 mg/ml)	Capsules: 5 mg/kg BW daily (with food—postprandial) Suspension: 3 mg/kg BW (fasting state) 50 mg daily (<20 kg BW) 100 mg daily (>20 kg BW) 2–4–6 weeks
Fluconazole (not licensed in tinea capitis/off-label use) Capsules (50 mg, 100 mg) Suspension (50 mg/10 ml)	5–6 mg/kg BW daily 8 mg/kg BW once weekly 3–6–12 weeks

daily application of antifungal therapy should be recommended until cure is achieved.

Surveillance Control

To prevent the spread of infection, screening of the infected person's family members and primary contacts should be obligatory. With regard to 'carrier state', all family members and other persons exposed to the affected individual should be treated with an antifungal shampoo. Clothing and hair care items used by the affected should not be shared by other persons. Haircutting procedures are strongly prohibited in infected persons.

There is evidence that infectious organisms like *M. canis* and *T. tonsurans* may be spread by contaminated fomites like toys, furniture and telephones with need for disinfection. A proven or reliable method to sterilize fomites has not been established.

In infections of zoophilic source, identification and treatment of the infected animal are of special concern.

After initiation of oral treatment regimens, children should be allowed to return to the kindergarden or school, only if *M. audouinii* infections quarantine is strictly followed [29].

10.2.3.2 Tinea Barbae (Syn. Ringworm of the Beard)

Ringworm of the beard and moustache areas of the face is a disease of the adult male and is mainly caused by zoophilic dermatophytes, *Trichophyton verrucosum* and *Trichophyton mentagrophytes* [30]. Patients affected are commonly farm workers with the infection retrieved by cattle ringworm. Ringworm of the beard may manifest as scaly, reddish, circular lesions up to highly inflammatory pustular folliculitis presenting features of a kerion with exudation and crusting. Hairs within the affected lesions are loose and easily considerably enlarged and painful. The lesions may persist over some months and settle spontaneously. Treatment of tinea barbae involves the use of oral terbinafine supplied by topical antimycotic preparations. Control of surveillance by the veterinarian is mandatory. Vaccines against *T. verrucosum* in cattle are available in many countries (Fig. 10.18).

10.2.3.3 Tinea of the Genitoinguinal Region (Tinea Genitalis)

Pubogenital tinea or tinea genitalis represents a rare type of dermatophytosis which, however, is increasingly observed [31]. The mons pubis is affected but also the outer regions to the penis shaft and the labia together with the groins. The infection may manifest from superficial erythrosquamous type to deep trichophytosis of kerion type with accompanying painful enlargement of the regional lymph nodes. Causative agents were mainly zoophilic dermatophytes (*M. canis, T. mentagrophytes, T. benhamiae, T. verrucosum*) with anthropophilic dermatophytes like *T. rubrum* being exceptionally observed by autoinoculation from undetected tinea unguium. Beside infected pets as the main source of infection, shaving procedures of the genital area seem to be

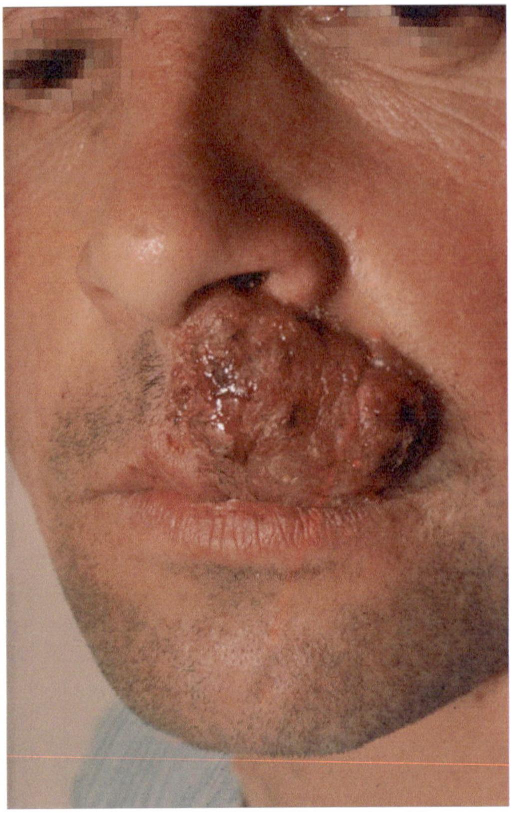

Fig. 10.18 Tinea barbae due to *Trichophyton verrucosum* in a farm worker

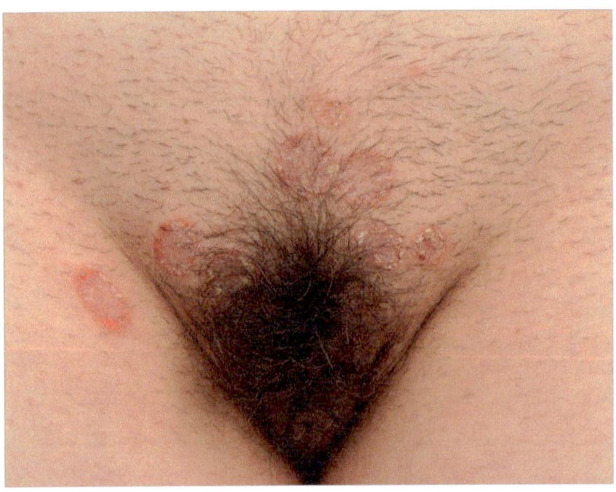

Fig. 10.19 Tinea genitalis with scaling and sharp marginated erythematous lesions due to *Microsporum canis*

the disposing factors explaining traumatic inoculation of infective agents. The infection needs systemic treatment with regard to the infectious organism (Figs. 10.19 and 10.20).

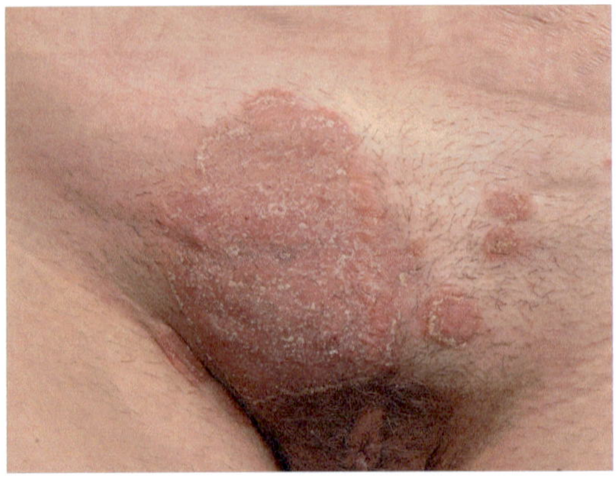

Fig. 10.20 Tinea genitalis due to *Trichophyton mentagrophytes*

10.2.4 Tinea Unguium (Onychomycosis)

Tinea unguium refers to dermatophyte infection of either fingernails or toenails. *Onychomycosis* is a broader term that includes nail infection by nondermatophytic moulds (NDM) and yeasts.

10.2.4.1 General Considerations

Fungal nail infections account for about one-third of all dermatophytoses and 50% of all nail disorders [32]. Fungal nail infection is of worldwide distribution with an estimated prevalence of 2–8%. According to the Foot Check Study, 23% of the European population suffers from pedal fungal infection with 12.4% prevalence in Germany [33].

The incidence of onychomycosis is inevitably going to rise, as industrialized societies are getting older.

In general toenails are more frequently infected than fingernails. In addition fungal nail infection is more prevalent in men and in individuals with other nail problems.

Tinea unguium is associated with tinea pedis in up to one-third of cases [34].

Many risk factors have been identified [35–37]:

Increasing age (approximately 20% of the population aged over 60 years and up to 50% of subjects aged over 70 years are reported to have onychomycosis)

Peripheral vascular disease
Periphery neuropathy
Occlusive footwear
Repeated nail trauma
Distorted nail surfaces
Slow nail growth
Foot deformities
Diabetes
Psoriasis vulgaris and psoriasis unguium
Immunosuppressive conditions (f.e. HIV infection)
Genetic predisposition (autosomal dominant pattern of inheritance in onychomycosis caused by *T. rubrum*)

10.2.4.2 Spread of Infection

Fungal nail infection is caused by interhuman transmission due to contact with exfoliated infected material, i.e. scalings or contaminated footwear or bathing units. All of the different morphological forms of dermatophytes have the potential to cause human infection, with the nonvegetative arthrospores (produced by fragmentation of hyphae) to be most suitable for the growth of dermatophytes in the nail-plate [38, 39].

10.2.4.3 Etiologic Agents in Onychomycosis

About 90% of fungal nail disease is caused by dermatophytes with the main organism *Trichophyton rubrum* and *Trichophyton interdigitale* (formerly *Trichophyton mentagrophytes*). Five to 10 percent of all onychomycosis are estimated to be caused by *Candida* species and about 2–11% by nondermatophyte moulds (NDM).

10.2.4.4 Classification According to Clinical Presentation [13]

Distal and Lateral Subungual Onychomycosis (DLSOM)

Fungal nail infections predominantly start at the distal free edge of the toenails as distal subungual onychomycosis. In the course of time, the pathogen slowly migrates from the hyponychium at the bottom side of the nail-plate proximally towards the matrix, resulting finally in DLOM. The nail appears thickened and hyperkeratotic with yellowish-brown discoloration. As time progresses, onycholysis sets in. Yellow streak represent dermatophytoma and point towards fungal matrix involvement. The most common causative agent is *T. rubrum* (Figs. 10.21 and 10.22).

Proximal Subungual Onychomycosis (PSOM)

Proximal subungual onychomycosis is quite rare. In this case the pathogen progresses from the proximal nail wall due to underlying tinea pedis onto the cuticle and later on onto the eponychium (the epithelium at the bottom side of the proximal nail wall). PSOM is a sign of immunodeficiency and may be seen in HIV-positive and AIDS patients. The association between PSOM and HIV is particularly striking in countries with high HIV prevalence, e.g. Sub-Saharan Africa. *T. rubrum* is usually the infectious organism of this kind of infection (Fig. 10.23).

White Superficial Onychomycosis (WSOM)

White superficial onychomycoses (leukonychia trichophytica) refer to a superficial dermatophyte infection of the nail-plate, mostly caused by *T. rubrum* but also *T. interdigitale*. In this infection a flat, bright white, plaque-like layer covers the nail-plate, sometimes affecting the entire nail surface.

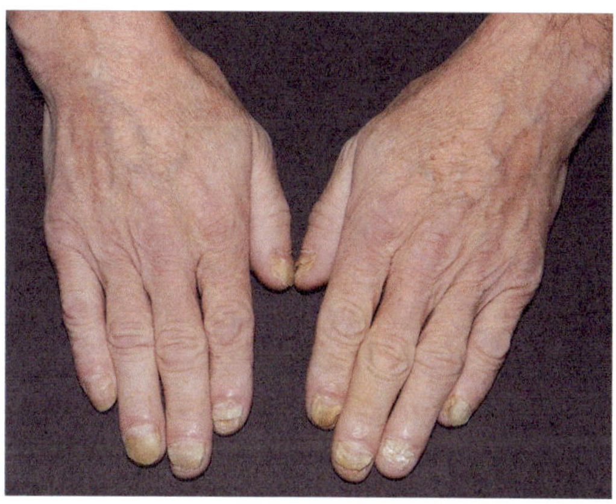

Fig. 10.21 Distal subungual onychomycosis presenting onycholysis due to *Trichophyton rubrum*

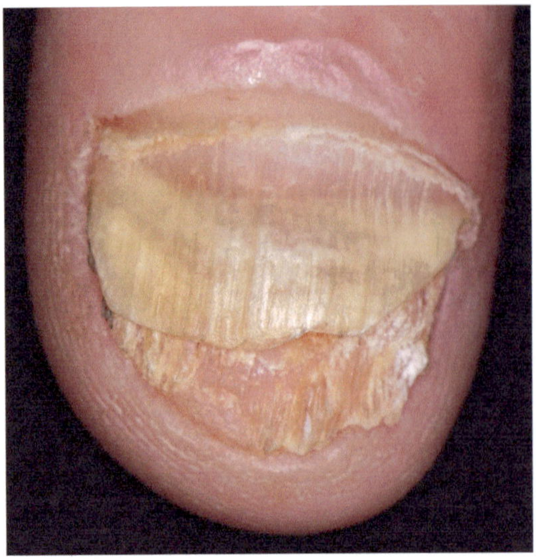

Fig. 10.22 Distal subungual onychomycosis presenting onycholysis due to *Trichophyton rubrum*

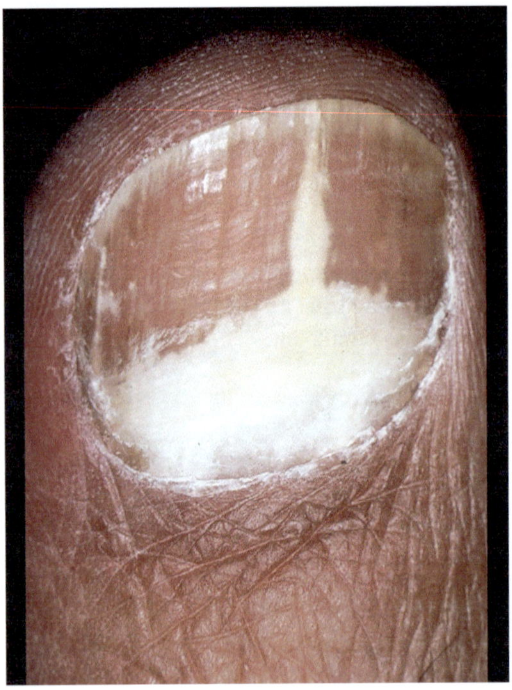

Fig. 10.23 Proximal subungual onychomycosis due to *Trichophyton rubrum*

Proximal white subungual onychomycosis (PWSOM) represents a special variant with white discoloration underneath the proximal part of the nail-plate and may be caused by *T. rubrum*, *T. schoenleinii* and *Epidermophyton floccosum*. Another special variant is black superficial onychomycosis caused by mould *Hendersonula toruloidea* (now renamed according current taxonomy as *Nattrassia mangiferae*).

Endonychial Onychomycosis (EOM)

Endonychial onychomycosis is a variant of nail infection with no subungual hyperkeratosis and no onycholysis. The nails are hyperkeratotically thickened and show white discoloration. This form of onychomycosis is caused by *T. soudanense* and is likely to be encountered in Africa.

Total Dystrophic Onychomycosis (TDOM)

Total dystrophic onychomycosis represents the most severe variant of onychomycosis and may be the final result of long-standing fungal nail infections. H. Grimmer coined the term 'glacier nail' in the 1960s. In this form the entire nail is mycotic and subsequently pushed upward by subungual hyperkeratoses, resulting in onycholysis. Yellow streaks, which mean longitudinal streaks medially or laterally frequently reaching the nail matrix, are characteristics for this type of onychomycosis [40].

In chronic mucocutaneous candidiasis, fingernails may become yeast-infected and appear as TDOM (Figs. 10.24 and 10.25) (Table 10.5) [41].

10.2.4.5 Onychomycosis by Nondermatophyte Moulds (NDM)

Nondermatophyte moulds account for about 5–11% of cases of onychomycoses [34].

Unlike dermatophytosis, these mould infections are not contagious and will not respond to the standard treatments for dermatophyte or *Candida* onychomycosis.

Causative Organisms

Various filamentous fungi other than dermatophytes have been isolated from abnormal nails [35, 42, 43].

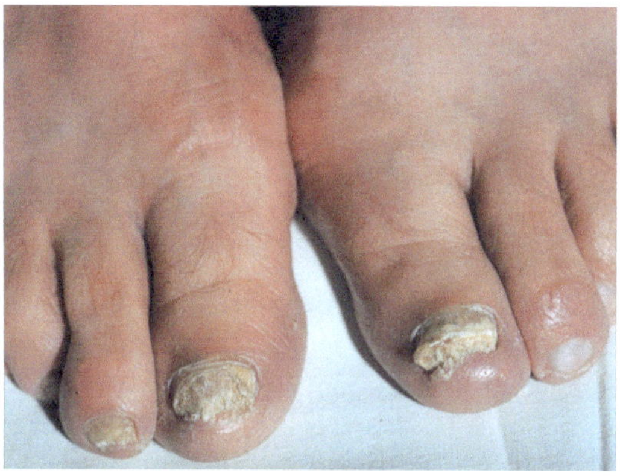

Fig. 10.24 Total dystrophic onychomycosis as result of long-standing nail infection

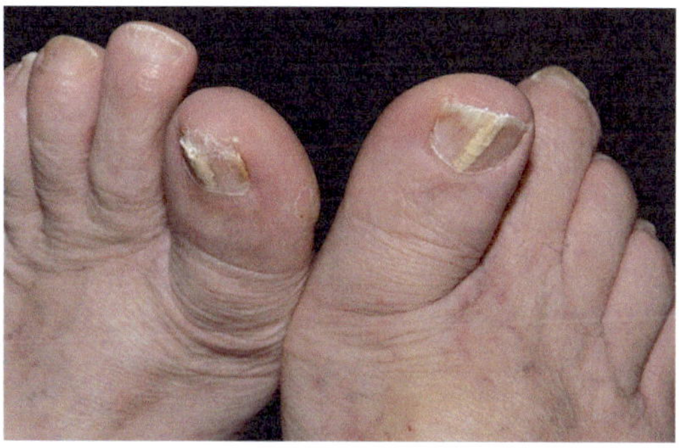

Fig. 10.25 Onychomycosis presenting yellow streaks

Table 10.5 Classification according to clinical presentation

Distal and lateral subungual OM	DLSO
Superficial white OM	SWO
Proximal subungual OM	PSO
Endonyx OM	EO
Total dystrophic OM	TDO
Mixed pattern OM	

Often these are casual, transient contaminants, and direct microscopic examination of nail clippings and scrapings is negative. However, environmental moulds that are found in soil or plant material are capable of causing nail infection. These moulds, with exception of *Neoscytalidium* species, are not keratinolytic, and they are generally considered to be secondary invaders rather than primary pathogens of the nail-plate [34].

The most common causative organism of NDM nail infection is *Scopulariopsis brevicaulis*, a ubiquitous soil fungus. Other causes of nail infections are *Neoscytalidium dimidiatum* (formerly called *Scytalidium dimidiatum* or *Hendersonula toruloidea*—causes black nail and skin infections in patients from tropics), *Sarocladium* (formerly *Acremonium*) species, *Aspergillus* species, *Fusarium* species and *Onychocola Canadensis* [44].

Mould infections of nails are most prevalent in older individuals, with men more commonly affected than women and toenails more frequently involved than fingernails. Similarly to dermatophyte onychomycosis, risk factors include increasing age, local trauma and immunosuppressive conditions such as diabetes mellitus or HIV infection [34].

NDM usually occur as secondary invaders in nails that have been previously been diseased or traumatized. This may account for the fact that these infections often affect only one nail [42].

Mould infections of nails have few specific clinical features and may present with onycholysis and hyperkeratosis like dermatophytic nail infection or with painful paronychia.

Suspicion of NDM onychomycosis [42]:

- Only one nail affected.
- Brown or black stained nails and subungual material.
- Previous antifungal treatment has failed on several occasions.
- Direct microscopic examination has been positive, but no dermatophyte has been isolated.
- No sign of associated skin infection (with exception of *Neoscytalidium dimidiatum*) (Figs. 10.26 and 10.27).

10.2.4.6 *Candida* Nail Infection

Candida infection accounts for 5–10% of all cases of onychomycosis [35].

Among the various species implicated, *C. albicans* and *C. parapsilosis* and *C. guilliermondii* are the most common causative agents.

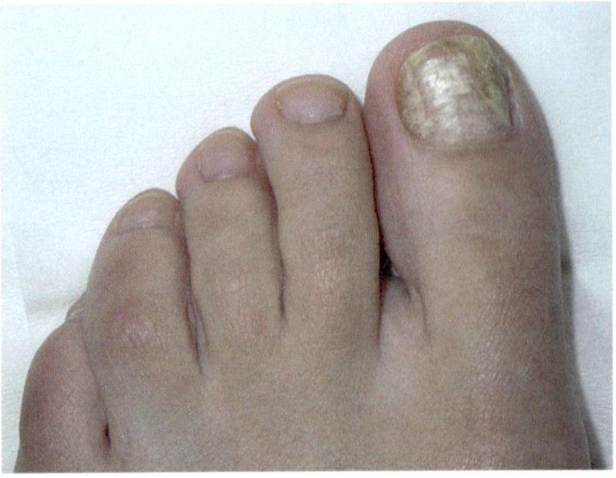

Fig. 10.26 Onychomycosis of the great toenail due to *Scopulariopsis brevicaulis*

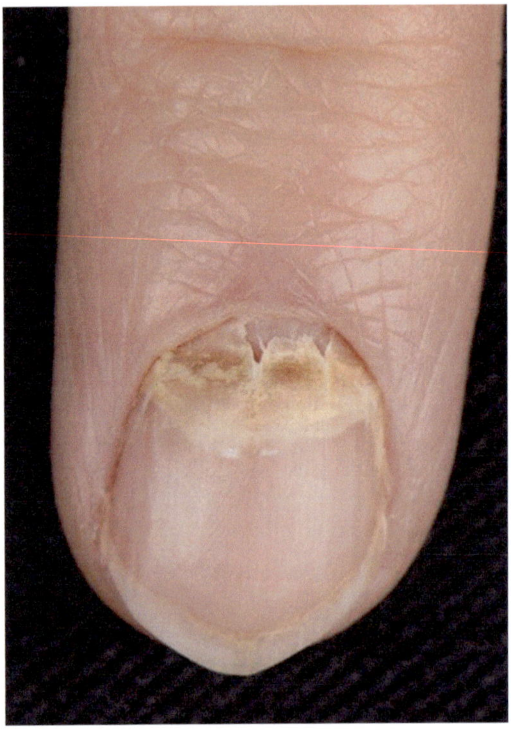

Fig. 10.27 Onychomycosis due to *Fusarium solani* presenting with proximal onycholysis

There are three forms of infection recognized: infection of the nail folds (or *Candida* paronychia), distal nail infection and total dystrophic onychomycosis.

Nail and nail fold infections with *Candida* (*Candida* paronychia) are more common in women than in men, with fingernails more commonly infected than toenails. These infections often occur in individuals whose occupations necessitate repeated immersion of the hands in water. The fingers mainly affected are the thumbs and middle fingers of the dominant hand. *Candida* paronychia usually starts in the proximal nail fold with erythematous and painful swelling followed by nail-plate involvement. The nail becomes more opaque with white, green or black discoloration and transverse or longitudinal furrowing or pitting. In the course of time, the nail-plate becomes friable and may become detached from the nail bed. Pressure on and movement of the nail are painful. Bacterial superinfection is common [34].

Distal *Candida* nail infection presents as onycholysis and subungual hyperkeratosis and must be distinguished from dermatophytosis. The fingernails are nearly always involved. Nearly all patients with this condition suffer from Raynaud's phenomenon or some other underlying vascular problem [45].

Total dystrophic onychomycosis caused by *Candida* is mainly seen in patients with chronic mucocutaneous candidiasis (CMCC) with gross thickening and hyperkeratosis of the nail-plate [34].

Nail and *Candida*:

- Women mostly infected
- Fingernails mainly infected
- Colonization more like than true infection
- Predisposing circumstances like repeated immersion
- Food allergy discussed (Figs. 10.28, 10.29 and 10.30)

10.2.4.7 Differential Diagnosis of Fungal Nail Disease

Many non-infectious conditions can produce nail changes that mimic onychomycosis

- Nail dystrophies following repetitive trauma
- Onychogryphosis
- Onycholysis
- Psoriasis
- Nail lichen
- Subungual malignant melanoma
- Yellow nail syndrome
- Darier's disease
- Ichthyotic conditions (f.e. KID syndrome, etc.)

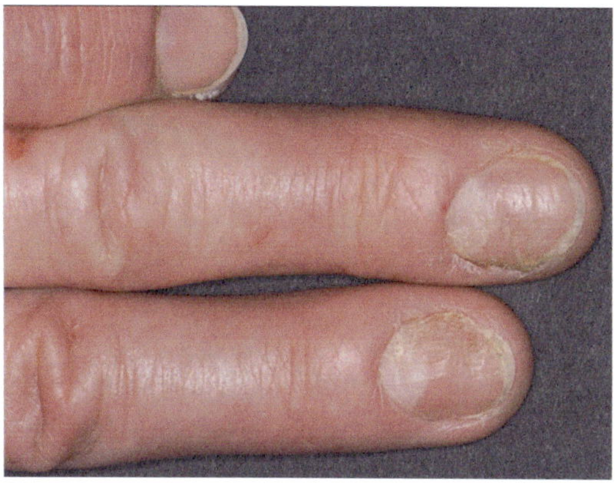

Fig. 10.28 *Candida* paronychia

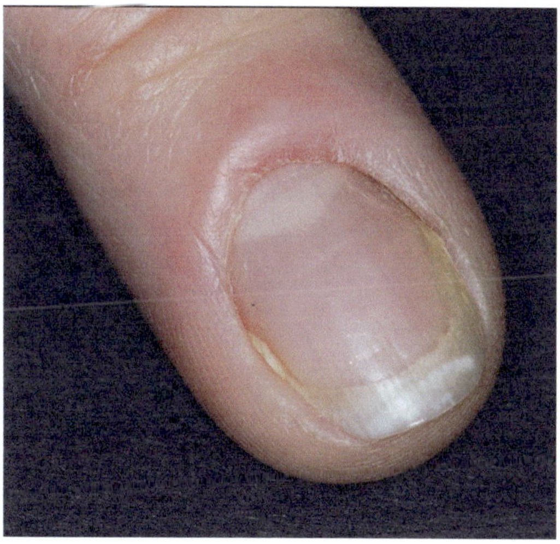

Fig. 10.29 *Candida* onycholysis

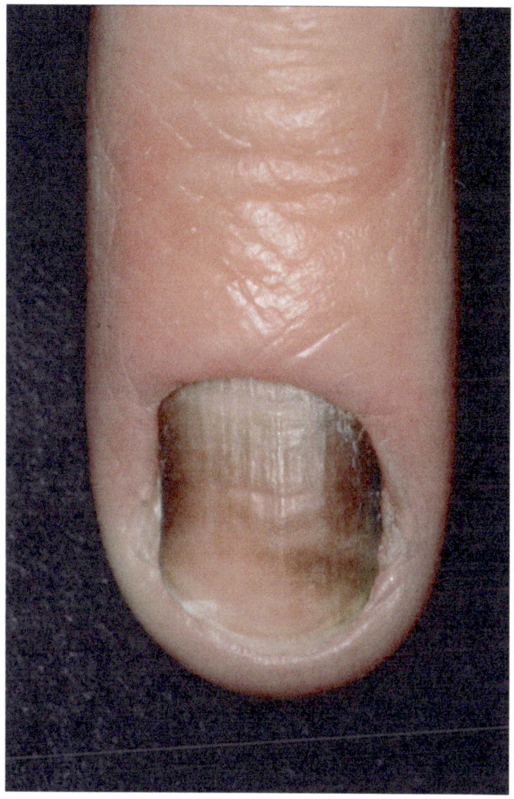

Fig. 10.30 *Candida* onychomycosis with *Candida* paronychia

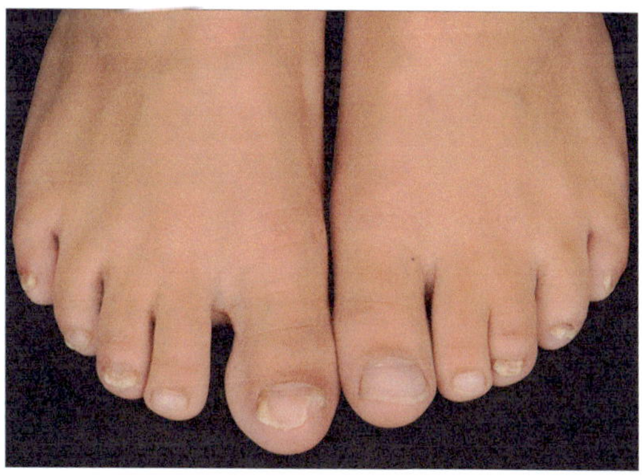

Fig. 10.31 Childhood onychomycosis in a 9-year-old boy

10.2.4.8 Childhood Onychomycosis

There has been a recent increase in childhood onychomycosis. The prevalence of childhood onychomycosis is between 0% and 2.6% [46].

Most cases of onychomycosis show pre-existing tinea pedis and a family history of pedal fungal infections, which means the infections have been transmitted by infected family members like the parents or grandparents. Physical activities like soccer and wearing of occlusive footwear are facilitative. Beside genetically determined predisposure for fungal nail infection, trisomy 21 is well known in children affected. The clinical picture of childhood onychomycosis resembles the same features as in adult infections with distal and lateral subungual onychomycosis being the most common picture, in addition to the infectious agents being the same (Fig. 10.31).

10.2.4.9 Onychomycosis in Athletes

Specific aspects of athletics such as repetitive nail injuries, increased sweating and increased exposure to infectious dermatophytes lead to a higher prevalence on fungal nail infection [47].

The key predisposing factors in sports persons are the intensity involved with sport (f.e. runners) and the sudden starting and stopping nature of specific activities as well as water sports and communal bathing.

10.2.4.10 Onychomycosis in Patients with Diabetes

Diabetics are almost three times more likely to develop onychomycosis than nondiabetics [48]. Approximately 34% of all diabetics have onychomycosis related to underlying risk factors like obesity, peripheral vascular disease and neuropathy and foot deformities. As in the general population in diabetic patients, *T. rubrum*, followed by *T. interdigitale* (formerly *T. mentagrophytes*), are the most common causative agents [49].

The types and frequency pattern of dermatophyte species in diabetic patients were similar to those in the immunocompetent group.

10.2.4.11 Diagnosis of Fungal Nail Infection

See Sect. 10.4, Diagnostic procedures.

10.2.4.12 Treatment

Onychomycosis can have a significant impact on the quality of life of patients by discomfort, difficulty in wearing footwear and walking, cosmetic embarrassment and lowered self-esteem [50–52].

Infected nails may serve as a reservoir of fungi with a potential for spread to the feet, hands and groin and to other family members. Another sequelae can be the disruption of the integrity of the skin leading to bacterial infections like cellulitis [53]. In the view of these aspects, treatment of fungal nail infection should be strongly considered.

With few exceptions in general, systemic therapy is compulsory to cure fungal nail infection, supported by topical treatment. The decision about other methods like surgical nail removal or nail avulsion by urea has to be drawn in attention in individual cases, which means in single nail onychomycosis. Laser treatment or photodynamic therapy (PDT) needs more experience and may be an option in the future.

Fungal-free nails are the goal of antifungal therapy in onychomycosis.

Topical treatment

- The efficacy of topically applied antifungal drugs is limited because the hard keratin and compact structure of the dorsal nail-plate act as a barrier against diffusion into and through the nail-plate. The concentration of topically administered drugs can drop by 1000 times from the outer to inner surface [54].
- The hydrophilic nature of the nail-plate also precludes absorption of lipophilic molecules with high molecular weight. These circumstances explain the limited role of monotherapy with topical antifungals with restriction to SWO and early DLSO [34].
- Terbinafine (topical formulation) [55]
- Amorolfine (morpholine) 5% lacquer—fungicidal against *C. albicans* and *T. mentagrophytes*
- Ciclopirox olamine (hydroxypyridone derivate) 8% lacquer—antifungal activity against *T. rubrum*, *S. brevicaulis* and *Candida* spp.
- Ciclopirox olamine and amorolfine are available in alcohol-based nail lacquers.
- Another ciclopirox olamine-containing nail lacquer has been available now for several years. Here, unlike the above-mentioned alcohol-based preparation, a film-forming agent is used as lacquer base. By binding to nail keratin, the water-soluble biopolymer hydroxypropyl chitosan (HPCS) allows for a better transport and release of ciclopirox olamine. The lacquer is applied once daily [56].

For successful application of antimycotic nail lacquer, onychomycosis should affect only up to 40% of the nail surface (an infestation level of <50% according to an international consensus conference) or a maximum of three out of ten affected toenails. The SPC for amorolfine-containing nail lacquer, however, lists onychomycosis with an involvement of <80% as indication.

Systemic Therapy

The main systemic drugs approved and widely used for the treatment of onychomycosis are the allylamine terbinafine and the triazole itraconazole. Griseofulvin is much less commonly used now given the higher efficacy and safety as well as compliance rates of the other systemic agents. Fluconazole represents a third-line therapy with restricted limitations, and in some countries, f.e. in the UK, it is not licensed for the treatment of onychomycosis [34].

Mainly with toenail onychomycosis, the rate of treatment failure with standard antifungal drugs is in the range of 25–40%, and this failure has been attributed to many aspects like poor patient compliance, low bioavailability, lack of drug penetration into the nail, drug resistance and poor nail growth [57].

New second-generation triazoles (f.e. voriconazole, posaconazole, ravuconazole, albaconazole, pramiconazole) recently are under development and may be of choice in refractory cases of onychomycosis.

Terbinafine is presently the only oral fungicidal antimycotic. It is detected in the nail within 1 week of starting therapy and persists for 6 months after the completion of treatment, as it has a long half-life [58]. Terbinafine has broad and potent fungicidal effects against dermatophytes, particularly *T. rubrum* and *T. interdigitale*, but has lower fungistatic activity against *Candida* species than the azoles [59]. The most common side effects are gastrointestinal, such as nausea, diarrhoea or taste disturbance, and dermatological events [60]. Serious side effects like hepatic toxicity are rare and occur mainly in patients with pre-existing liver disease; therefore systemic terbinafine is not recommended in those patients [61].

The efficacy and safety of terbinafine for the treatment of onychomycosis have been widely studied with different dosage—schedules with continuous dosing being superior to pulsing regimens (Table 10.6).

Itraconazole is active against a broad range of fungi including yeasts, dermatophytes and some nondermatophyte moulds. Like terbinafine it penetrates the nail quickly and is detectable in the nail as early as 7 days after starting therapy and persists in the nails for up to 6–9 months after treatment discontinuation [58]. The most common side effects including headache and gastrointestinal upset and asymptomatic liver function abnormalities are observed in 1.9–3% of patients [62]. Itraconazole can be administered in continuous or pulsing dosing regimens (Table 10.6).

Table 10.6 Systemic treatment of onychomycosis

Terbinafine	250 mg daily 6 weeks in fingernail infection 12–16 weeks in toenail infection
Itraconazole	*Continuous schedule* 200 mg daily for 12 weeks *Pulsing schedule* 400 mg daily for 1 week per month 2 pulses in fingernail infection 3 pulses (or more) in toenail infection
Fluconazole	150–450 mg per week 3 months in fingernail infection At least 6 (-10) months in toenail infection

Onychomycoses is associated with high recurrence rates (40–70%) [63]. The term 'recurrence' suggests both relapse and reinfection: in treatment relapse, infection is not completely cured and returns and in reinfection cure of fungal nail disease is followed by a new infection by the same or a different organism. Nail thickness (>2 mm), slow outgrowth, severe onycholysis and dermatophytoma are considered the most common reasons for recurrence and should raise attention to the outcome of antifungal therapy.

- Oral antimycotic agents are indicated for cure [64].
- Management requires correct mycological identification.
- Risk-to-benefit ratio of onychomycosis treatment should be assessed.
- Terbinafine is drug of choice in tinea unguium.
- Triazoles (itraconazole, fluconazole) in candidal and NDM onychomycosis.

10.2.5 Tinea Incognita (Steroid-Modified Tinea)

In tinea incognita (=tinea atypica), i.e. unrecognized tinea, cutaneous dermatophytosis is not considered as differential diagnosis. By definition, tinea incognita is a dermatophyte infection that has lost its typical clinical appearance due to the unjustified use of topical corticosteroids or calcineurin inhibitors [65].

Groin, lower legs, the face and the hands are mostly affected, with clinical lesions of dermatophyte infections being misdiagnosed as eczema, psoriasis and facial dermatoses. Due to the use of corticosteroids, typical aspects of the dermatophytosis are modified, i.e., the raised margin is diminished, scaling is lost and inflammation may be reduced to few nondescript nodules of bruise-like brownish discoloration. In the course of time due to chronic steroid treatment atrophy, telangiectasia in the axillae and groins striae may develop. The history of tinea incognita is characteristic—whereas discontinuation causes relapses, the patient continues the use of steroids, despite cure may not be achieved [66].

Special features of tinea incognita are Majocchi's granuloma, *Malassezia* folliculitis (formerly called *Pityrosporum* folliculitis) and Ofuji's syndrome. Majocchi's granuloma is defined to a deep-seated dermatophytosis, mainly as granulomatous folliculitis, following trauma, such as shaving as well as long-standing natural or therapeutic occlusion or topical steroid treatment. Treatment requires recognition; KOH testings have to be done to prove the nature of infection. In general systemic antifungals have to be administered (f.e. itraconazole or terbinafine for a three to four weeks duration), accompanied by topical treatment regimen.

Clues for diagnosis of tinea incognita:

- Long-standing treatment by corticosteroids with regular relapse after treatment discontinuation
- Misleading clinical features due to corticosteroid modification [67]
- Face, groin and hands mostly affected (Fig. 10.32)

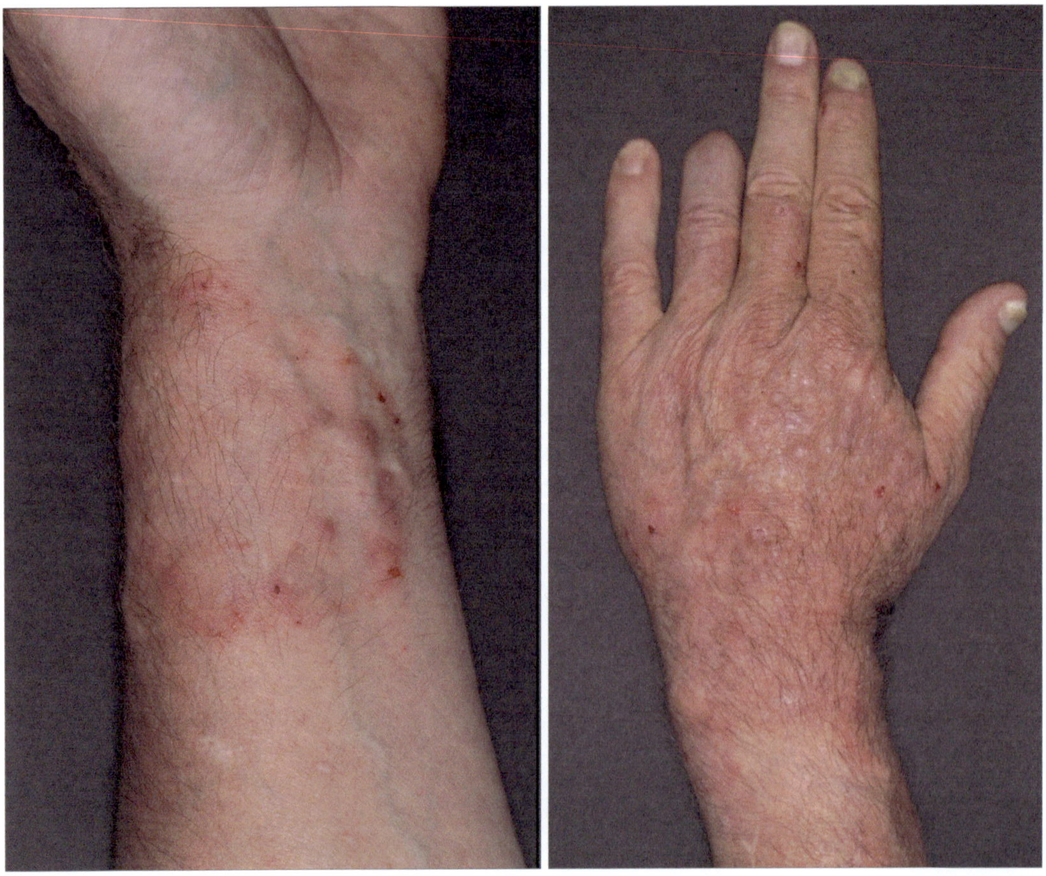

Fig. 10.32 Tinea incognita due to *Trichophyton rubrum* following autoinoculation by fungal infection of the toenails

10.3 Yeast Infections

10.3.1 Etiologic Agents

Yeasts are unicellular fungi that are reproduced by the process of budding in which daughter cells are produced from parents by outpouching of the cell membrane and wall, migration of cytoplasma into the new structure that formed and then separation from the parent cell [45].

The most frequently isolated causative agents in superficial infections are *Candida* species, *Cryptococcus neoformans* and the lipophilic yeasts of the genus *Malassezia*. In addition to *Candida albicans*, the genus *Candida* includes over 100 species, some of which (*C. stellatoidea*, *C. africana*, *C. dubliniensis*, *C. tropicalis*, *C. parapsilosis*, *C. guilliermondii*, *C. krusei*, *C. kefyr* (formerly *C. pseudotropicalis*), *C. zeylanoides*, *C. glabrata*, etc.) occasionally cause human disease.

10.3.2 Superficial Candidiasis

Candidiasis is an infection most commonly caused by the yeast *Candida albicans* or other species of *Candida*. Most common are superficial infections of the mucous membranes and skin, giving entrance to invasive infections by dissemination. Humans carry yeast fungi in the gastrointestinal tract, from the mouth to rectum as part of the normal commensal flora. The vagina may also be colonized by yeasts without any signs of infection. By contrast, *Candida* species are not permanent members of the normal flora of the skin but can transiently colonize some areas like fingers and body folds. In given predisposition colonization can proceed to true infection.

10.3.2.1 Skin Infections by *Candida* Species

Cutaneous candidiasis predominantly affects intertriginous areas, i.e. groins, abdominal skin folds, inframammary skin but also interdigital spaces. Skin infections caused by yeasts are typically characterized by erythematous (bright red to purple-red), erosive, dry, scaly, sometimes macerated lesions. It often has an irregular edge and satellite papules and pustules that develop beyond the margin. Where the webspaces of the toes or the fingers are affected, marked maceration with a thick white horny layer is usually prominent. In interdigital candidiasis of the toe webs, Gram-negative bacteria are often co-pathogens beside *Candida*. Non-intertriginous areas characteristically display erythemato-squamous lesions with collaret-like scaling. Soreness and burning itch are usual [13, 45].

The development of superficial candidiasis in general needs predisposing factors to manifest. Obese subjects as well as diabetics, immunosuppression, serious illness, the age group of the elderly and early infants are predisposed for these infections. With regard to immunosuppression, interdigital mycoses by *C. albicans* may be indicative of full-blown AIDS in areas with high HIV prevalence, e.g. in sub-Saharan Africa. Differential diagnosis of candidiasis includes tinea (dermatophytosis), contact dermatitis, seborrheic dermatitis, bacterial infections and inverse psoriasis. *Candida* may also contaminate any of these conditions and lead to secondary infection.

Diaper Candidiasis (Napkin candidiasis)
Candida albicans is commonly isolated from the moist skin of the buttocks and genitalia of the infant but is more prevalent where the skin is infected by nappy rash [68]. This special form of cutaneous candidiasis is marked by maceration and erosion, yet also whitish patches and desquamation. In addition fringed irregular borders and satellite lesions are indicative for the infection. Wet and warm surroundings are a predisposing factor, aggravated by urine acting as irritant. Similar lesions can be found in elderly, bedridden and incontinent patients [69].

In recalcitrant cases with *Candida* infection, acrodermatitis enteropathica (zinc deficiency syndrome) should be drawn in attention.

Nodular or granulomatous candidiasis of the napkin area (syn. granuloma gluteale infantum) is a syndrome that represents a peculiar reaction to *Candida* infection. This kind of napkin eruption is characterized by the development of bluish or brownish nodules. Beside *Candida* topical steroids are probably an important etiological factor. The true nature of this condition has not yet been elucidated [70, 71].

Treatment

With regard to treatment, underlying localized and general predisposing and susceptibility factors should be considered. In skin infections drying and ventilation are of highest importance. In many cases topical therapy alone is sufficient, but considerations should always be given to the reduction of the *Candida* reservoir in the mouth and the gut, not at least with respect to prophylactic reasons [72].

The polyene antibiotics (f.e. nystatin) and the group of imidazoles (clotrimazole, miconazole, econazole, ketoconazole, flutrimazole, etc.) are highly effective against *Candida* spp. and most other yeast pathogens. Development of resistance against these groups is *up to now not* observed.

- Mind localized and general predisposing factors.
- Topical steroids may modify the inflammatory changes.
- Topical antimycotic treatment (azoles, nystatin) alone usually sufficient.
- With recurrent infections oral therapy with a polyene or triazole should be considered (Figs. 10.33, 10.34 and 10.35).

10.3.2.2 Mucocutaneous Candidiasis

- Oral candidiasis—see Chap. 4
- Genital candidiasis
  - *Candida* vulvovaginitis—see Chap. 4
  - *Candida* balanitis (balanoposthitis candidomycetica)

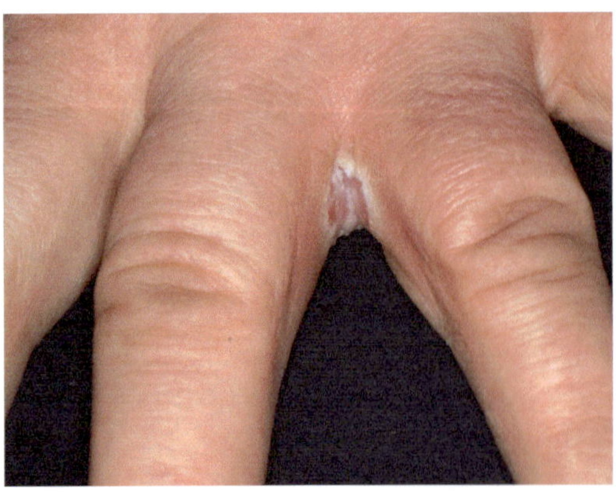

Fig. 10.33 Candidal infections of interdigital spaces ('erosio interdigitalis blastomycetica') arising from prolonged water exposure of the hands

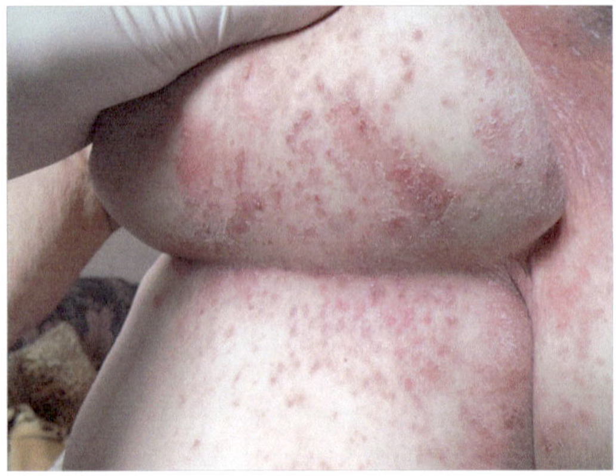

Fig. 10.34 Intertriginous candidiasis ('*Candida* intertrigo') in the inframammary folds

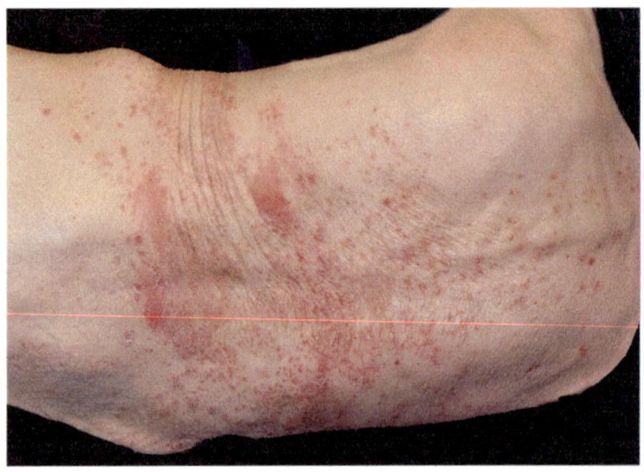

Fig. 10.35 Cutaneous widespread candidiasis in a bedridden elderly

The skin of the glans penis, especially in the uncircumcised, may sometimes be colonized by *Candida* asymptomatically [73]. When *Candida* balanitis develops, it presents with transient tiny papules and white pustules or vesicles and rupture, leaving a peeling edge. Soreness, itching and irritation may be of subjective complaints. Exacerbation of the condition after intercourse is common. In more severe and chronic cases, the inflammatory changes become persistent over the glans and the prepuce. When *Candida* balanitis develops, usually either abundant vaginal *Candida* carriage (symptomless) or frank vulvovaginitis in the sexual partner may be found. It is worth considering diabetes where persistent lesions spread beyond the genitalia. Concerning the situation with a contracted prepuce (phimosis), the need of circumcision has to be drawn in attention.

Treatment

- Topical antimycotic treatment (azoles, nystatin) usually satisfactory.
- Rule out susceptibility factors (phimosis, diabetes, etc.).
- Screening of the sexual partner (s) and appropriate treatment.
- Exclude differential diagnoses, like psoriasis inversa, balanitis simplex, herpes genitalis, balanitis plasmacellularis Zoon (Fig. 10.36).

10.3.2.3 *Candida* and the Nail

See Sect. 10.2.4.6.

10.3.3 Pityriasis Versicolor

Pityriasis versicolor is a mild chronic infection of the skin caused by *Malassezia* spp. (formerly *Pityrosporum ovale sive orbiculare*). The condition is characterized by discrete discoloured or depigmented areas mainly on the upper trunk, back, chest, shoulders and upper arms.

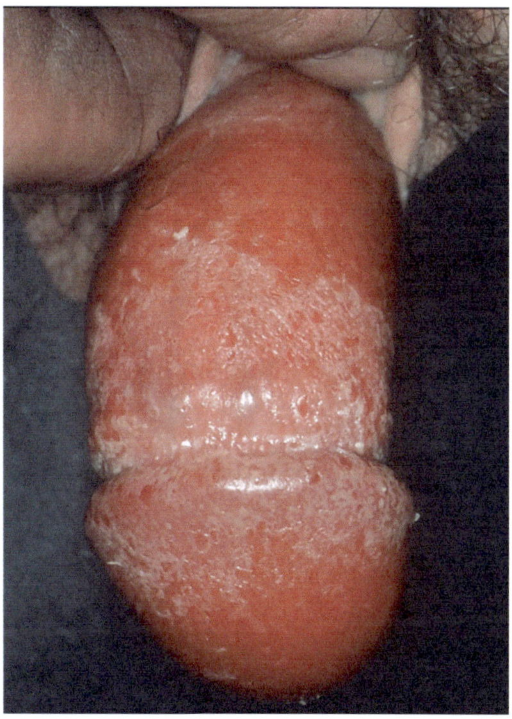

Fig. 10.36 *Candida* balanitis

The disease typically starts with brownish-red, macular, coalescing, apparently non-scaly lesions and is defined as 'pityriasis versicolor rubra'. In the course of time, the lesions spread in a map-like fashion without sharp demarcation. Except in children and dark-skinned people in tropical countries, pityriasis versicolor never affects the face. By tangential scraping the skin with a wooden scapula or scalpel bran-like scaling may be evoked (shaving phenomenon).

'Pityriasis versicolor alba' presents the white pseudochromatic variant of pityriasis versicolor. This depigmentation is caused by dicarboxylic acids, such as azelaic acid produced by *Malassezia* spp., which may competitively inhibit tyrosinase and perhaps have a direct cytotoxic effect on hyperactive melanocytes [74].

10.3.3.1 Skin and *Malassezia*

The lipophilic yeast fungus *Malassezia* spp. is the only fungal genus or species which is part of the physiological human microbiome, beside in other warm-blooded animals [75].

Today, at least 14 different *Malassezia* species are known, of which 8 have been isolated from human skin. Most of them can only be identified using molecular biological techniques. In pityriasis versicolor, *M. globosa* is predominantly found in 62.5% of patients, followed by *M. sympodialis* [76, 77].

Colonization by these species is particularly dense in the scalp, upper trunk and flexures. Pityriasis versicolor appears to represent a shift in the balance between host and resident flora in which mycelial forms develop [45]. Multiple factors contribute to the change and include genetically determined host susceptibility factors, climate and immune competence [78, 79].

Likewise *Malassezia* folliculitis and seborrheic dermatitis are conditions contributed to Malassezia yeasts. Whereas in seborrheic dermatitis or scaling of the scalp, dandruff, *Malassezia* yeasts are found in large quantities in the scales of patients, in *Malassezia* folliculitis yeasts may be found by means of histology within the body of the follicles. Lesions are itchy papules and pustules diffusely scattered on the shoulders and back [45].

Beside these conditions *Malassezia* allergens should be considered as the trigger of 'Head-Neck'-type atopic dermatitis [76, 80].

10.3.3.2 Treatment

The topical azole antifungals but also the allylamine terbinafine and the hydroxypyridone antifungal agent ciclopirox olamine work well, with ketoconazole, selenium sulphide or zinc pyrithione shampoos being available for washings. Alternatively, itraconazole is effective in a total dose of 800–1000 mg (given over 7 days, e.g. 100 mg twice daily for 1 week) but may be subject to extensive disease. Repigmentation may take several months and should not be interpreted as treatment failure. In some patients who are unresponsive to conventional treatments with frequent relapsing episodes, narrow-band UV-B phototherapy may be effective [45, 81, 82].

- Scalp, upper trunk and the flexures are colonized by *Malassezia* spp.
- Topical and oral azoles first-line drugs in pityriasis versicolor.
- Repigmentation takes several months (Figs. 10.37, 10.38 and 10.39).

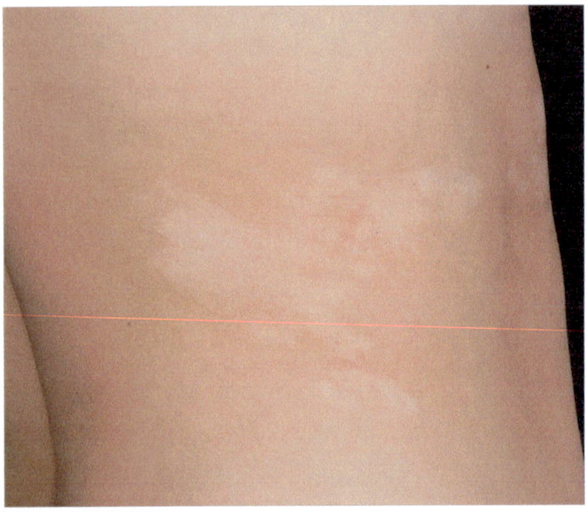

Fig. 10.37 Pityriasis versicolor presenting finely scaling hypopigmented lesions

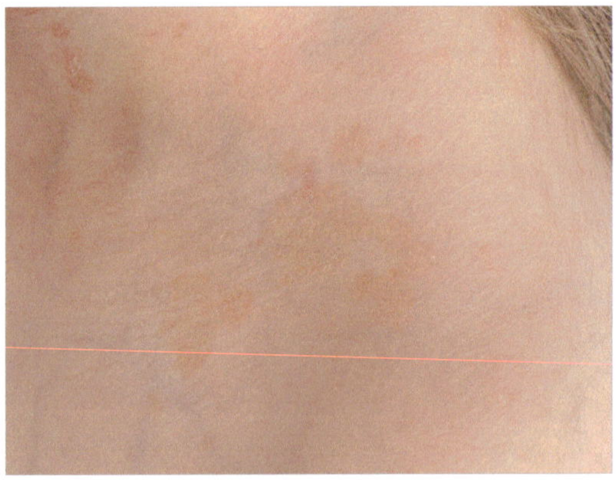

Fig. 10.38 Pityriasis versicolor on the neck in a child

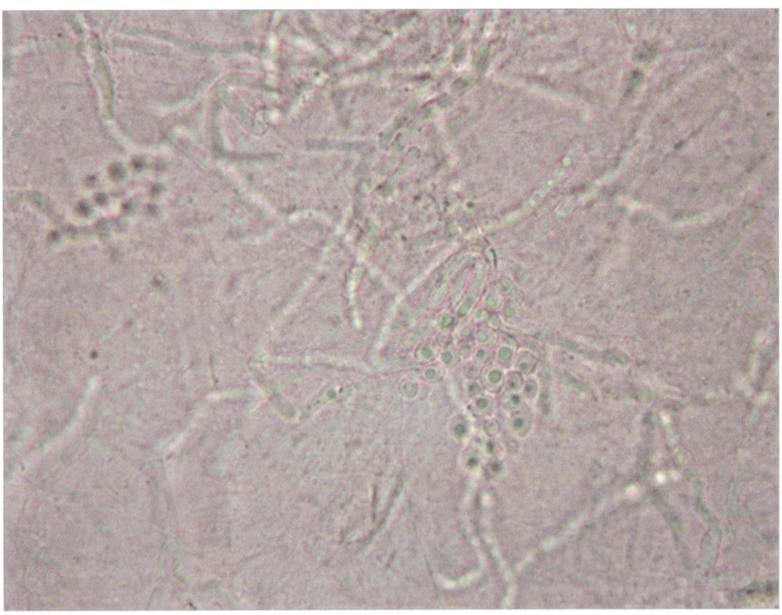

Fig. 10.39 Microscopic examination of KOH-treated skin scrapings: *Malassezia* yeasts (spherical yeasts and short hyphae =pseudomycelia)

10.4 Diagnostic Procedures

Diagnostic procedures in fungal infections comprise sampling of material, microscopy, cultivation proceedings and molecular methods (PCR) for detection of fungal pathogens. In general topical antimycotic treatment may be started if microscopic findings are positive.

10.4.1 Diagnostic Sampling

Apart from skin scrapings, samples include hair roots in cases of suspected tinea capitis and nail clippings in cases of suspected onychomycosis. Skin scrapings should be taken by a scalpel or curette from the lesional border, whereas hair roots may be collected by epilation tweezers. Additional methods like the hairbrush technique (in scaling tinea capitis or for screening exams among family members) or swab sampling (in purulent infections) are other techniques for diagnostic sampling.

10.4.2 Microscopic Preparations

The KOH (potassium hydroxide) examination using 20% KOH represents the simplest method to detect fungi in skin scales, nails and hair roots microscopically. Tetraethylammonium hydroxide (TEAH) may be used alternatively for immediate determination of fungal elements mainly in nail clippings. The diagnostic sensitivity may be partially insufficient, especially in onychomycosis. The most sensitive method of microscopic detection of fungi in skin scales, nail clippings, hair roots, hair as well as Scotch tape preparations is fluorescent staining with optical brighteners (diaminostilbene). These substances bind to chitin, the main cell wall component of fungi. Currently available stains are Blankophor® or Calcofluor® test solutions that are prepared with 20% KOH. Using fluorescent microscopy, spores, yeast cells, hyphal fragments and arthrospores (=disintegrating mycelium) may be differentiated [13].

10.4.3 Cultural Dermatophyte Detection

As fungi are heterotrophic microorganisms, culture media contain organic nutrients required for growth and reproduction, among them a carbon source (glucose), a nitrogen source (peptone, meat extract), water, vitamins and antibiotics.

Every sample should be inoculated onto two culture media, one of them containing cycloheximide (Actidion®) to suppress mould growth. Cultures should be incubated at a temperature of 26–32 °C, optimally at 28 °C, for 3–4 weeks and visually checked for fungal growth twice weekly. For slow-growing dermatophytes (*T. verrucosum* or *T. violaceum*), the incubation period should be extended to 5–6 weeks.

The selective dermatophyte agar according to Taplin is a selective but at the same time also differentiation medium because the addition of cycloheximide allows for selective growth of dermatophytes on this cultural medium. Dermatophytes produce alkaline metabolites that alkalize the initially acidic cultural medium, causing the indicator phenol red to turn from yellow to red, thus signalling dermatophyte growth.

The differentiation of dermatophytes, yeasts and moulds is predicated on macroscopic (upper and bottom side of colonies as well as pigmentation) and microscopic characteristics (formation of macro- and microconidia) as well as biochemical properties. Quite frequently, cultural detection fails (sensitivity roughly 70% in onychomycosis) because of pretreatment with topical or systemic antifungals. Thus, vital fungi are already inhibited in vivo, preventing them from growing in vitro [13].

10.4.4 Molecular Detection of Dermatophytes [13]

Nucleic acid amplification techniques (NAAT) are more and more used for direct examination of dermatophytes in clinical samples, e.g. *T. rubrum* and *T. interdigitale*. NAAT are also used as culture confirmation tests for identification of rare dermatophytes like *T. verrucosum*. Today, singleplex and multiplex quantitative real-time PCR (qRT-PCR) assays for the detection of the most common dermatophytes including rare dermatophyte species like *T. verrucosum* in clinical specimens are available.

Ohst et al. from Germany developed a modular singleplex quantitative real-time PCR (qRT-PCR) assay for the detection of the most common dermatophytes in clinical specimens [83]. This qRT-PCR assay is based on single-tube reactions with TaqMan probes. *T. rubrum* (75.6%) and *T. interdigitale* (16.9%) were the most frequently detected dermatophytes. Some less common dermatophytes, among them *M. canis*, *Epidermophyton floccosum*, *T. benhamiae* and *T. verrucosum*, were detected, too. It was concluded that the qRT-PCR assay allows a specific and sensitive detection of relevant dermatophytes at low cost in a short time.

A dermatophyte-specific single-tube real-time PCR assay based on internal transcribed sequences was developed for rapid detection and identification of 11 species within the 3 dermatophyte genera *Trichophyton*, *Microsporum* and *Epidermophyton* in nail, skin and hair samples within a few hours [84].

Sequencing of the ITS region of the rDNA is used for culture confirmation of rare dermatophytes [85, 86].

References

1. Gruby D (1841) Memoire sur une vegetation qui constitue la vraie teigne. C R Acad Sci 13:72–75
2. Seeliger HPR (1985) The discovery of *Achorion schoenleinii*. Mykosen 28:161–182
3. Castellani A (1910) Observations on new species of epidermophyton found in tinea cruris. Br J Dermatol 22:147–150
4. Rippon JW (1985) The changing epidemiology and emerging patterns of dermatophyte species. Curr Top Med Mycol 1:208–234
5. De Hoog GS, Dukik K, Monod M, Packeu A, Stubbe D, Hendrickx M, Kupsch C, Stielow B, Freeke J, Göker M, Rezaei-Matehkolaei A, Mirhendi H, Gräser Y (2017) Toward a novel multilocus phylogenetic taxonomy for the dermatophytes. Mycopathologia 182:5–31
6. Nenoff P, Uhrlaß S, Schulze I, Koch D, Rahmig N, Hipler UC, Krüger C (2017) Tinea capitis and onychomycosis due to Trichophyton soudanense in siblings from Angola – successful treatment with fluconazole. Case reports in Germany and review of the literature. Hautarzt. https://doi.org/10.1007/s00105-018-4155-0
7. Uhrlaß S, Schroedl W, Mehlhorn C, Krüger C, Hubka V, Maier T, Gräser Y, Paasch U, Nenoff P (2018) Molecular epidemiology of *Trichophyton quinckeanum* – a zoophilic dermatophyte on the rise. J Dtsch Dermatol Ges 16(1):21–32
8. English M (1962) The saprophyte growth of keratinophilic fungi on keratin. Sabouraudia 2:115–130
9. Dahl MV (1987) Immunological resistance to dermatophyte infection. Adv Dermatol 2:305–320
10. Dahl MV, Randall C (1986) Polymorphnuclear leukocytes, compliment and Trichophyton rubrum. J Invest Dermatol 86:138–141
11. Swan JW, Dahl MV, Coppo PA, Hammerschmidt DE (1983) Compliment activation by Trichophyton rubrum. J Invest Dermatol 80:156–158
12. Elewski BE (1998) The superficial mycoses, the dermatophytoses, and select dermatomycosies. In: Cutaneous fungal infections, Sec. Edt. Blackwell Science, Malden, p 13–20
13. Nenoff P, Krüger C, Schaller J, Ginter-Hanselmayer G, Schulte-Beerbühl R, Tietz HJ (2014) Mycology – an update. Part 2: dermatomycoses: clinical picture and diagnostics. J Dtsch Dermatol Ges 12(9):749–777
14. Wan SJ, Lara-Corrales I (2018) An unresponsive rash to topical steroids: tinea incognito. Arch Dis Child 103(1):3
15. Seebacher C, Bouchara JP, Mignon B (2008) Updates on the epidemiology of dermatophyte infections. Mycopathologia 166:335–352
16. Nenoff P, Fischer S, Schulze I, Krüger C (2017) Trichophyton rubrum syndrome and tinea incognita under immunosuppressive treatment with leflunomide and fumaric acid esters in patients with rheumatoid arthritis and psoriasis vulgaris. Akt Dermatol 43:346–353
17. Masri-Fridling GD (1996) Dermatophytosis of the feet. Dermatol Clin Cutaneous Mycol 14(1):33–40
18. Mayser P (2012) Mykosen im Bereich der Leistenhaut von Händen und Füßen. Haut 23:2–6
19. Ferguson L, Fuller LC (2017) Spectrum and burden of dermatophytes in children. J Infect 74(Suppl 1):S54–S60
20. Chen W, Mempel M, Traidl-Hofmann C et al (2010) Gender aspects in skin diseases. JEADV 24(12):1378–1385
21. Zaraa I, Hawilo A, Trojjet S et al (2012) Tinea capitis in infants in their first 2 years of life: a 12-year study and a review of the literature. Dermatol Online J 18(7):16
22. Ginter-Hanselmayer G, Weger W, Ilkit M, Smolle J (2007) Epidemiology of tinea capitis in Europe: current state and changing patterns. Mycoses 50(Suppl 2):6–13
23. Wiegand C, Mugisha P, Mulyowa GK, Elsner P, Hipler UC, Gräser Y, Uhrlaß S, Nenoff P (2016)

Trichophyton violaceum – Haupterreger der Tinea capitis bei Kindern im Mbarara Regional Referral Hospital in Uganda. Hautarzt 67:712–717
24. Ilkit M, Gümral R, Saracli MA, Burgut R (2011) Trichophyton tonsurans scalp carriage among wrestlers in a national competition in Turkey. Mycopathologia 172(3):215–222
25. Kawachi Y, Ikegami M, Takase T, Otsuka F (2010) Chronically recurrent and disseminated tinea faciei/corporis - autoinoculation from asymptomatic tinea capitis carriage. Pediatr Dermatol 27:527–528
26. Silverman RA (1998) Pediatric mycoses-Tinea capitis. In: Cutaneous fungal infections, Sec. Edt. Blackwell Science, London, p 268–270
27. Nenoff P, Süß A, Staubach P, Anemüller A, Renner R, Uhrlaß S, Krüger C, Ginter-Hanselmayer G (2017) Tinea capitis bei Flüchtlingen und Migranten. Dtsch Dermatol 65(3):199–206
28. Chen X et al (2016) Systemic antifungal therapy for tinea capitis in children: an abridged cochrane review. J Am Acad Dermatol 76:368–374. https://doi.org/10.1002/14651858.CD004685.pub3
29. Fuller LC, Barton RC, Mohd Mustapa MF et al (2014) British Association of Dermatologists' guidelines for the management of Tinea capitis 2014. Br J Dermatol 171:454–463
30. Wollina U, Hansel G, Uhrlaß S, Krüger C, Schönlebe J, Hipler UC, Nenoff P (2017) Deep facial mycosis in a diabetic patient caused by Trichophyton verrucosum – a case report and review of the literature. Mycoses 61(3):152–158
31. Ginter-Hanselmayer G, Nenoff P, Kurrat W, Propst E, Durrant-Finn U, Uhrlaß S, Weger W (2016) Tinea im Genitalbereich. Eine diagnostische und therapeutische Herausforderung. Hautarzt 67(9).689–699
32. Burns T, Breathnach S, Cox N, Griffiths C (2010) Rook's textbook of dermatology, 8th edn. Wiley-Blackwell, Chichester
33. Nenoff P, Ginter-Hanselmayer G, Tietz HJ (2012) Fungal nail infections-an update: part 2-Prevalence, epidemiology, predisposing conditions, and differential diagnosis. Hautarzt 63(19):30–38
34. Ameen M, Lear JT, Madan V, Mohd Mustapa MF, Richardson M (2014) British Association of Dermatologist's guidelines for the management of onychomycosis 2014. Br J Dermatol 171(5):937–958. https://doi.org/10.1111/bjd.13358
35. Richardson MD, Warnock DW (2012) Fungal infection: diagnosis and management, 4th edn. Wiley-Blackwell, Chichester
36. Faergemann J, Correia O, Nowicki R, Ro BI (2005) Genetic predisposition- understanding underlying mechanisms of onychomycosis. J Eur Acad Dermatol Venereol 19:17–19
37. Tsentemeidou A, Vyzantiadis TA, Kyriakou A, Sotiriadis D, Patsatsi A (2017) Prevalence of onychomycosis among patients with nail psoriasis who are not receiving immunosuppressive agents: Results of a pilot study. Mycoses 60(12):830–835
38. Richardson MD, Edward M (2000) Model systems for the study of dermatophytes and non-dermatophyte invasion of human keratin. In: Kushwaha RKS, Guarro J (eds) Biology of dermatophytes and other keratinophilic fungi. Revista Iberoamericana de Micologia, Bilbao, pp 115–121
39. Yazdanparast SA, Barton RC (2006) Arthroconidia production in Trichophyton rubrum and a new ex vivo model of onychomycosis. J Med Microbiol 55:1577–1581
40. Seebacher C, Müller J (2011) 50 Jahre Deutschsprachige Mykologische Gesellschaft. Ein Rückblick auf die Gründungsveranstaltung am 15. Januar 1961 in Essen. Mykol Forum 1/11:6–11
41. Manz M, Scholz GH, Willgerodt H et al (2002) Autoimmun polyglandular syndrome (APS) type I and Candida onychomycosis. Eur J Dermatol 12:283–286
42. Gupta AK, Drummond-Main C, Cooper EA et al (2012) Systemic review of nondermatophyte mould onychomycosis: diagnosis, clinical types, epidemiology, and treatment. JAAD 66:494–502
43. Hwang SM, Suh MK, Ha GY (2012) Onychomycosis due to nondermatophytic moulds. Ann Dermatol 24:175–180
44. Nenoff P, Schorlemmer B, Uhrlaß S, Baunacke A, Baunacke A, Friedrichs C, Iffländer J, Syhre E, Schneider A, Krüger C, Maier T (2016) Onychocola canadensis Sigler in onychomycosis: a new dermatophyte-like mould in Germany. Hautarzt 67(9):739–749
45. Hay RJ (1996) Yeast infections. In: Thiers BH, Elgart ML (eds) Dermatologic clinics-cutaneous mycology, vol 14, Issue 1. W.B. Saunders, Philadelphia, pp 113–124
46. Ginter-Hanselmayer G, Weger W, Smolle J (2008) Onychomycosis: a new emerging infectious disease in childhood population and adolescents. Report on treatment experience with terbinafine and itraconazole in 36 patients. J Eur Acad Dermatol Venereol 22:470–475
47. Field LA, Adams BB (2008) Tinea pedis in athletes. Int J Dermatol 47:485–492
48. Al-Mutairi N, Eassa BI, DA A-R (2010) Clinical and mycological characteristics of onychomycosis in diabetic patients. Acta Dermatovenerol Croat 18:84–91
49. Romano C, Massai L, Asta F, Signorini AM (2001) Prevalence of dermatophytic skin and nail infections in diabetic patients. Mycoses 44:83–86
50. Elewski BE (2000) Onychomycosis. Treatment, quality of life, and economic issues. Am J Clin Dermatol 1:19–26
51. Szepietowski JC, Reich A (2009) Stigmatisation in onychomycosis patients: a population-based study. Mycoses 52:343–349
52. Thomas J, Jacobson GA, Narkowicz CK et al (2010) Toenail onychomycosis: an important global disease burden. J Clin Pharm Ther 35:497–519
53. Tan JS, Joseph WS (2004) Common fungal infections of the feet in patients with diabetes mellitus. Drugs Aging 21:101–112

54. Stuttgen G, Bauer E (1982) Bioavailability, skin- and nail-penetration of topically applied antimycotics. Mykosen 25:74–80
55. Hartmane I, Dervenice A, Mailland F et al (2013) Evaluation of safety profile, pharmacokinetics, and clinical benefit of an innovative terbinafine transungual solution (p-3058): a phase I study in patients with mild-to-moderate distal subungual onychomycosis. JAAD 68(Suppl. 1):AB105
56. Iorizzo M, Ilona H, Derveniece A, Mikazans I (2015) Ciclopirox 8% HPCH nail lacquer in the treatment of mild-to-moderate onychomycosis: a randomized, double-blind amorolfine controlled study using a blinded evaluator. Skin Appendage Disord 1:134–140
57. Hay RJ (2001) The future of onychomycosis therapy may involve a combination of approaches. Br J Dermatol 145(Suppl. 60):S3–S8
58. Dubruyne D, Coquerel A (2001) Pharmacokinetics of antifungal agents in onychomycoses. Clin Pharmacokinet 40:441–472
59. Bueno JG, Martinez C, Zapata B et al (2010) In vitro activity of fluconazole, itraconazole, voriconazole and terbinafine against fungi causing onychomycosis. Clin Exp Dermatol 35:658–663
60. Hall M, Monka C, Krupp P, O'Sullivan D (1997) Safety of oral terbinafine: results of a postmarketing surveillance study in 25,884 patients. Arch Dermatol 133:1213–1219
61. O'Sullivan DP, Needham CA, Bangs A et al (1996) Postmarketing surveillance of oral terbinafine in the U.K.: report of a large cohort study. Br J Clin Pharmacol 42:559–565
62. Gupta A, Lambert J, Revuz J, Shear N (2001) Update on the safety of itraconazole pulse therapy in onychomycosis and dermatomycoses. Eur J Dermatol 11:6–10
63. Singal A, Khanna D (2011) Onychomycosis: diagnosis and management. Indian J Dermatol Venereol Leprol 77:659–572
64. Wollina U, Nenoff P, Haroske G, Haenssle H (2016) The diagnosis and treatment of nail disorders. Dtsch Ärztebl Intern 113:509–518
65. Verma SB (2017) A closer look at the term "tinea incognito": a factual as well as grammatical inaccuracy. Indian J Dermatol 62(2):219–220
66. Champion RH, Burton JL, Ebling FJG (1994) Steroid-modified tinea. In: Rook's textbook of dermatology, 5th edn. Blackwell, Oxford
67. Verma S, Hay RJ (2015) Topical steroid-induced Tinea pseudoimbricata: a striking form of tinea incognito. Int J Dermatol 54(5):e192–e193
68. Rebora A, Leyden JJ (1981) Napkin (diaper) dermatitis and gastrointestinal carriage of Candida albicans. Br J Dermatol 105:551–555
69. Fölster-Holst R, Buchner M, Proksch E (2011) Diaper dermatitis. Hautarzt 62:699–709
70. Keiichi U, Nakayasu K, Takaishi Y (1973) Kaposi sarcoma-like granuloma on diaper dermatitis. Arch Dermatol 107:605–607
71. Tappeiner J, Pfleger L (1971) Granuloma gluteale infantum. Hautarzt 22:383–388
72. Roberts SOB (1980) Antifungal chemotherapy. Wiley, Chichester, pp 225–383
73. Odds FC (1988) Candida and candidosis. Bailliere Tindall, London
74. Mayser P, Preuss J (2012) Pityriasis versicolor-Aktuelles zu einer alten Erkrankung. Hautarzt 63:859–867
75. Jo JH, Deming C, Kennedy EA, Conlan S, Polley EC, Ng WL, Segre JA, Kong HH, NISC Comparative Sequencing Program (2016) Diverse human skin fungal communities in children converge in adulthood. J Invest Dermatol 136(12):2356–2363
76. Nenoff P, Krüger C, Mayser P (2015) Cutaneous Malassezia infections and Malassezia associated dermatoses: an update. Hautarzt 66(6):465–484
77. Prohic A, Jovovic Sadikovic T, Krupalija-Fazlic M, Kuskunovic-Vlahovljak S. Malassezi Burke RC (1961) Tinea versicolor. Susceptibility factors and experimental infections in human beings. J Invest Dermatol 36:398; Prohic A, Jovovic Sadikovic T, Krupalija-Fazlic M, Kuskunovic-Vlahovljak S. Malassezi Burke RC (2016) A species in healthy skin and in dermatological conditions. Int J Dermatol 55(5):494–504
78. Burke RC (1961) Tinea versicolor. Susceptibility factors and experimental infections in human beings. J Invest Dermatol 36:398
79. Sparber F, LeibundGut-Landmann S (2017) Host responses to Malassezia spp. in the mammalian skin. Front Immunol 8:614
80. Darabi K, Hostetler SG, Bechtel MA, Zirwas M (2009) The role of Malassezia in atopic dermatitis affecting the head and neck of adults. JAAD 60:125–136
81. Gupta AK, Lyons DC (2014) Pityriasis versicolor: an update on pharmacological treatment option. Expert Opin Pharmacother 15(12):1707–1713
82. Balevi A, Üstüner P, Kaksi SA, Özdemir M (2017) Narrow-band UV-B phototherapy: an effective and reliable treatment alternative for extensive and recurrent pityriasis versicolor. J Dermatol Treat 9:1
83. Ohst T, Kupsch C, Gräser Y (2016) Detection of common dermatophytes in clinical specimens using a simple quantitative real-time TaqMan polymerase chain reaction assay. Br J Dermatol 174(3):602–609
84. Bergmans AM, van der Ent M, Klaassen A et al (2010) Evaluation of a single-tube real-time PCR for detection and identification of 11 dermatophyte species in clinical material. Clin Microbiol Infect 16(6):704–710
85. Uhrlaß S, Mayser P, Schwarz R, Koch D, Krüger C, Korfmann I, Nenoff P (2017) Dermatomycoses due to Nannizzia praecox (formerly Microsporum praecox) in Germany - case reports and review of the literature. Mycopathologia 183(2):391–398
86. Wiegand C, Mugisha P, Mulyowa GK, Elsner P, Hipler UC, Gräser Y, Uhrlaß S, Nenoff P (2017) Identification of the causative dermatophyte of tinea capitis in children attending Mbarara Regional Referral Hospital in Uganda by PCR-ELISA and comparison with conventional mycological diagnostic methods. Med Mycol 55(6):660–668

Part III

Special Issues

11 Infection Control to Reduce Invasive Fungal Infections

Magda Diab-El Schahawi

A combination of antifungal stewardship and environmental infection control strategies

In this chapter you will learn about:

- Susceptible patient groups at risk for invasive fungal infection (IFI)
- Prevention of invasive fungal infection
- Need for antifungal stewardship programs
- Environmental infection control strategies to prevent IFI during construction work in the hospital setting

Substantial progress in diagnostic and therapeutic medical procedures over the past century has helped increase longevity in the industrialized world. Progress in oncological treatment options and successful human organ as well as hematopoietic stem cell transplantation can be counted as some of the biggest achievements of modern medicine. With the development of more effective immunosuppressive drugs, organ transplants have become an accepted treatment for a growing number of otherwise incurable diseases. Longer survival of transplant recipients has at the same time greatly increased the number of immunocompromised patients. These patients are typically at greater risk of acquiring infections caused by the so-called opportunistic organisms (bacterial, viral, or fungal) whose virulence is low in immunocompetent patients. In a recent study, Martin et al. found that fungal microorganisms as cause of sepsis have greatly increased in the United States between 1979 and 2000 [1]. Associated morbidity and mortality of these infections are substantial and make them an emerging public health issue [2, 3]. Also the overall incidence of invasive fungal infections is estimated to be increasing affecting mostly oncological patients and transplant recipients [4]. Neutropenic patients, for example, are at increased risk for invasive filamentous fungal infections, while non-neutropenic multimorbid patients in the intensive care unit harboring multiple lifesaving invasive devices are at increased risk for endogenous yeast infections. The types of fungal infection occurring in susceptible patients depend not only on the host's underlying disease, i.e., their net state of immunosuppression, but also on their epidemiological exposure and/or colonization with opportunistic fungi.

Comprising about a quarter of the earth's biomass, fungi can survive in hostile environments. They can be found ubiquitous in nature and their overall diversity is considerable. Fungi are a group of eukaryotic microorganisms with approximately 300,000 species of fungi described in the literature. Fewer than 200 fungal species have been reported as human pathogens that can cause infections [5]. From an infection control point of view, we will concentrate in this chapter

M. Diab-El Schahawi
Department of Infection Control and Hospital Epidemiology, Medical University of Vienna, Vienna, Austria
e-mail: magda.diab-elschahawi@meduniwien.ac.at

E. Presterl (ed.), *Clinically Relevant Mycoses*, https://doi.org/10.1007/978-3-319-92300-0_11

on two medically relevant species of fungi, i.e., yeast and mold. Yeasts are single-celled fungi that reproduce by budding, whereas molds occur in filaments, so-called hyphae and grow by apical extension.

Candida species is the most prominent representative of opportunistic human pathogens belonging to the yeast family. Even though *Candida* species constitutes a part of the mycoflora of the normal human gastrointestinal tract and vagina, they may cause systemic infection in immunocompromised situations [6]. More than 90% of invasive infections are caused by *Candida albicans*, *Candida glabrata*, *Candida parapsilosis*, *Candida tropicalis*, and *Candida krusei*, each of them exhibiting unique antifungal susceptibility spectra [7]. Invasive fungal infections are severe and life-threatening complications in the immunocompromised or seriously ill patient populations. *Candida* species are the cause of nosocomial sepsis, septic shock, and lethal disseminated infection in critically ill patients admitted to the intensive care unit (ICU), rising over the past decade to the fourth most common pathogen causing nosocomial bloodstream infections in the United States [8]. Most nosocomial candidemia is thought to be endogenous, acquired through prior colonization acting as the source. The increasing frequency rate of serious *Candida* hospital infections in intensive care patients has multifactorial causes, including more increasing usage of intravascular catheters, broad-spectrum antibiotics, extensive surgery, and immunosuppression for neoplastic disease or allograft preservation. Despite the availability of potent antifungal agents, the mortality rate from invasive *Candida* infection is up to 65%. Valerio and colleagues used an antifungal adequacy score to evaluate antifungal prescriptions in their study population of 100 inpatients in a tertiary care institution receiving systemic antifungal therapy. They could show that almost half of overall antifungal prescriptions needed improvement with regard to need and drug selection and duration of antifungal therapy, deducing the urgent need for antifungal stewardship programs [9]. Therefore any hospital-wide antimicrobial stewardship program should include antifungal agents with regard to the prevention of IFD. Choice of antifungal agents for the management of IFDs should be guided by local epidemiology, thereby emphasizing the need for surveillance.

Human infections with environmental fungi are increasingly reported in the literature. Recently there has been an epidemiological shift in hematopoietic stem cell transplant recipients. The incidence of invasive mold infections is rising [10]. Kontoyiannis DP and colleagues found in their prospective surveillance for invasive fungal infections in hematopoietic stem cell transplant recipient (2001–2006) that invasive molds were the commonest fungi causing invasive fungal infection (IFI) and had also a high crude mortality within 90 days after diagnosis [10]. Mold species are the most frequent environmental fungal pathogens associated with invasive fungal disease in susceptible patients. They include *Scedosporium*, *Fusarium*, *Mucor*, and *Aspergillus* species with the latter still remaining the most prevalent cause of invasive mold infections in the immunocompromised host. *Aspergillus* spp. are saprophytic filamentous fungi that can be found ubiquitous in the environment. Their spores are capable of resisting dry, adverse environmental conditions where they can survive a long time. The conidia may travel long distances as airborne particles and are inhaled by humans [11]. For healthy individuals mold is not considered to be a health hazard. However for immunosuppressed individuals, mold could result in adverse health effects. Pulmonary infections arising by local tissue invasion do only occur if an incresaed host susceptibility is present.

Fungal contamination in the health-care environment has been reported to be a hazard to immunocompromised individuals. Dust production during construction work, renovation, or demolition activities within the hospital or in close surrounding areas has been reported as cause of nosocomial aspergillus outbreaks. Such activities are likely to increase the concentration of airborne fungal spores. Bouza and colleagues [12] sampled the air in and around their hospital main building before, during, and after demolition work of the maternity hospital complex situated directly opposite their main hospital building. During the demolition period, a significant increase of colony-forming fungal units was found as expected in the ambient air surrounding the hospital site but also in non-protected internal air samples. Other publications could demonstrate a potential relationship between the proximity of construction sites and the timely increased occurrence of invasive fungal infections in immunocompromised patients [13–16]. In the case of construction in and around health-care facilities, transmission to at-risk patients is of particular concern. The role of the inanimate environment in health-care facilities should always be considered in disease transmission when immunocompromised patients are involved. Protective measures are therefore necessary when it comes to hospital construction, especially in areas where susceptible patients are concerned.

Environmental infection control strategies as well as a close cooperation with the engineering departments regulating water, air, and medical device processing need to be an integral part of the health-care-associated infection control manual in order to prevent hospital-acquired infections due to the inanimate environment.

11.1 Baseline Infection Control Measures

- Cleaning and disinfection of the inanimate environment: compilation of all disinfection requirements including the appropriate use of cleaners and disinfectants summarized in a disinfection plan.
- Reprocessing of medical equipment (e.g., disinfection, sterilization, automated endoscope washer disinfector).
- Adherence to hospital-wide water quality standards with the establishment of an interdisciplinary water safety plan. Water used in health-care facilities needs to be monitored regularly for its quality.
- Adherence to hospital-wide ventilation standards with a focus on specialized care environments (e.g., airborne infection isolation rooms, protective isolation rooms, or operating rooms) and diligent maintenance of air filtration systems. Insufficient maintenance of ventilation systems has been shown to be a potential source of airborne outbreaks of aspergillosis in susceptible patient groups [17, 18].

Even though mold is not considered to be a health hazard for healthy individuals, it could result in adverse health effects in immunocompromised individuals. These patient groups are at increased risk of fungal infections which is of particular importance when it comes to building, renovation, and construction work in and around the hospital, as detailed earlier. Since airborne fungal spores can travel significant distances, preventive measures will have also to include all works in the immediate vicinity or within the boundary of the health-care facility. Early and sustained involvement of the infection control team in the planning process is essential and will lead to minimizing of potential infection risks. Before a new building project is started, the infection control team (ICT) needs to be involved early in the planning stage in order to perform a risk assessment to define the magnitude of necessary control measures [16]. This risk assessment has to account for the type of planned construction activity as well as for the involved patient groups. Fungal spores may also be dispersed during refurbishment activities considered at low-risk dust generation such as ceiling openings or recarpeting. Ideally renovation and construction work should be planned during periods without patient treatment (e.g., during ward maintenance closures). However sudden events with acute damage may warrant immediate refurbishment action, which needs to be closely supervised by the infection control team regarding infection prevention. The initial risk appraisal has to assess whether the ward can stay open during the time of the construction activities. Depending on the local structural circumstances (layout of the ward and surrounding departments), patients might have to be transferred to another ward altogether until construction work is finished and the ward is cleared/reopened for clinical use by the infection control department. Depending on the scope of the project, ICT needs to determine to what extent immunocompromised patients may be at risk for exposure to fungal spores from dust or water aerosols generated during the project. ICT needs to decide if patients whose rooms are adjacent to work zones need to be relocated, depending on their immune status, to an alternative ward during the construction phase, or if they can stay in place, the necessary infection control measures need to be defined. During the ongoing construction work, the infection control team should ensure implementation of infection control measures and closely supervise the adherence to established preventive measures, including a monitoring checklist. It is important to keep written records of summary statements of the infection control team's activities and recommendations for documentation purposes. Enhanced surveillance measures should be established before, during, and after high-risk activities such as a construction period to ensure the timely identification of outbreaks [19].

Preventive infection control measures necessary during construction or renovation periods described in this chapter are largely based on expert opinions as there is a lack of randomized controlled studies. Nevertheless the underlying principle recommendations are integral part of many international guidelines [20–22].

To prevent invasive fungal disease (IFD) in susceptible patient groups in health-care institutions, it is necessary to avoid patient's exposure to dust, stagnant water, and damp areas.

Therefore it is strongly recommended that:

- The area where renovation/construction/refurbishment work takes place needs to be tightly insulated from patient care areas.
- Access to these areas where mold contamination is known or suspected should be restricted.
- If access is unavoidable, personal protective equipment must be worn.
- Hands, skin, and clothing must be kept clean and free from mold-contaminated dust at any time.

Health-care workers and personnel coming in close contact with susceptible patients must equally adhere to above recommendations and change clothes if contact with fungal spores cannot be excluded.

11.2 Dust Protection Measures

During the planning phase of the construction project, an interdisciplinary team including representatives of the ICT should as far as possible determine special routes, corridors, and elevators designated for the construction crew only. Otherwise dust-producing work needs to be scheduled during low patient frequency periods in the outpatient setting or in phases according to vacancies after patient discharge and before readmission of new patients.

The routine building dust control measures may not be sufficient for the control of fungal spore release during construction work in the hospital setting; therefore, the following measures to limit dust exposure of patients and personnel should be considered [21]:

- Dust protection boundaries should encompass floor-to-ceiling barriers that completely enclose the work area.
- Windows and other sources of outside air intrusion in areas accommodating susceptible patients should be sealed to minimize ingress of dust and fungal spores generated by nearby building work.
- Negative air pressure should be maintained in construction areas adjacent to patient-care zones.
- Increase frequency of environmental cleaning services during construction work using methods to avoid dust generation such as wet-wiping tools.
- Transport debris in sealed containers with tightly fitting lids, or cover debris with a wet sheet.
- The removal of debris by chutes is liable to produce airborne fungal spores. The use and positioning of chutes should therefore be carefully considered.
- Try always to establish passageways/routes restricted to the construction crew and their import and export of relevant materials, in order to avoid transporting debris through

patient-care areas and minimize dust dispersion.
- Intermittent storage for clinical equipment and clean linen in daily use should be dry, clean, and dust protected.

If air-handling systems are in place, their proper operation needs to be verified before start of the construction phase and monitored regularly. The integrity of instituted construction barriers, window sealings, and door closure needs to be equally monitored on a regular base.

11.3 Water Damage Control

Water damage after leaks or water intrusion increases the likelihood of fungal growth in buildings/hospitals and therefore equally poses a threat to the immunocompromised patient population. It is estimated that humidity remaining for more than 48 h will generally support mold growth. Therefore the early start of remediation work is essential in order to prevent exposure to mold and resulting mold-related health effects. The only way to control mold growth is to identify the cause of the water damage and remediate it. Regardless of the original source of water damage, all wet materials must be identified and removed within 48 h, and replacement should only be allowed once the source of the water damage is located and repaired and the underlying structures are declared by an expert to be thoroughly dry. Additional assessment of the origin of the water damage is necessary for determining further actions. Either clean water (e.g., broken drinking water appliance) is involved or the so-called gray water (e.g., broken toilet). In the latter case, the water is most likely contaminated with fecal microorganisms and warrants additional decontamination/disinfection action. Interdisciplinary management of water leakages or water intrusion within the facility is therefore needed. Remediation activities need to follow the preventive measures discussed in the dust protection section of this chapter. Standardized air sampling procedures can be used to help detect hidden mold if no visible signs of mold can be identified, but contamination is still suspected due to the typical musty smell of mold. It should also be used to monitor progress of remediation work after water damage in areas hosting susceptible patient groups.

11.4 Environmental Sampling

Natural outdoor levels of environmental fungal spores vary seasonally, depending on weather conditions. Indoor concentration of particles and mold is influenced by various factors such as existing ventilation systems and their maintenance state, indoor activity, and cleaning frequency. No uniform recommendations regarding routine microbiologic air sampling before, during, or after construction in and around hospital wards are available. In general routine environmental microbiologic sampling is only advised when sampling results can be applied directly to infection-control decisions and to ensure quality assurance purposes. Because of the ubiquitous occurrence of environmental fungi causing invasive fungal disease in susceptible patients as well as the indefinite incubation period, disease causality is difficult to attribute, and the value of environmental sampling is being argued. Nevertheless, in hospital wards with functioning and correctly maintained ventilation systems, i.e., closed windows, fungal colony count measured at the beginning of the day directly after correct ward cleaning should be close to zero; otherwise either cleaning procedures were not efficacious or a fungal source should be considered. Preliminary determination of baseline values of fungal colony count for the concrete high-risk area using standardized air sampling procedures is advised before the construction phase starts. High-volume air samplers are recommended for this purpose rather than settle plates, as fungal spores can remain suspended in the air for very long periods [23]. Active environmental surveillance by initiating prospective longitudinal fungal microbiological surveillance during the whole construction activity to monitor background fungal colony count should follow for infection prevention and quality assurance purposes. Sudden rises in fungal colony count may signal a problem and warrant further investigation to identify potential areas for correction or improvement, followed by prompt corrective measures to eliminate potential fungal point sources or routes of entry.

11.5 Training and Education

It is very important to educate patient groups at risk for invasive fungal infections about their increased susceptibility and the necessary infection control measures. Accordingly special education of healthcare workers and on-site construction workers needs to raise awareness of the exceptional risk situation of invasive fungal infections in susceptible patient groups, focusing on possible airborne transmission routes associated with construction projects and dispersal of fungal spores during such activities. Methods to control the dissemination of fungal spores need to be emphasized.

11.6 Summary Statement

Patients at risk for invasive fungal disease are not anymore confined to special wards but can increasingly be found in every part of the healthcare environment. The types of fungal infection occurring in susceptible patients depend not only on the host's underlying disease but also on their epidemiological exposure. Data on IFI are still probably underestimated due to the lack of sensitivity of current detection methods as well as differences in diagnostic definitions used for invasive mold infections. On the other hand, the development of new diagnostic microbiological tools for fungal identification broadens our understanding of the role of "newly" recognized fungi in IFI [24]. The prevention of endogenous as well as exogenous invasive fungal infections in susceptible patient groups therefore necessitates a combination of antifungal stewardship with environmental infection control strategies.

References

1. Martin GS, Mannino DM, Eaton S, Moss M (2003) The epidemiology of sepsis in the United States from 1979 through 2000. N Engl J Med 348:1546–1554
2. Dasbach EJ, Davies GM, Teutsch SM (2000) Burden of aspergillosis-related hospitalizations in the United States. Clin Infect Dis 31:1524–1528
3. Gudlaugsson O, Gillespie S, Lee K, Vande Berg J, Hu J, Messer S, Herwaldt L, Pfaller M, Diekema D (2003) Attributable mortality of nosocomial candidemia, revisited. Clin Infect Dis 37:1172–1177
4. Wisplinghoff H, Bischoff T, Tallent SM, Seifert H, Wenzel RP, Edmond MB (2004) Nosocomial bloodstream infections in US hospitals: analysis of 24,179 cases from a prospective nationwide surveillance study. Clin Infect Dis 39(3):309–317
5. Brandt ME, Warnock DW (2003) Laboratory aspects of medical mycology. In: Dismukes WE, Pappas PG, Sobel JD (eds) Clinical mycology. Oxford University Press, New York, pp 1–22
6. Sardi JCO, Scorzoni L, Bernardi T, Fusco-Almeida AM, Mendes Giannini MJS (2013) Candida species: current epidemiology, pathogenicity, biofilm formation, natural antifungal products and new therapeutic options. J Med Microbiol 62:10–24
7. Pfaller MA, Diekema DJ (2007) Epidemiology of invasive candidiasis: a persistent public health problem. Clin Microbiol Rev 20(1):133–163
8. Cantón E, Espinel-Ingroff A, Peman J, del Castillo L (2010) In vitro fungicidal activities of echinocandins against Candida metapsilosis, C. orthopsilosis, and C. parapsilosis evaluated by time-kill studies. Antimicrob Agents Chemother 54:2194–2197
9. Valerio M, Rodriguez-Gonzalez CG, Muñoz P, Caliz B, Sanjurjo M, Bouza E, COMIC Study Group (Collaborative Group on Mycoses) (2014) Evaluation of antifungal use in a tertiary care institution: antifungal stewardship urgently needed. J Antimicrob Chemother 69(7):1993–1999
10. Kontoyiannis DP, Marr KA, Park BJ, Alexander BD, Anaissie EJ, Walsh TJ, Ito J, Andes DR, Baddley JW, Brown JM, Brumble LM, Freifeld AG, Hadley S, Herwaldt LA, Kauffman CA, Knapp K, Lyon GM, Morrison VA, Papanicolaou G, Patterson TF, Perl TM, Schuster MG, Walker R, Wannemuehler KA, Wingard JR, Chiller TM, Pappas PG (2010) Prospective surveillance for invasive fungal infections in hematopoietic stem cell transplant recipients, 2001–2006: overview of the transplant-associated infection surveillance network (TRANSNET) database. Clin Infect Dis 50(8):1091–1100
11. Denning DW (1998) Invasive aspergillosis. Clin Infect Dis 26(4):781–803

12. Bouza E, Peláez T, Pérez-Molina J, Marín M, Alcalá L, Padilla B, Muñoz P, Adán P, Bové B, Bueno MJ, Grande F, Puente D, Rodríguez MP, Rodríguez-Créixems M, Vigil D, Cuevas O, Team AS (2002) Demolition of a hospital building by controlled explosion: the impact on filamentous fungal load in internal and external air. J Hosp Infect 52(4):234–242
13. Burwen DR, Lasker BA, Rao N, Durry E, Padhye AA, Jarvis WR (2001) Invasive aspergillosis outbreak on a hematology-oncology ward. Infect Control Hosp Epidemiol 22(1):45–48
14. Vonberg RP, Gastmeier P (2006) Nosocomial aspergillosis in outbreak settings. J Hosp Infect 63(3):246–254
15. Srinivasan A, Beck C, Buckley T, Geyh A, Bova G, Merz W, Perl TM (2002) The ability of hospital ventilation systems to filter Aspergillus and other fungi following a building implosion. Infect Control Hosp Epidemiol 23(9):520–524
16. Berger J, Willinger B, Diab-Elschahawi M, Blacky A, Kalhs P, Koller W, Assadian O, Aichberger KJC et al (2011) Effectiveness of preventive measures for hemato-oncologic patients undergoing stem cell transplantation during a period of hospital construction. Am J Infect Control 39(9):746–751
17. Anderson K, Morris G, Kennedy H, Croall J, Michie J, Richardson MD, Gibson B (1996) Aspergillosis in immunocompromised paediatric patients: associations with building hygiene, design, and indoor air. Thorax 51(3):256–261
18. Ruutu P, Valtonen V, Tiitanen L, Elonen E, Volin L, Veijalainen P, Ruutu T (1987) An outbreak of invasive aspergillosis in a haematologic unit. Scand J Infect Dis 19(3):347–351
19. Chang CC, Ananda-Rajah M, Belcastro A, McMullan B, Reid A, Dempsey K, Athan E, Cheng AC, Slavin MA (2014) Consensus guidelines for implementation of quality processes to prevent invasive fungal disease and enhanced surveillance measures during hospital building works, 2014. Intern Med J 44(12b):1389–1397
20. Sehulster L, Chinn RYW, Arduino MJ, Carpenter J, Donlan R, Ashford D et al (2003) Guidelines for environmental infection control in health-care facilities. Recommendations of CDC and the Healthcare Infection Control Practices Advisory Committee (HICPAC). American Society for Healthcare Engineering/American Hospital Association, Chicago
21. Department of Health Estates and Facilities (UK) (2013) Health building note 00-09: infection control in the built environment UK. Department of Health, London
22. National Disease Surveillance Centre (Ireland) (2002) National guidelines for the prevention of nosocomial invasive aspergillus during construction/renovation activities. NDSC, Dublin
23. Morris G, Kokki MH, Anderson K, Richardson MD (2000) Sampling of aspergillus spores in air. J Hosp Infect 44(2):81–92
24. Roilides E (2016) Emerging fungi causing human infection: new or better identified? Clin Microbiol Infect 22(8):660–661

12 Pediatric Invasive Fungal Infections

Andreas Groll, Romana Klasinc, and Luigi Segagni-Lusignani

Invasive fungal infections occur in neonates and children with compromised immune system or in critical condition. Infections in these patients are due to *Candida*, *Aspergillus*, and other, less common opportunistic fungi.

12.1 Invasive *Candida* Infections

Invasive *Candida* infections are the most frequent fungal infections in pediatric patients and occur in similar settings as in adults. Accordingly, pediatric populations at risk are those with granulocytopenia due to chemotherapy for hemato oncological diseases, with immunosuppression following transplantation or for inflammatory diseases, and those with life-threatening conditions requiring intensive care. Specific risk factors for children admitted to the intensive care unit (ICU) include severe underlying diseases, prolonged stay in the ICU, use of broad-spectrum antibacterial agents, the presence of central venous catheters, mechanical ventilation, dialysis, status post-organ transplantation, and major surgery. *Candida* species were the 4th most frequent pathogen isolated in children and neonates in the European prevalence survey on health-care associated infections [1], and in a propensity analysis conducted in the USA, candidemia in pediatric patients was associated with a mean 21.1-day increase in length of hospital stay and a mean increase in total per-patient hospital charges of 92,266 dollars [2, 3]. *Candida albicans* accounts for approximately half of all invasive *Candida* infections, followed by *C. parapsilosis, C. glabrata, C. tropicalis,* and other non-albicans *Candida* spp. [4, 5]. Mortality rates in invasive *Candida* infection range between 10 and 25% but increase substantially in granulocytopenic patients and in patients admitted to the ICU [2, 3, 6–9]. Independent risk factors of mortality are organ site *Candida* infection, persistent candidemia, and failure to remove the vascular catheter [10].

Two groups of pediatric patients are at particular risk for invasive *Candida* infections (Fig. 12.1):

- Premature neonates with very low and extremely low birth weight who may develop candidemia and other forms of invasive candidiasis
- Immunocompromised patients with indwelling central venous catheters undergoing intensive chemotherapeutic regimens resulting in profound and prolonged granulocytopenia

A. Groll (✉)
Infectious Disease Research Program, Center for Bone Marrow Transplantation and Department of Pediatric Hematology/Oncology, University Children's Hospital Münster, Münster, Germany
e-mail: grollan@ukmuenster.de

R. Klasinc · L. Segagni-Lusignani
Department of Infection Control and Hospital Epidemiology, Medical University of Vienna, Vienna, Austria

E. Presterl (ed.), *Clinically Relevant Mycoses*, https://doi.org/10.1007/978-3-319-92300-0_12

Fig. 12.1 Pediatric populations at risk to develop opportunistic invasive fungal diseases

- Acute myeloid leukemia (AML)
- Acute lymphatic leukemia (ALL) if granulocytopenic and on steroids
- Recurrent leukemia (AML and ALL)

- Allogeneic hematopoietic stem cell transplantation
  - during granulocytopenia until engraftment
  - during augmented immunosuppression for GVHD

- Very low and extremely low birth weight
- Treatment for life-threatening problems in the ICU

... chronic granulomatous disease; chronic lung disease/ cystic fibrosis; lung- and heart/lung-, liver-, and small bowel/pancreas transplantation; decompensated metabolic diseases

12.1.1 Invasive *Candida* Infections in Low Birth Weight Premature Neonates

12.1.1.1 Illustrative Case

A preterm girl after cesarean section in the 26th week of gestation was transferred from the neonatal ward to the intensive care unit (ICU) because of new fever, increased laboratory markers of inflammation, respiratory instability, intermittent bradycardia, and hypotension. Antimicrobial therapy with ampicillin and gentamicin was changed to piperacillin-tazobactam and vancomycin. An abdominal X-ray made due to increasing abdominal distension with livid discoloration revealed free intraabdominal air and the decision for a laparotomy was made. The intraoperative findings were consistent with necrotizing enterocolitis and multiple perforations that were resected with subsequent placement of a bidirectional colostomy. Blood cultures obtained on the day of the procedure and an intraoperative smear showed growth of *C. albicans*. All indwelling catheters and tubes were immediately replaced and appropriate antifungal treatment was initiated.

In the last two decades, the survival rate of premature neonates has increased substantially. The risk of infection increases with the gestational age and the birth weight. Per definition, neonates with a birth weight ≥1250 g to <1500 g are classified as low birth weight infants (LBWI), those with a birth weight ≥1000 g to <1250 g as very low birth weight infants (VLBWI) and those with a birth weight of <1000 g as extremely low birth weight infants (ELBWI). Care in specialized neonatal intensive care units (NICUs) provides a survival in ELBWI of up to 33% for infants born at 23 weeks and 65% for infants born at 24 weeks gestation [11].

ELBWI are most at risk to acquire invasive *Candida* infection because the barrier function of their skin and mucosal membranes and all arms of innate and acquired immunity are not yet fully developed. Further risk factors include vaginal colonization of the mother with vaginal delivery, which may result in early onset invasive infection. Another entity is late-onset invasive *Candida* infection that occurs after 2–3 weeks of life. Risk factors for this entity include early gestational age (<26 gestational week), long-term antimicrobial therapy, treatment with glucocorticosteroids, long-term mechanical ventilation, parenteral nutrition, invasive procedures, invasive devices for life-support (central venous catheters, peripheral venous catheters), and abdominal surgery [12, 13].

Of note, between 4.8% and 10% of all VLBWI are found to be colonized with *Candida* spp. post-partum; within the following 4 weeks, up to 25% of these infants become colonized by horizontal [14, 15]. Vaginal colonization with *Candida* spp. during pregnancy is found in 25–30% of women, and 70–85% of colonized mothers transmit *Candida* spp. to their infants; as a consequence, 22–24% of all neonates are already colonized or infected at birth. Prenatal topical antifungal treatment of pregnant women may reduce vaginal *Candida* colonization from 25% to 7%, leading to a decrease in the colonization rate of the newborns from 20% to 3% [16]. Accordingly, treatment of maternal vaginal candidiasis prior to delivery is recommended in the literature as it may prevent subsequent neonatal colonization [17]. The German Society of Gynaecology and Obstetrics recommends screening by doing a vaginal culture at the 34th gestational week and at least week before the calculated delivery a local antifungal treatment is applied. If there is imminent premature delivery, the vaginal antifungal treatment should be administered earlier [18].

The clinical signs and symptoms of invasive *Candida* infections in neonates are not specific. Early onset or congenital invasive candidiasis is rare but life threatening. It may present initially as oral or anogenital thrush or disseminated dermatitis and develop into overt sepsis with deterioration of respiratory function and apnoea, instability of circulation and temperature, abdominal distention, irritability, and lethargy.

Invasive *Candida* infections occur in association with prolonged stays at the intensive care units and represent the third-leading cause of late-onset invasive sepsis in VLBWI [19–21]. Recent data suggests a decreasing incidence of invasive candidiasis in the NICU, and this is thought to be related to an increased use of antifungal prophylaxis and empirical antifungal therapy, as well as a decreased use of broad-spectrum antibacterial agents [22, 23].

12.1.2 Invasive *Candida* Infections in Children and Adolescents

12.1.2.1 Illustrative Case

An 11-year-old-girl was hospitalized and treated with chemotherapy after placement of a port-a-cath because of chordoma. Unfortunately, progressive disease was diagnosed shortly before the end of treatment in the form of a diffuse leptomeningeal and ventricular spread of tumor cells. Following a cycle of intensive second-line chemotherapy and continuing treatment with dexamethasone for increased intracranial pressure, the patient developed fever during granulocytopenia and received empirical treatment with broad-spectrum antibacterial agents. While initial blood cultures remained sterile, a specimen from the indwelling urinary catheter and blood cultures obtained several days after admission because of persisting fever grew Candida dubliniensis. The patient was placed on appropriate antifungal treatment and the catheter was surgically removed at 30 h after the report of the positive blood culture.

The clinical syndromes of invasive candidiasis in older children are similar to those in adults. *Candida* spp. are important causes of health-care associated infections in pediatric cancer patients receiving treatment for hematological malignancies, in pediatric allogeneic hematopoietic stem cell transplant recipients, and in children and adolescents with indwelling central venous catheters. Severe sepsis and/or septic shock eventually develops in approximately 30%, and mortality ranges between 10 and 25% and reaches 50% in patients admitted to the intensive care unit. Invasive candidiasis is also a clinically important syndrome in solid organ transplant recipients with incidence rates of 5–15% in patients with liver, small bowel, and pancreas transplantation [24, 25]. Candidemia occurs in cancer patients with neutropenia, in critically ill patients with prolonged hospitalization in the intensive care unit, in those with abdominal surgery, "short gut" syndrome, and total parenteral nutrition, and is found usually in conjunction with an indwelling central venous catheter [26]. Acute disseminated candidiasis with hemodynamic and inflammatory signs of sepsis and metastatic skin lesions may follow candidemia. *C. glabrata* and *C. tropicalis* are more frequent in children with hematological malignancies than in other patients probably due to the increased use of azoles and amphotericin B in these patients.

Chronic disseminated candidiasis (hepatosplenic candidiasis) is a well-established syndrome that occurs in children with hematological malignancies during and after recovery from neutropenia. It is characterized by persistent fever and upper abdominal pain as well as increased inflammatory indices, alkaline phosphatase, and gamma-glutamyltransferase but not transaminases. Ultrasounds, MRI may reveal "bull's eye" shaped small abscesses throughout the liver and spleen. The disease can last weeks to months despite appropriate antifungal therapy and is maintained by an ineffective inflammatory response [24].

12.1.3 Organ- or Tissue-Specific *Candida* Infections

12.1.3.1 Meningoencephalitis

Candidemia in neonates may be associated with meningoencephalitis in as many as 25% of the cases. In contrast, it is rarely diagnosed in older children with malignancies. Symptoms include signs and symptoms of sepsis but also any kind of central nervous symptoms. If there is any suspicion of central nervous infection, cerebrospinal fluid shall be obtained for inflammatory markers and culture. However, the culture from the cerebrospinal fluid (CSF) is frequently negative, and abnormal CSF findings and the blood culture positivity for *Candida* are diagnostic [24]

Chorioretinitis and endophthalmitis occur usually due to hematogenous seeding of *Candida* during candidemia. Fundoscopy reveals yellow-white, fluffy patch retinitis with indistinct border. Although treatment of endophthalmitis usually consists of vitrectomy and instillation of amphotericin B, use of systemic antifungal therapy alone may be curative depending on the extent of the disease. However, loss of vision may occur [24].

12.1.3.2 *Candida* Endocarditis

Candida endocarditis is rare but usually very serious with a high likelihood of a fatal outcome. Surgical removal of the affected valve should be attempted if possible. Most cases occur in children with congenital or acquired heart disease. Prolonged use of broad-spectrum antibiotics along with central venous catheters has been identified as predisposing factors. In patients with persistent fever and persistent candidemia, endocarditis should always be ruled out by appropriate studies [27, 28].

12.1.3.3 *Candida* Pneumonia

The presence of *Candida* spp. in respiratory specimens usually is colonization when the patient is intubated, mechanically ventilated, and receiving broad-spectrum antibacterial agents. Candida invading the lung parenchyma (bronchopneumonia) is rare and usually seen only at autopsy. *Candida* involvement may occur in the form of septic metastases in patients with acute or chronic disseminated candidiasis [29].

12.1.3.4 Urinary Tract Infection

Urinary tract infection can present as cystitis, pyelonephritis, or as fungal balls within the kidneys. In addition to urine culture, ultrasound and MRI scans facilitate diagnosis of these syndromes. Fungal balls are usually refractory to antifungal therapy and in some refractory cases may require surgery.

12.1.3.5 Peritonitis

Peritonitis may occur in children with end stage renal insufficiency, who are on continuous ambulatory peritoneal dialysis (CAPD), and usually presents with abdominal pain and low-grade fever. Peritoneal fluid neutrophil count is increased and its culture may be positive for *Candida* spp. Peritonitis may also occur following prolonged intraabdominal procedures or following bowel perforation and may be associated with fungemia [24].

12.1.3.6 Osteoarticular Infections

Osteoarticular infections are relatively rare and predominantly occur in neonates. In neonates, *Candida* can infect the bone and the joint simultaneously (osteoarthritis) and the infection is almost always hematogenous. In older children infection occurs either hematogenously or through contiguous spread of the organism, and it can be either osteomyelitis or arthritis. The most frequent bones affected are femur, humerus, then vertebra/ribs, whereas the joints frequently affected are knee, hip, and shoulder. Spondylodiscitis is a specific form of osteomyelitis that requires particularly careful surgery in conjunction with antifungal therapy [30].

12.1.3.7 Skin Manifestations

Skin manifestations are the typical erythematous, maculopapular lesion of cutaneous *Candida* infection. Most commonly these lesions are found around the mouth, perianal region, and at the perineum. However, they may occur anywhere on the skin. They need to be distinguished from septic metastases that may be observed as sequelae of candidemia (acute disseminated candidiasis).

12.1.4 Chronic Mucocutaneous Candidiasis

12.1.4.1 Illustrative Case

A 3-year-old girl was referred to the Immunology service for a long-standing history of aphthous stomatitis and diaper rash with incomplete resolution upon topical treatment. The remainder of her past medical history was unremarkable except for the fact that the diagnosis of chronic mucocutaneous candidiasis in her father. Physical examination was significant for marked oropharyngeal candidiasis and chronic dermatitis in the diaper area but no apparent lesions at the remaining skin, the nails, and hair. Swabs taken from the oral mucosa and the perianal region grew *C. albicans*, and molecular genetics revealed a heterozygous mutation in the STAT1-gene. Mucosal candidiasis was rapidly controlled by systemic treatment with fluconazole. Three years after diagnosis, the patient is managed with continuous oral amphotericin and systemic treatment with fluconazole on demand.

Chronic mucocutaneous candidiasis (CMC) is characterized by persistent and recurrent infection of mucous membranes, skin, and nails predominantly by *C. albicans*. Most commonly, CMC is diagnosed before the age of 3 with persistent or recurrent diaper rash or oral *Candida* infection, but the condition may be first recognized at a later age and even in adulthood. The clinical presentation includes erosion and inflammation of the mucous membranes of the mouth and the esophagus; inflammation of the edges of the mouth (perleche) and vulvovaginal candidiasis are also common. The mucous membranes are covered with white or cream-colored film (thrush); in vaginitis there is a typical creamy white discharge. Affected nails are thickened, miscolored, and fragile with frequent co-infections by dermatophytes [31]. Despite chronic-recurrent and often extensive superficial infections, patients with CMC do not have a general predisposition to develop invasive candidiasis.

CMC is linked to a couple of congenital de novo or inherited immunodeficiencies. Impaired functions of interleukin-17 and/or errors in its pathway have been recognized as major contributor to CMC. Patients with autosomal dominant hyper-IgE syndrome or autosomal recessive autoimmune polyendocrinopathy syndrome 1 display various phenotypes that include CMC as common feature. Casanova et al. identified loss-of-function mutations of the IL17F, IL-17 receptor A (IL17RA), IL17RC, and actin-related gene 1 (ACT1) genes in patients with isolated CMC, of whom some are also linked to staphylococcal or mycobacterial infections [32]. In addition, many patients with inherited CMC were found to carry STAT1 gain-of-function mutations [33].

Diagnosis of CMC in children is based on a history of recurrent, progressive, or treatment-resistant oral *Candida* infection (thrush) and/or *Candida* diaper dermatitis. However, thrush and diaper dermatitis are very common in infants, and observing the clinical course and excluding any risk factors and other conditions that contribute to *Candida* infection are always indicated before an inherited immunodeficiency is to be considered and the patient is referred to a center for rare diseases where specific diagnostic testing is available.

12.1.5 Evaluation of the Patient

Microscopy and culture of appropriate specimens remain the gold standards of mycological diagnosis. Successful management of invasive *Candida* infections relies on early recognition and rapid initiation of effective treatment [25].

Whereas blood cultures are state of the art for diagnosis of candidemia, however, only 50% or fewer of autopsy-proven cases of invasive candidiasis can be detected by this method in adults [34]. In neonates, the estimated sensitivity of blood cultures to detect *Candida* is not higher than 50–75%, and even in children below 2 kg of body weight, at least 2–4 mL of blood should be obtained [35]. Since candidemia occurs intermittently, blood cultures should be taken at least at two different occasions. Furthermore, since candidemia is often associated with meningoencephalitis, cerebrospinal fluid should be examined when candidemia is suspected or confirmed in a neonate.

When an organism has grown in culture, it must be identified to the species level especially when it is derived from a sterile site. Testing of susceptibility to antifungal agents is necessary for strains isolated from sterile sites. Some of the non-albicans isolates, such as *C. krusei* and a large proportion of *C. glabrata*, are not susceptible to fluconazole. *C. parapsilosis* may exhibit high MIC values for echinocandins (although this usually is not clinically important), and *C. lusitaniae* may be resistant to amphotericin B [24].

Hematologic parameters (white blood cell and platelet counts), C-reactive protein, interleukin-6, procalcitonin, and other biomarkers are also used to predict infection in neonates and critically ill children, but all of them lack sensitivity and specificity in the diagnosis of *Candida* infection. The sensitivities and specificities of fungal antigens (mannan, glucan) are between 40–90 and 60–100%, respectively, but their clinical correlation is poorly defined as is the role of PCR-based methods, although performance parameters are reported to be as high as 100% in select studies. Thus, antigen markers and PCR-based methods are not currently recommended for routine use in pediatric patients [24, 25]. To distinguish colonization from invasive disease often is challenging. In candiduria, consideration of clinical parameters, removal of a urine catheter and repeat urine culture, ultrasound of kidneys, and blood cultures should be used to decide whether the presence of *Candida* in the urine is a sign of invasive disease. Similarly, interpretation of *Candida* growth in endotracheal tube secretion cultures requires consideration of the presence of lung opacities and other indices of lung inflammation. Almost always it does not correspond to lung infection by *Candida* [24].

Imaging is an important tool and guided by clinical findings. Ultrasound of heart, liver, spleen, kidneys, or neonatal brain is a very useful and immediately available diagnostic tool and yields reliable results. In addition, MRI is helpful for diagnosing osteoarticular infections and brain abscesses as well as other organ infections in cases, where ultrasound findings are unclear. Finally, ophthalmological examination is a reliable tool for diagnosis of chorioretinitis or endophthalmitis and is required in all cases of candidemia prior to the stop of antifungal therapy.

12.1.6 Antifungal Agents for Management of Invasive Candidiasis

Important considerations when choosing the antifungal agent and the mode of application include the localization of the infection, the severity of the disease, impairment of liver and renal functions, previous exposure to antifungal agents, identified *Candida* species, and local or institutional patterns of resistance [25, 36]. Currently, four classes of systemic antifungal agents are available and approved for management of fungal infections in neonates, children, and adolescents: polyenes, triazoles, echinocandins, and flucytosine (Table 12.1) [37].

The class of polyenes includes natamycin, nystatin, amphotericin B deoxycholate (DAMB), amphotericin B lipid complex (ABLC), and liposomal amphotericin B (LAMB). All amphotericin B formulations are intravenously administered and are fungicidal against most *Candida* species, with the possible exception of *Candida guilliermondii* and *Candida lusitaniae*. Natamycin and nystatin are available only for topical applications. For decades, conventional amphotericin B (DAMB) has been the cornerstone of antifungal treatment; nevertheless, its use is limited by relevant glomerular and tubular renal toxicity and

Table 12.1 Pediatric dosages of systemic antifungal agents used for management of invasive fungal diseases[a]

	Daily dosage per age group[a]			
Agent	13–18 years	2–12 years	1–24 months	Neonates
Amphotericin B deoxycholate	1–1.5 mg/kg IV QD	1–1.5 mg/kg IV QD	1–1.5 mg/kg IV QD	1–1.5 mg/kg IV QD
Liposomal Amphotericin B	3 (-5) mg/kg IV QD	3 (-5) mg/kg IV QD	3 (-5) mg/kg IV QD	3 (-5) mg/kg IV QD
Amphotericin B Lipid Complex	5 mg/kg IV QD	5 mg/kg IV QD	5 mg/kg IV QD	5 mg/kg IV QD
5-Flucytosine[b]	50 mg/kg IV/PO TID	50 mg/kg IV/PO TID	50 mg/kg IV/PO TID	50 mg/kg IV/PO TID
Fluconazole	12 mg/kg IV/PO QD	12 mg/kg IV/PO QD	12 mg/kg IV/PO QD	12 mg/kg IV/PO QD
Itraconazole suspension[b]	2.5 mg/kg PO BID	2.5 mg/kg PO BID	n/a	n/a
Voriconazole[b]	4 mg/kg (d 1:6) IV BID 200–300 mg PO BID	8 mg/kg (d 1:9) IV BID 9 mg/kg PO BID	n/a n/a	n/a n/a
Posaconazole[b]	300 mg IV QD (d1: 300 BID) 300 mg PO QD (d1: 300 BID)	n/a n/a	n/a n/a	n/a n/a
Isavuconazole	n/a	n/a	n/a	n/a
Caspofungin	50 mg/m^2 (d1: 70) IV QD	50 mg/m^2 (d1: 70) IV QD	50 mg/m^2 (d1: 70) IV QD	25 mg/m^2 (d1: 70) IV QD
Micafungin	100–200 mg IV QD	2–4 mg/kg IV QD	2–4 mg/kg IV QD	(4)–10 mg/kg IV QD

[a]For detailed indications, please refer to the text. *IV* intravenous, *PO* oral, *QD* once daily, *BID* twice daily, *TID* three times daily, *n/a* no sufficient data

[b]Therapeutic drug monitoring strongly advised

infusion-related reactions of fever, chills, and rigor. ABLC and LAMB show less nephrotoxicity than DAMB, while infusion-related adverse effects are substantially less with LAMB only. Since the disposition of the three formulations in neonates and other pediatric patients is not different from that in adults, they can be dosed at similar weight-based dosages as in adults. The overall spectrum of adverse effects is likewise similar, with the potential exception for better renal tolerance in children that is most likely age-related. Whereas DAMB and LAMB have approved first-line indications for treatment of invasive candidiasis, ABLC is approved as second-line alternative only [36].

The currently available systemic antifungal triazoles encompass fluconazole, itraconazole, voriconazole, posaconazole, and isavuconazole. All triazoles are fungistatic against *Candida* spp., which is a limiting factor in critically ill patients: In direct comparisons with the fungicidal echinocandins, trends for better outcomes were consistently noted for the echinocandin. The triazoles are effective against *C. albicans*, while non-*C. albicans* spp. show increasing resistance to fluconazole, a fact that is believed to be related to the wide use of this agent as antifungal prophylaxis. Fluconazole exhibits no activity against *C. krusei* and variable activity against *C. glabrata*. The so-called second generation triazoles (voriconazole, posaconazole, and isavuconazole) have a wider therapeutic range including *C. glabrata*, *C. krusei,* and many filamentous fungi with varying degrees of cross-resistance. Although the triazoles are considered safe and well-tolerated drugs, liver enzyme elevation is a common side effect; serious hepatotoxicity including hepatic failure may occur but is rare. The triazoles are metabolized through cytochrome P450 isoenzymes and caution should be implemented with the concomitant use of other drugs sharing the same metabolic pathways. Due to a high degree of intra- and interindividual pharmacokinetic variability, therapeutic drug monitoring (TDM) is recommended for itraconazole, voriconazole, and posaconazole suspension [36]. Whereas the use of itraconazole, posaconazole, and isavuconazole for treatment of invasive candidiasis is not supported by appropriate clinical trials, fluconazole and voriconazole are approved for prevention and treatment on invasive *Candida* infections. Nevertheless, voriconazole (approved in subject 2 years and older) plays a minor role for treatment of invasive candidiasis due to inconsistent exposure and need for TDM. In contrast, fluconazole is approved in children of all ages, has an excellent safety profile, and displays favorable pharmacokinetics with excellent penetration into the CSF and the urine. Of note, based on pharmacokinetic/pharmacodynamic considerations, the maximum approved pediatric dose should be used for treatment of invasive candidiasis [36].

The echinocandins (anidulafungin, caspofungin, and micafungin) are available as parenteral compounds and are fungicidal against most *Candida* spp., including azole-resistant strains. They all display excellent tissue penetration, with the exception of the CSF, the eyes, and the urinary tract, and they can be dosed once daily. Echinocandins are mostly metabolized by the liver, but are not processed to a greater extent by the cytochrome 450 enzyme system, resulting in a low potential for drug interactions. The echinocandins are very well tolerated by both liver and kidney with few if any relevant adverse events, and are approved for first-line treatment of invasive candidiasis in adults (all), children, and neonates (caspofungin and micafungin). While data for neonates are quite limited for caspofungin, solid preclinical and clinical data exists for micafungin with a sound pharmacokinetic/pharmacodynamic rationale for use of high doses in neonates to consider the high frequency of *Candida* meningoencephalitis in this population [25, 36].

Flucytosine has excellent oral bioavailability and organ distribution including the CSF, and demonstrates broad antifungal activity against *Candida* spp. Because of rapid emergence of resistance, it is only used as part of combination therapy with amphotericin B, with potential indications in complicated invasive *Candida* infections. The compound is approved in children at similar weight-based doses as in adults. Its main indication is induction treatment of cryptococcal meningoencephalitis in combination with DAMB or LAMB [36].

12.1.7 Options for Treatment of Documented *Candida* Infections

Options for first-line therapy of candidemia and most other forms of invasive candidiasis approved by the FDA and/or the EMA for all pediatric age groups include liposomal amphotericin B (LAMB; 3 mg/kg QD IV), fluconazole (FCZ; 12 mg/kg QD IV), caspofungin (CAS; 50 mg/msqu QD IV; day 1: 70 mg/msqu; max.: 70 mg QD; neonates: 25 mg/msqu QD), and micafungin (MICA; <40 kg: 2–4 mg/kg QD IV; ≥40 kg: 100–200 mg QD; premature neonates at risk to develop meningoencephalitis: 10 mg/kg QD) (Table 12.1) [5, 25, 36, 38].

Criteria for selecting the initial regimen include the clinical status of the patient, organ impairment, concomitant medications, pretreatment with antifungal agents, the *Candida* species isolated, and its resistance pattern: Patients who have received azole prophylaxis are hemodynamically instable or granulocytopenic, who are colonized with *C. glabrata* or *C. krusei*, or are admitted at institutions with a high frequency of these organism should receive a polyene or echinocandin upfront [25, 36]. As outcome depends critically on the prompt initiation of appropriate antifungal chemotherapy, risk-based, preemptive approaches have been proposed for adult ICU patients; however, no data exist for pediatric patients.

Amphotericin B lipid complex (ABLC; 5 mg/kg QD IV; approval status) and voriconazole (VCZ; children 2–11 years and adolescents 12–14 years weighing <50 kg: 2 × 8 mg/kg IV (day 1: 2 × 9 mg/kg); adolescents 12–14 years weighing >50 kg and those 15 years and beyond: 2 × 4 mg/kg IV (2 × 6 mg day 1); cave interactions; adverse events and need for TDM) are options for second-line therapy or when additional coverage for molds is required [25, 36, 39, 40]. Due to its inferior safety profile in comparison to newer agents, the use of deoxycholate amphotericin B (1 mg/kg QD IV) is controversial in subjects beyond the neonatal age.

Similar to adults, central venous catheters should be removed promptly if feasible. Neutropenic patients should receive colony-stimulating factors (G-CSF or GM-CSF, respectively), and in patients on immunosuppressive therapy, steroids should be reduced, discontinued, or replaced. Follow-up blood cultures should be taken in order to assess treatment efficacy. Treatment should last at least 14 days after documented clearance of infection from the bloodstream and resolution of symptoms, in the absence of dissemination. Following clearance of the bloodstream and clinical stabilization, oral consolidation with fluconazole is feasible for susceptible isolates. Fundoscopy is mandatory prior to end of treatment to rule out endophthalmitis [25, 36].

Treatment of invasive candidiasis of deep tissues and compartments other than blood is ill defined. It is based mostly on pharmacological considerations such as a cidal mode of action and water-solubility and experiences from small case series [25, 36]. Therapy usually lasts longer and can extend to months. The degree of immunosuppression and the presence of foreign material, such as prosthetic valves, influence the duration and efficacy of treatment, while in many cases surgical intervention might be warranted. In most cases of deep-seated *Candida* infections, treatment options include fluconazole in stable patients or LAMB alone or in combination with flucytosine. Echinocandins present an option with the exception of CNS and eye infections due to unsatisfactory penetration. Fluconazole consolidation therapy after clinical improvement is recommended in many cases [24].

Distinction between infection and colonization is essential in candiduria and *Candida* isolation from respiratory secretions. Isolated candiduria usually needs no antifungal therapy and removal of predisposing factors (i.e., urinary catheter) is sufficient. If invasive disease is suspected, treatment as for candidemia is proposed. Based on their excretion into the urine, fluconazole and amphotericin B deoxycholate with or without the addition of flucytosine are the most appropriate agents for susceptible urinary tract infections. Isolation of *Candida* spp. in respiratory tract secretions represents colonization in virtually all cases and no antifungal therapy is required.

For CNS infections such as meningitis, meningoencephalitis, or infections related to foreign bodies, i.e., shunts, AMB preparations (conventional amphotericin B (1 mg/kg QD) or liposomal amphotericin B (5 mg/kg QD)), due to their sufficient CNS penetration, are the drugs of choice, preferentially in combination with flucytosine (100 mg/kg and day in 3–4 divided doses IV). Fluconazole (12 mg/kg QD IV) can also be used, alone or in combination with flucytosine. In the case of an infected shunt, it is very important that the foreign body is removed. The duration of therapy is at least 21 days [24]. Treatment of endophthalmitis often requires combination therapy with fluconazole or LAMB and flucytosine and long-term follow-up. Voriconazole is an alternative agent with good ocular penetration. Intravitreal amphotericin B or voriconazole are occasionally necessary for the treatment of endophthalmitis [24].

Candida endocarditis requires liposomal amphotericin B or an echinocandin usually in combination for several weeks. Early surgery is necessary in most cases. The advent of the new antifungal agents and the use of combination therapy has improved outcome [25].

In hepatosplenic candidiasis, prolonged therapy is required and the addition of corticosteroids might be beneficial, as an inflammatory reaction is the main driver of its pathogenesis and clinical disease. Peritonitis due to *Candida* spp. in patients on CAPD usually requires both systemic administration of fluconazole or LAMB and removal of the peritoneal catheter. Local infusions of amphotericin B may cause chemical peritonitis and may be painful. An echinocandin or voriconazole may replace LAMB based on species identification and MIC values [24].

For oropharyngeal and genital infections, topical treatment with azoles and/or polyenes is usually sufficient. If local therapy is not sufficient, systemic administration of an azole (fluconazole or itraconazole) is required. For esophagitis, systemic therapy with fluconazole is advised with echinocandins and LAMB as alternative agents. For chronic mucocutaneous candidiasis (CMC), topical azoles and/or polyenes are often effective but may need to be given continuously due to the propensity for recurrent infection in most patients. However, topical therapies are not effective for nail infections. For these and other more recalcitrant infections or exacerbations, systemic use of antifungal triazoles such as fluconazole and itraconazole is indicated. Treatment failure may be due to emergence of resistance (rare) and superinfection by other pathogens (dermatophytes; Staphylococci). Novel therapies based on the underlying mechanisms of the immunodeficiency are conceivable for the future but not yet available [33].

12.1.8 Prophylaxis in High-Risk Patients

Due to high morbidity and mortality, antifungal prophylaxis has been recommended in high-risk patients both in neonates and in children.

In NICUs with a high prevalence of invasive candidiasis, prophylaxis is recommended for all neonates with a birth weight <1000 g. Fluconazole 3 or 6 mg/kg 2 times per week is administered IV or orally. This policy leads to reduction in *Candida* colonization as well as fungal infection, but no to change in overall mortality; concerns of emergence of resistant species have not been substantiated [41–45]. In NICUs with a lower incidence of invasive candidiasis (i.e., <2%) for neonates with birth weight <1000 g who have risk factors (i.e., central venous catheters, use 3rd generation cephalosporins and carbapenems) for the development of invasive candidiasis, fluconazole 3 or 6 mg/kg 2 times per week iv or orally is recommended on an individual basis [24].

Recommendations for the prevention of invasive candidiasis in immunocompromised children are largely extrapolated from studies performed in adults with concomitant pharmacokinetic data and models in children. Antifungal prophylaxis should be implemented in allogeneic stem cell transplant recipients with neutropenia (<500 cell/mm^3); liver and pancreas transplant recipients; and possibly PICU patients in institutions with high rate of candidiasis (>10%), who have prior colonization with *Candida* in multiple body sites, total parenteral nutrition, exposure to broad-spectrum antimicrobial agents for >3 days especially those with antianaerobic activity, vancomycin, carbapenems, and others; and those with multiple abdominal surgeries [24, 25].

Prophylactic FCZ (8–12 mg/kg QD) remains a standard in antifungal prophylaxis post-allogeneic hematopoietic stem cell transplantation (HSCT) due to its marked effect on long-term outcome. Alternatives may include the use of VCZ or micafungin (1 mg/kg QD). In patients with graft-vs.-host disease (GVHD) and increased immunosuppression, posaconazole has been shown to prevent invasive fungal infections and invasive aspergillosis [46]. In adults with AML/MDS, posaconazole had a significant impact on the frequency of invasive fungal infections and invasive aspergillosis coupled with an overall survival benefit [47]. Limited data in children >12 years of age suggest no differences in pharmacokinetics as compared to adults. Therefore, as a practical approach, posaconazole tablets may be given to children with high-risk hematological malignancies or augmented immunosuppression for GVHD >12 years of age, and voriconazole in younger children. Alternatives include the intermittent administration of LAMB (1 mg/kg QOD) or micafungin (1 mg/kg QD) [36].

12.1.9 Empiric Therapy in High-Risk Patients

Empiric therapy is the administration of antifungal treatment in patients with clinical signs or laboratory indications of fungal infection. While colonization with *Candida* does not require therapy, if a patient is colonized at multiple sites (possibly at least 2) and has nonspecific signs of infection, he may be in need for empiric antifungal therapy. Clinical scoring systems of prediction of candidemia are used in adults, but they have not been validated in children. A clinical prediction rule for children in PICU, based on combinations of various risk factors most important of which were the presence of a central venous catheter, malignancy, use of vancomycin for >3 days in the prior 2 weeks, and receipt of agents against anaerobic organisms for >3 days in the prior 2 weeks, has been suggested [7]. As a first choice empiric treatment in non-neutropenic children fluconazole (12 mg/kg QD) or echinocandins can be used.

Empirical antifungal therapy is an established standard of care in high-risk hemato-oncological patients with prolonged neutropenia (absolute neutrophil count <500/≥10 days) and refractory or new fever that provides targeted prevention in a high-risk setting. Agents approved by the FDA and/or the EMA for this indication in pediatric patients of all age groups include LAMB (1–3 mg/kg QD) and CAS (50 mg/msqu QD; day 1: 70 mg/msqu; max.: 70 mg QD) (Maertens PIDJ Pediatric CAS vs. LAMB; [36, 48]).

12.2 Invasive *Aspergillus* Infections

12.2.1 Instructive Case

A 5-year-old profoundly granulocytopenic boy with newly diagnosed acute lymphoblastic leukemia was started on induction chemotherapy consisting of high-dose prednisone, vincristine, daunorubicin, and PEG-asparaginase. In week three, he developed a new onset of moderate pain in the right lateral chest wall upon deeper inspiration while on empirical antibacterial therapy for persisting fever. A low dose chest CT was ordered and revealed several up to 1 cm in diameter rounded lesions. Because he appeared less alert and complained also of slight headaches, the CT was followed a few hours later by cranial magnetic resonance imaging (MRI) that showed several smaller embolic lesions. The patient was immediately placed on voriconazole plus caspofungin at age-appropriate dosages. A bronchoscopy and antigen testing were performed, which revealed *Aspergillus fumigatus* in bronchoalveolar (BAL) fluid and *Aspergillus* galactomannan antigen in BAL fluid and serum. Unfortunately, while in stable respiratory and neurological condition, the boy died a few days later from peracute pulmonary hemorrhage in the pediatric oncology unit.

Filamentous fungi of the order *Aspergillus* may cause a broad spectrum of conditions in children, including pulmonary hypersensitivity reactions, saprophytic colonization of pathologic airway structures, and life-threatening invasive infections predominantly of the lung with or without dissemination in patients with congenital or acquired deficiencies in host defenses. Most cases of human disease are caused by *Aspergillus fumigatus*, followed by *Aspergillus flavus*, and, less commonly, *Aspergillus nidulans*, *Aspergillus niger*, and *Aspergillus terreus*. Aspergilli are predominantly saprophytes, growing on dead or decaying matter in the environment; the usual portal of entry is the respiratory tract through inhalation of *Aspergillus conidia* [8, 9, 36, 49].

12.2.1.1 Invasive Aspergillosis in Immunocompromised Children

The most important clinical risk factors for invasive *Aspergillus* infections include prolonged and profound granulocytopenia (<500 neutrophil granulocytes/µl for ≥10 days) and functional deficiencies of neutrophil granulocytes and macrophages. T-cell dependent, acquired defense mechanisms are involved but appear to be of limited epidemiological relevance. Nonimmunological factors also are important and include damage to protective surfaces of skin and mucosa and co-morbidities such as cytomegaloviral diseases.

Based on data obtained prior to the existence of prophylactic or preemptive antifungal therapy, the risk of developing invasive aspergillosis is highest in children with acute myeloid leukemia and recurrent leukemias (25%), acute lymphoblastic leukemia (approx. 5%), post-allogeneic hematopoietic stem cell transplantation (HSCT) during the time until engraftment, during augmented immunosuppression for GVHD and profound T-cell deficiency (approximately 10% each), following liver transplantation (up to 10%), and lung and heart-lung transplantation (up to 30%, including tracheobronchial aspergillosis). Patients with chronic granulomatous disease (CGD) have a cumulative lifetime infection rate of up to 40%. Sporadic cases have been reported in children without one of these conditions receiving treatment in the ICU, in patients with chronic destructive lung diseases and in premature neonates (Fig. 12.1).

Invasive pulmonary aspergillosis is the most frequent entity with dissemination predominantly to the central nervous system (CNS) in approximately 30% of cases. Fever, cough, and dyspnea, although nonspecific and not obligatory, represent the main symptoms; pleuritic chest pain and potentially life-threatening hemoptysis may occur in granulocytopenic patients, particularly during the time of granulocyte recovery. Tracheobronchial forms of invasive aspergillosis also may occur and have been reported predominantly in non-granulocytopenic, immunocompromised patients. CNS aspergillosis should be considered in immunocompromised patients with acute onset of focal or diffuse neurological signs and symptoms. Facial swelling, facial pain, black or brownish nasal secretions, proptosis, and cranial nerve abnormalities are suggestive of invasive paranasal sinus infection. Primary cutaneous or gastrointestinal aspergillosis is a rare clinical entity whose symptoms are determined by the site and the extent of the infection.

The outcome of invasive aspergillosis is mostly dismal, particularly following allogeneic HSCT, and after liver transplantation. Case fatality rates at 3 months post-diagnosis outside of the setting of clinical registration trial may be well above 50% with worse prognosis in patients with persisting granulocytopenia or immunosuppression, CNS involvement, and major hemorrhage [8, 9, 36, 49].

12.2.1.2 Approaches to Diagnosis

Early recognition and rapid initiation of effective treatment are paramount for control of invasive aspergillosis. Knowledge of epidemiology, risk factors and populations at risk, a careful history, and a meticulous physical examination provide guidance for a targeted imaging and further workup. Identification of the causative agent and resistance testing should always be attempted. While microscopy and culture obtained from the clinically affected site remain the gold standard, technical problems in obtaining a specimen, the time of culturing and negative results are limiting factors; with 50% sensitivity, the diagnostic yield of histology also is unsatisfactory. Given this background, detection of fungal cell wall antigens and DNA in blood and other tissues may enhance the diagnosis of invasive aspergillosis.

Low dose computed tomography imaging is a sensitive screening method of pulmonary mold infections. However, CT findings that are deemed characteristic in adults appear to be of lesser utility in children, particularly in non-hematological patients. Therefore, any non-diffuse pulmonary CT finding in a high-risk patient needs to be considered to indicate invasive mold infection and should prompt further diagnostic work up. Galactomannan (GM), a heteropolysaccharide of the cell wall of *Aspergillus* spp., is released into the extracellular fluid during cell wall turnover and hyphal growth and can be detected by an enzyme immunoassay (EIA). Studies performed in adults show a high sensitivity and specificity of the GM assay in serum in granulocytopenic patients with hematological malignancies or following allogeneic HSCT, and usefulness for early diagnosis in conjunction with serial CT-imaging. Data generated in children compare favorably to the studies of GM testing in adults. Limitations to the assay are false-positive results due to cross-reacting polysaccharides and a decreased sensitivity of the assay in patients receiving prophylactic antifungal compounds. The GM assay also has high diagnostic utility for analysis of BAL fluid in suspected pulmonary aspergillosis and may be useful in the CSF in individual cases of CNS-disease. The use of PCR on diagnostic aspirates or tissue biopsies may be helpful in individual cases [8, 9, 36, 50].

12.2.1.3 Options for Treatment of Invasive Aspergillosis

Options for first-line therapy approved by the FDA and/or the EMEA include voriconazole (VCZ; children 2–11 years and adolescents 12–14 years weighing <50 kg: 2 × 8 mg/kg IV (day 1: 2 × 9 mg/kg); adolescents 12–14 years weighing >50 kg and those 15 years and beyond: 2 × 4 mg/kg IV (2 × 6 mg day 1); cave interactions; adverse events and need for TDM) and liposomal amphotericin B (LAMB; 3 mg/kg QD IV) (Table 12.1). Criteria for selecting one of these agents include organ impairment, concomitant medications, availability of TDM, the type of preceding antifungal treatment, and the local epidemiology [36, 51, 52].

Approved second-line options are ABLC (5 mg/kg QD) and CAS (50 mg/msqu QD; day 1: 70 mg/msqu; max.: 70 mg QD). While itraconazole, isavuconazole, and posaconazole are not approved in pediatric patients, the use of DAMB is no longer appropriate due to inferior outcomes in a randomized first-line trial. Based on solid preclinical and limited clinical data, VCZ currently is recommended for *A. terreus* infections and infections affecting the CNS. Dose escalation of LAMB to 10 mg/kg QD for the initial 14 days of treatment was not beneficial in a randomized comparative trial; similarly, the combination of VCZ with an echinocandin (anidulafungin) was not superior in terms of overall mortality at week six relative to treatment with VCZ alone and can therefore not generally be recommended [53].

Similar to adults, adjunctive surgical interventions need consideration in skin and soft tissue infections, sinus infections, impending erosion of pulmonary arteries, and in operable CNS and lung lesions. G-CSF or GM-CSF, respectively, is indicated in neutropenic patients, and reduction, discontinuation, or replacement of steroids in immunosuppressed patients. The duration of therapy is individual and determined by the clinical and microbiological response. Clinical stabilization and at least a partial response provided, treatment can be consolidated with oral therapies [8, 9, 36, 52, 54].

12.2.1.4 Prophylaxis and Empirical Therapy

Primary chemoprophylaxis of invasive aspergillosis may be indicated in high-risk populations with incidence rates of close to 10% or higher. These include patients receiving intensive chemotherapy for acute leukemia and patients following allogeneic HSCT, particularly when immunosuppression is augmented for GVHD. Based on pivotal clinical trials conducted in adults [46, 47] and similar pharmacokinetics, posaconazole tablets may be given to children >12 years of age, and voriconazole in younger children. Alternatives include the intermittent administration of LAMB (1 mg/kg QOD) or micafungin (1 mg/kg QD) [36]. This practical algorithm, however, requires careful attention to contraindications, drug interactions, and adverse events as appropriate clinical trials in pediatric patients are lacking.

Empirical antifungal therapy is an established standard of care in hemato-oncological patients with prolonged neutropenia (ANC <500/≥10 days) and refractory or new fever that provides targeted prevention in a high-risk setting. Agents approved by the FDA and/or the EMEA and recommended for this indication in pediatric patients of all age groups include LAMB (1–3 mg/kg QD) and CAS (50 mg/msqu QD; day 1: 70 mg/msqu; max.: 70 mg QD) [36, 48].

12.3 Less Common Invasive Opportunistic Fungal Infections

12.3.1 Instructive Case

A 6-year-old profoundly neutropenic girl with recurrent metastatic nephroblastoma had an accidental minor trauma at home, resulting in a laceration on the scalp requiring surgical suture. The next day, she was admitted with new fever. She remained febrile despite administration of empirical antibacterial treatment and developed severe headaches, increasing swelling and liquid discharge from the wound. Surgical debridement and biopsies were done on day 12. Histology revealed invasive hyphal growth, and cultures white/cream-colored colonies with aerial mycelium identified as Coprinopsis cinerea, a rare environmental mold, by gene sequence analysis (ITS1/ITS2). The girl made a complete recovery with LAMB 3 mg/kg/d for six days until neutrophil recovery on HD 18, followed by posaconazole (100/200 mg PO QD alternating) for a total of 66 days.

A large number of biologically diverse filamentous fungi can cause invasive disease in susceptible hosts (Fig. 12.1). Among these organisms, mucormycosis is mostly airborne and requires breakdown of phagocytic functions or protective surfaces. In a review of 157 pediatric cases of zygomycosis, most patients presented with cutaneous or gastrointestinal disease, followed by rhinocerebral and pulmonary disease. Among 59 reported cases of neonatal zygomycosis, the majority occurred in premature infants. Gastrointestinal and cutaneous diseases were more frequent than in older patients. Rates of disseminated disease (56%) and mortality (64%) were exceedingly high, indicating that zygomycosis is associated with an extremely poor prognosis in neonates. *Fusarium* infections may be similar to invasive aspergillosis, but frequently presents with fungemia and disseminated skin and soft tissue lesions. Infection due to Trichosporon asahii in neutropenic patients and neonates mimic invasive candidiasis with fungemia and disseminated infection and carries a high mortality. Cryptococcosis appears to be an infrequent opportunistic infection; in HIV-infected children, the estimated 10-year prevalence is 1% [49, 54–59]. Management of cryptococcal meningoencephalitis includes the combination of amphotericin B and flucytosine for induction and maintenance treatment with fluconazole (Perfect IDSA guideline). Whereas the echinocandins have no useful activity as single agents against less frequent opportunistic fungi, limited and uncontrolled data indicate an important role of amphotericin B, posaconazole, isavuconazole, and voriconazole (cave: inactive against the mucorales). Treatment of these infections is an interdisciplinary challenge and needs to be individualized based on the patient's presentation and response to treatment [60–62].

References

1. Zingg W, Hopkins S, Gayet-Ageron A, Holmes A, Sharland M, Suetens C, Almeida M, Asembergiene J, Borg MA, Budimir A, Cairns S, Cunney R, Deptula A, Berciano PG, Gudlaugsson O, Hadjiloucas A, Hammami N, Harrison W, Heisbourg E, Kolman J, Kontopidou F, Kristensen B, Lyytikäinen O, Märtin P, McIlvenny G, Moro ML, Piening B, Presterl E, Serban R, Smid E, Sorknes NK, Stefkovicova M, Sviestina I, Szabo R, Tkadlecova H, Vatcheva-Dobrevska R, VerjatTrannoy D (2017) Health-care-associated infections in neonates, children, and adolescents: an analysis of paediatric data from the European Centre for Disease Prevention and Control point-prevalence survey. Lancet Infect Dis 17(4):381–389
2. Zaoutis TE, Argon J, Chu J, Berlin JA, Walsh TJ, Feudtner C (2005) The epidemiology and attributable outcomes of candidemia in adults and children hospitalized in the United States: a propensity analysis. Clin Infect Dis 41(9):1232–1239
3. Zaoutis TE, Coffin SE, Chu JH, Heydon K, Zhao H, Greves HM, Walsh TJ (2005) Risk factors for mortality in children with candidemia. Pediatr Infect Dis J 24(8):736–739
4. Baptista MI, Nona J, Ferreira M, Sampaio I, Abrantes M, Tome MT, Neto MT, Barroso R, Serelha M, Virella D (2016) Invasive fungal infection in neonatal intensive care units: a multicenter survey. J Chemother 28(1):37–43
5. Zaoutis TE, Prasad PA, Localio AR, Coffin SE, Bell LM, Walsh TJ, Gross R (2010) Risk factors and predictors for candidemia in pediatric intensive care unit patients: implications for prevention. Clin Infect Dis 51(5):e38–e45
6. Roilides E, Kadiltsoglou I, Zahides D, Bibashi E (1997) Invasive candidosis in pediatric patients. Clin Microbiol Infect 3(2):192–197
7. Zaoutis T (2010) Candidemia in children. Curr Med Res Opin 26(7):1761–1768
8. Tragiannidis A, Fegeler W, Rellensmann G, Debus V, Müller V, Hörnig-Franz I, Siam K, Pama ZD, Jürgens H, Groll AH (2012a) Candidaemia in a European Paediatric University Hospital: a 10-year observational study. Clin Microbiol Infect 18:E27–E30

9. Tragiannidis A, Roilides E, Walsh T, Groll AH (2012) Invasive aspergillosis in children with acquired immunodeficiencies. Clin Infect Dis 54(2):258–267
10. Pasqualotto AC, de Moraes AB, Zanini RR, Severo LC (2007) Analysis of independent risk factors for death among pediatric patients with candidemia and a central venous catheter in place. Infect Control Hosp Epidemiol 28(7):799–804
11. Stoll BJ, Hansen NI, Bell EF, Walsh MC, Carlo WA, Shankaran S, Laptook AR, Sanchez PJ, Van Meurs KP, Wyckoff M, Das A, Hale EC, Ball MB, Newman NS, Schibler K, Poindexter BB, Kennedy KA, Cotten CM, Watterberg KL, D'Angio CT, DeMauro SB, Truog WE, Devaskar U, Higgins RD (2015) Trends in care practices, morbidity, and mortality of extremely preterm neonates, 1993-2012. JAMA 314(10):1039–1051
12. Benjamin DK Jr, Ross K, McKinney RE Jr, Benjamin DK, Auten R, Fisher RG (2000) When to suspect fungal infection in neonates: A clinical comparison of Candida albicans and Candida parapsilosis fungemia with coagulase-negative staphylococcal bacteremia. Pediatrics 106(4):712–718
13. Saiman L, Ludington E, Pfaller M, Rangel-Frausto S, Wiblin RT, Dawson J, Blumberg HM, Patterson JE, Rinaldi M, Edwards JE, Wenzel RP, Jarvis W (2000) Risk factors for candidemia in neonatal intensive care unit patients. The National Epidemiology of Mycosis Survey Study Group. Pediatr Infect Dis J 19(4):319–324
14. Hammarskjold F, Mernelius S, Andersson RE, Berg S, Hanberger H, Lofgren S, Malmvall BE, Petzold M, Matussek A (2013) Possible transmission of Candida albicans on an intensive care unit: genotype and temporal cluster analyses. J Hosp Infect 85(1):60–65
15. Pfaller MA (1996) Nosocomial candidiasis: emerging species, reservoirs, and modes of transmission. Clin Infect Dis 22(Suppl 2):S89–S94
16. Schnell JD (1977) The epidemiology and prophylaxis of mycoses in perinatology. Contrib Microbiol Immunol 4:40–45
17. Kaufman DA (2010) Challenging issues in neonatal candidiasis. Curr Med Res Opin 26(7):1769–1778
18. Mendling W, Friese K, Mylonas I, Weissenbacher ER, Brasch J, Schaller M, Mayser P, Effend I, Ginter-Hanselmayer G, Hof H, Cornely O, Ruhnke M (2015) Vulvovaginal candidosis. Guideline of the German Society of Gynecology and Obstretrics. Geburtshilfe Frauenheilkd. 75:342–354
19. Leibovitz E (2012) Strategies for the prevention of neonatal candidiasis. Pediatr Neonatol 53(2):83–89
20. Manzoni P, Farina D, Leonessa M, d'Oulx EA, Galletto P, Mostert M, Miniero R, Gomirato G (2006) Risk factors for progression to invasive fungal infection in preterm neonates with fungal colonization. Pediatrics 118(6):2359–2364
21. Manzoni P, Mostert M, Leonessa ML, Priolo C, Farina D, Monetti C, Latino MA, Gomirato G (2006) Oral supplementation with Lactobacillus casei subspecies rhamnosus prevents enteric colonization by Candida species in preterm neonates: a randomized study. Clin Infect Dis 42(12):1735–1742
22. Aliaga S, Clark RH, Laughon M, Walsh TJ, Hope WW, Benjamin DK, Kaufman D, Arrieta A, Benjamin DK Jr, Smith PB (2014) Changes in the incidence of candidiasis in neonatal intensive care units. Pediatrics 133(2):236–242
23. Kelly MS, Benjamin DK Jr, Smith PB (2015) The epidemiology and diagnosis of invasive candidiasis among premature infants. Clin Perinatol 42(1):105–117 viii-ix
24. Roilides E, Antachopoulos C, Groll AH, Walsh TJ (2017) Chapter 39: candidiasis. In: Succinct pediatrics: evaluation and management for infectious diseases and dermatologic disorders. American Academy of Pediatris, Elk Grove Village, pp 435–452
25. Hope WW, Castagnola E, Groll AH, Roilides E, Akova M, Arendrup MC, Arikan-Akdagli S, Bassetti M, Bille J, Cornely OA, Cuenca-Estrella M, Donnelly JP, Garbino J, Herbrecht R, Jensen HE, Kullberg BJ, Lass-Florl C, Lortholary O, Meersseman W, Petrikkos G, Richardson MD, Verweij PE, Viscoli C, Ullmann AJ, E. F. I. S. Group (2012) ESCMID* guideline for the diagnosis and management of Candida diseases 2012: prevention and management of invasive infections in neonates and children caused by Candida spp. Clin Microbiol Infect 18(Suppl 7):38–52
26. Blyth CC, Chen SC, Slavin MA, Serena C, Nguyen Q, Marriott D, Ellis D, Meyer W, Sorrell TC (2009) Not just little adults: candidemia epidemiology, molecular characterization, and antifungal susceptibility in neonatal and pediatric patients. Pediatrics. 123(5):1360–1368
27. Noyola DE, Fernandez M, Moylett EH, Baker CJ (2001) Ophthalmologic, visceral, and cardiac involvement in neonates with candidemia. Clin Infect Dis 32(7):1018–1023
28. Tissieres P, Jaeggi ET, Beghetti M, Gervaix A (2005) Increase of fungal endocarditis in children. Infection 33(4):267–272
29. Meersseman W, Lagrou K, Spriet I, Maertens J, Verbeken E, Peetermans WE, Van Wijngaerden E (2009) Significance of the isolation of Candida species from airway samples in critically ill patients: a prospective, autopsy study. Intensive Care Med 35(9):1526–1531
30. Gamaletsou MN, Kontoyiannis DP, Sipsas NV, Moriyama B, Alexander E, Roilides E, Brause B, Walsh TJ (2012) Candida osteomyelitis: analysis of 207 pediatric and adult cases (1970–2011). Clin Infect Dis. 55(10):1338–1351
31. Kirkpatrick C (1993) Chronic mucocutaneous candidiasis. In: Bodey GP (ed) Candidiasis. Raven Press, New York, pp 167–184
32. Casanova JL (2015) Severe infectious diseases of childhood as monogenic inborn errors of immunity. Proc Natl Acad Sci U S A 112(51):E7128–E7137
33. Pilmis B, Puel A, Lortholary O, Lanternier F (2016) New clinical phenotypes of fungal infections in special hosts. Clin Microbiol Infect 22(8):681–687

34. Berenguer J, Buck M, Witebsky F, Stock F, Pizzo PA, Walsh TJ (1993) Lysis-centrifugation blood cultures in the detection of tissue-proven invasive candidiasis. Disseminated versus single-organ infection. Diagn Microbiol Infect Dis 17(2):103–109
35. Cuenca-Estrella M, Verweij PE, Arendrup MC, Arikan-Akdagli S, Bille J, Donnelly JP, Jensen HE, Lass-Florl C, Richardson MD, Akova M, Bassetti M, Calandra T, Castagnola E, Cornely OA, Garbino J, Groll AH, Herbrecht R, Hope WW, Kullberg BJ, Lortholary O, Meersseman W, Petrikkos G, Roilides E, Viscoli C, Ullmann AJ, E. F. I. S. Group (2012) ESCMID* guideline for the diagnosis and management of Candida diseases 2012: diagnostic procedures. Clin Microbiol Infect 18(Suppl 7):9–18
36. Groll AH, Castagnola E, Cesaro S, Dalle JH, Engelhard D, Hope W, Roilides E, Styczynski J, Warris A, Lehrnbecher T, Fourth European Conference on Infections in Leukaemia; Infectious Diseases Working Party of the European Group for Blood Marrow Transplantation (EBMT-IDWP); Infectious Diseases Group of the European Organisation for Research and Treatment of Cancer (EORTC-IDG); International Immunocompromised Host Society (ICHS); European Leukaemia Net (ELN) (2014) Fourth European Conference on Infections in Leukaemia (ECIL-4): guidelines for diagnosis, prevention, and treatment of invasive fungal diseases in paediatric patients with cancer or allogeneic haemopoietic stem-cell transplantation. Lancet Oncol 15(8):e327–e340
37. Katragkou A, Roilides E (2011) Best practice in treating infants and children with proven, probable or suspected invasive fungal infections. Curr Opin Infect Dis. 24(3):225–229
38. Queiroz-Telles F, Berezin E, Leverger G, Freire A, van der Vyver A, Chotpitayasunondh T, Konja J, Diekmann-Berndt H, Koblinger S, Groll AH, Arrieta A (2008) Micafungin versus liposomal amphotericin B for pediatric patients with invasive candidiasis: substudy of a randomized double-blind trial. Pediatr Infect Dis J 27(9):820–826
39. Wiley JM, Seibel NL, Walsh TJ (2005) Efficacy and safety of amphotericin B lipid complex in 548 children and adolescents with invasive fungal infections. Pediatr Infect Dis J 24(2):167–174
40. Walsh TJ, Lutsar I, Driscoll T, Dupont B, Roden M, Ghahramani P, Hodges M, Groll AH, Perfect JR (2002) Voriconazole in the treatment of aspergillosis, scedosporiosis and other invasive fungal infections in children. Pediatr Infect Dis J 21(3):240–248
41. Kaufman D, Boyle R, Hazen KC, Patrie JT, Robinson M, Donowitz LG (2001) Fluconazole prophylaxis against fungal colonization and infection in preterm infants. N Engl J Med 345(23):1660–1666
42. Kaufman D, Boyle R, Hazen KC, Patrie JT, Robinson M, Grossman LB (2005) Twice weekly fluconazole prophylaxis for prevention of invasive Candida infection in high-risk infants of <1000 grams birth weight. J Pediatr 147(2):172–179
43. Kicklighter SD, Springer SC, Cox T, Hulsey TC, Turner RB (2001) Fluconazole for prophylaxis against candidal rectal colonization in the very low birth weight infant. Pediatrics. 107(2):293–298
44. Manzoni P, Stolfi I, Pugni L, Decembrino L, Magnani C, Vetrano G, Tridapalli E, Corona G, Giovannozzi C, Farina D, Arisio R, Merletti F, Maule M, Mosca F, Pedicino R, Stronati M, Mostert M, Gomirato G, Italian Task Force for the Study and Prevention of Neonatal Fungal Infections; Italian Society of Neonatology (2007) A multicenter, randomized trial of prophylactic fluconazole in preterm neonates. N Engl J Med. 356(24):2483–2495
45. Manzoni P, Leonessa M, Galletto P, Latino MA, Arisio R, Maule M, Agriesti G, Gastaldo L, Gallo E, Mostert M, Farina D (2008) Routine use of fluconazole prophylaxis in a neonatal intensive care unit does not select natively fluconazole-resistant Candida subspecies. Pediatr Infect Dis J. 27(8):731–737
46. Ullmann AJ, Lipton JH, Vesole DH, Chandrasekar P, Langston A, Tarantolo SR, Greinix H, Morais de Azevedo W, Reddy V, Boparai N, Pedicone L, Patino H, Durrant S (2007) Posaconazole or fluconazole for prophylaxis in severe graft-versus-host disease. N Engl J Med 356(4):335–347
47. Cornely OA, Maertens J, Winston DJ, Perfect J, Ullmann AJ, Walsh TJ, Helfgott D, Holowiecki J, Stockelberg D, Goh YT, Petrini M, Hardalo C, Suresh R, Angulo-Gonzalez D (2007) Posaconazole vs. fluconazole or itraconazole prophylaxis in patients with neutropenia. N Engl J Med. 356(4):348–359
48. Maertens JA, Madero L, Reilly AF, Lehrnbecher T, Groll AH, Jafri HS, Green M, Nania JJ, Bourque MR, Wise BA, Strohmaier KM, Taylor AF, Kartsonis NA, Chow JW, Arndt CA, DePauw BE, Walsh TJ (2010) A randomized, double-blind, multicenter study of caspofungin versus liposomal amphotericin B for empiric antifungal therapy in pediatric patients with persistent fever and neutropenia. Pediatr Infect Dis J 29(5):415–420
49. Groll AH, Antachopoulos C, Roilides E, Walsh TJ (2017) Chapter 38: aspergillosis. In: Succinct pediatrics: evaluation and management for infectious diseases and dermatologic disorders. American Academy of Pediatris, Elk Grove Village, pp 425–434
50. Lehrnbecher T, Robinson PD, Fisher BT, Castagnola E, Groll AH, Steinbach WJ, Zaoutis TE, Negeri ZF, Beyene J, Phillips B, Sung L (2016) Galactomannan, β-D-glucan, and polymerase chain reaction-based assays for the diagnosis of invasive fungal disease in pediatric cancer and hematopoietic stem cell transplantation: a systematic review and meta-analysis. Clin Infect Dis 63(10):1340–1348
51. Herbrecht R, Denning DW, Patterson TF, Bennett JE, Greene RE, Oestmann JW, Kern WV, Marr KA, Ribaud P, Lortholary O, Sylvester R, Rubin RH, Wingard JR, Stark P, Durand C, Caillot D, Thiel E, Chandrasekar PH, Hodges MR, Schlamm HT, Troke PF, de Pauw B (2002) Voriconazole versus amphoteri-

cin B for primary therapy of invasive aspergillosis. N Engl J Med 347(6):408–415

52. Ullmann A, Aguado JM, Arikan S, Denning D, Groll A, Lagrou K, Lass-Florl C, Lewis R, Muñoz P, Verweij P, Warris A, Akova M, Arendrup MC, Barnes R, Blot S, Bouza E, Brüggemann RJM, Buchheidt D, cadranel J, Chakrabarti A, Cuenca-Estrella M, Dimopoulos G, Gangneux J-P, Garbino J, Heinz W, Herbrecht R, Kibbler C, Klimko N, Kullberg B-J, Lange C, Lehrnbecher T, Loeffler J, Lortholary O, Maertens J, Cornely O (2018) Diagnosis and management of aspergillus diseases: executive summary of the 2017 ESCMID-ECMM-ERS guideline. Clin Microbiol Infect 24(Suppl. 1):e1–e38
53. Cornely OA, Maertens J, Bresnik M, Ebrahimi R, Ullmann AJ, Bouza E, Heussel CP, Lortholary O, Rieger C, Boehme A, Aoun M, Horst HA, Thiebaut A, Ruhnke M, Reichert D, Vianelli N, Krause SW, Olavarria E, Herbrecht R, AmBiLoad Trial Study Group (2007) Liposomal amphotericin B as initial therapy for invasive mold infection: a randomized trial comparing a high-loading dose regimen with standard dosing (AmBiLoad trial). Clin Infect Dis. 44(10):1289–1297
54. Dornbusch HJ, Manzoni P, Roilides E, Walsh TJ, Groll AH (2009) Invasive fungal infections in children. Pediatr Infect Dis J 28(8):734–737
55. Walsh TJ, Karlsson MO, Driscoll T, Arguedas AG, Adamson P, Saez-Llorens X, Vora AJ, Arrieta AC, Blumer J, Lutsar I, Milligan P, Wood N (2004) Pharmacokinetics and safety of intravenous voriconazole in children after single- or multiple-dose administration. Antimicrob Agents Chemother 48(6):2166–2172
56. Walsh TJ, Teppler H, Donowitz GR, Maertens JA, Baden LR, Dmoszynska A, Cornely OA, Bourque MR, Lupinacci RJ, Sable CA, dePauw BE (2004) Caspofungin versus liposomal amphotericin B for empirical antifungal therapy in patients with persistent fever and neutropenia. N Engl J Med 351(14):1391–1402
57. Zaoutis TE, Roilides E, Chiou CC, Buchanan WL, Knudsen TA, Sarkisova TA, Schaufele RL, Sein M, Sein T, Prasad PA, Chu JH, Walsh TJ (2007) Zygomycosis in children: a systematic review and analysis of reported cases. Pediatr Infect Dis J. 26(8):723–727
58. Roilides E, Zaoutis TE, Walsh TJ (2009) Invasive zygomycosis in neonates and children. Clin Microbiol Infect. 15(Suppl 5):50–54
59. Gonzalez CE, Shetty D, Lewis LL, Mueller BU, Pizzo PA, Walsh TJ (1996) Cryptococcosis in human immunodeficiency virus-infected children. Pediatr Infect Dis J. 15(9):796–800
60. Cornely OA, Arikan-Akdagli S, Dannaoui E, Groll AH, Lagrou K, Chakrabarti A, Lanternier F, Pagano L, Skiada A, Akova M, Arendrup MC, Boekhout T, Chowdhary A, Cuenca-Estrella M, Freiberger T, Guinea J, Guarro J, de Hoog S, Hope W, Johnson E, Kathuria S, Lackner M, Lass-Flörl C, Lortholary O, Meis JF, Meletiadis J, Muñoz P, Richardson M, Roilides E, Tortorano AM, Ullmann AJ, van Diepeningen A, Verweij P, Petrikkos G, European Society of Clinical Microbiology and Infectious Diseases Fungal Infection Study Group; European Confederation of Medical Mycology (2014) ESCMID and ECMM joint clinical guidelines for the diagnosis and management of mucormycosis 2013. Clin Microbiol Infect 20(Suppl 3):5–26
61. Chowdhary A, Meis JF, Guarro J, de Hoog GS, Kathuria S, Arendrup MC, Arikan-Akdagli S, Akova M, Boekhout T, Caira M, Guinea J, Chakrabarti A, Dannaoui E, van Diepeningen A, Freiberger T, Groll AH, Hope WW, Johnson E, Lackner M, Lagrou K, Lanternier F, Lass-Flörl C, Lortholary O, Meletiadis J, Muñoz P, Pagano L, Petrikkos G, Richardson MD, Roilides E, Skiada A, Tortorano AM, Ullmann AJ, Verweij PE, Cornely OA, Cuenca-Estrella M, European Society of Clinical Microbiology and Infectious Diseases Fungal Infection Study Group; European Confederation of Medical Mycology (2014) ESCMID and ECMM joint clinical guidelines for the diagnosis and management of systemic phaeohyphomycosis: diseases caused by black fungi. Clin Microbiol Infect 20(Suppl 3):47–75
62. Tortorano AM, Richardson M, Roilides E, van Diepeningen A, Caira M, Munoz P, Johnson E, Meletiadis J, Pana ZD, Lackner M, Verweij P, Freiberger T, Cornely OA, Arikan-Akdagli S, Dannaoui E, Groll AH, Lagrou K, Chakrabarti A, Lanternier F, Pagano L, Skiada A, Akova M, Arendrup MC, Boekhout T, Chowdhary A, Cuenca-Estrella M, Guinea J, Guarro J, de Hoog S, Hope W, Kathuria S, Lortholary O, Meis JF, Ullmann AJ, Petrikkos G, Lass-Flörl C, European Society of Clinical Microbiology and Infectious Diseases Fungal Infection Study Group; European Confederation of Medical Mycology (2014) ESCMID and ECMM joint guidelines on diagnosis and management of hyalohyphomycosis: Fusarium spp., Scedosporium spp. and others. Clin Microbiol Infect 20(Suppl 3):27–46

13 Special Issue: Fungal Infection in Patients with Organ Transplantation

Stephan Eschertzhuber

13.1 Introduction

The ubiquitous presence of fungal spores leads to a continuous contact of inner and outer body surfaces to these potential pathogens. The immunological defense system of healthy individuals effectively protects the body against fungal infections. But an impairment of the immunologic system is one of the main factors, which makes patients prone to suffer from fungal colonization and topic or invasive fungal infections. Immunocompromised patients are found in the settings of hematological or solid cancer diseases, human immunodeficiency virus (HIV) infection, stem cell transplantation, solid organ transplantation (SOT), and neonatology as well as prolonged intensive care dependency after major trauma, surgery, or burns.

13.2 Solid Organ Transplantation (SOT)

Each year over 120,000 organ transplantations were performed worldwide. Due to high surgical expertise and a steady progress in the management of possible transplant candidates as well as of transplant recipients, the constantly improving outcomes of organ transplantations led to a common acceptance of more liberal indications for these lifesaving procedures. Subsequently the number of transplant recipients, suffering from severe comorbidities, belonging to extreme age groups, exhibiting an increased immunological risk profile, or simply undergoing re-transplantation, is tremendously rising. Despite a more individualized and closely monitored immunosuppressive therapy, the recipients of organ grafts are prone to infections. The combination of the impairment of the immune status, major surgery, intensive care dependency, extracorporeal organ replacement therapy, and a preexisting chronic illness is responsible that posttransplant infections are still one main cause of mortality in these patients. Also donor-derived fungal infections are described; their incidence is very low [1]. Between 2005 and 2011, only 31 confirmed transmissions of donor-derived fungal infection were reported in the USA. In the same time period, almost 200,000 organ transplantations were performed in the USA [2].

Among SOT recipients the overall 1-year cumulative incidence of invasive fungal infections (IFI) is 5.6% [3]. Invasive candidiasis (IC) is the most frequent IFI and is diagnosed in 1.9–4.0% of all SOT patients during the first 12 months after transplantation [4]. About 50% of these fungal infections were caused by *Candida albicans*, followed by *C. glabrata*, and less frequent by *C. krusei* and *C. guilliermondii* [4]. The incidence of invasive aspergillosis (IA) in SOT is 0.65–15% [3, 5]. To a far lesser extent,

S. Eschertzhuber
Anesthesia and Intensive Care, Medical University Innsbruck, Innsbruck, Austria
e-mail: stephan.eschertzhuber@i-med.ac.at

E. Presterl (ed.), *Clinically Relevant Mycoses*, https://doi.org/10.1007/978-3-319-92300-0_13

IFI are caused by *Cryptococcus* spp., non-*Aspergillus* molds, *Mucormycetes*, or other rare fungi.

The time of onset of IFI in SOT mostly follows a specific pattern depending on the etiologic fungus and the transplanted type of organ. Whereas IC occurs early after transplantation (median, 179 days after transplantation), IA shows a more delayed onset (median, 400 days after transplantation) [6]. Infections due to *Cryptococcus* spp., *Mucormycetes*, and other rare fungi generally occur later after SOT. It is important to keep in mind that these time patterns are not valid in the setting of re-transplantation.

In SOT recipients the diagnosis of fungal infections is hindered by several influencing factors. On one hand the typical immunologic response to pathogens is depressed by the immunosuppressive therapy, and on the other hand, the surgical trauma during implantation or the rejection of the transplanted graft causes reactions like fever and/or an increase of inflammatory markers. The broad use of antibiotics and of antifungal prophylaxis interferes with the results of antigen or (1-3)-β-D-glucan tests. Also high-resolution computer tomography, PCR-based diagnostics, and galactomannan assays may be helpful in certain clinical situations; definitive diagnosis can only be achieved by blood cultures or cultures of sterile tissue, liquid, and biopsy samples.

13.2.1 Immunosuppressive Therapy in SOT

To achieve the necessary grade of host tolerance to protect the transplanted organ against rejection, a combination of different immunosuppressive agents is applied. At the time of transplantation, the induction therapy is facilitated by the use of corticosteroids, polyclonal antibodies (i.e., antithymocyte globulins), or monoclonal antibodies (i.e., basiliximab, alemtuzumab, etc.). Mostly the immunosuppressive maintenance therapy consists of three pillars: the concomitant application of corticosteroids, calcineurin inhibitors (cyclosporin A, tacrolimus), and proliferation inhibitors (azathioprine, mycophenolate acid, mTOR inhibitors) is widely used to reduce side effects and provoke sufficient immunosuppression. In the case of rejection episodes, corticosteroids, antithymocyte globulins, or murine monoclonal anti-CD3 antibodies (OKT3) are in use to save the transplanted graft.

Corticosteroids suppress the production of pro-inflammatory cytokines as prostaglandins, tumor necrosis factor (TNF-α), interleukins (IL-1, IL-2, IL-6), and many others. Calcineurin inhibitors (CNI) block the production of IL-2 and in consequence the activation of B-cells and T-cells. The proliferation of these cells as well as the DNA synthesis of other proliferating cells is markedly impaired by agents like mycophenolate or azathioprine [7].

All these mechanisms to prevent rejection of a transplanted organ interfere with the ability of the human body to protect itself from infection and invasion of pathogens like bacteria, viruses, and fungus.

Many interactions between immunosuppressive agents and concomitant administered medications are well known. In the context of fungal infections, the effect of azoles in SOT is of special importance. All azoles cause increased levels of calcineurin inhibitor serum concentrations. Therefore the dosage of calcineurin inhibitors has to be adjusted. With exception of isavuconazole, all azoles cause a prolongation of the QT time, an effect that is intensified by concomitant administration of tacrolimus. Because liver transplant recipients exhibit a high incidence of QT-time prolongation, the described effect is of special interest in this patient population.

13.2.2 Kidney Transplantation

Despite the longest waiting time for organ transplantation and the dependency on renal replacement therapy (RRT), sometimes over many years, recipients of a renal graft have the lowest incidence of invasive fungal infections (IFI) compared to all other SOT groups. The onset of IFI occurs in kidney transplantation typically late. A delay of more than 2 years between transplantation and the diagnosis of an IFI is not uncommon

[6, 8]. Over 90% of observed IFI are due to *Candida* spp. The overall incidence of IFI in these patients is stated with 1.3% [3]. The incidence of invasive aspergillosis (IA) is as low as 0.7% [9]. Typically invasive infections only occur in highly immunosuppressed patients and in the setting of re-transplantation or are facilitated by other infective or surgical complications and prolonged intensive care dependency. Although the incidence of IFI in kidney transplantation is low, the mortality of these infections exceeds 75%. Nevertheless universal antifungal prophylaxis in the setting of kidney transplantation is not recommended [10].

More frequent than from IFI, the kidney recipients suffer from candiduria, with an incidence of 3–11% [11]. The treatment of candiduria consists, besides the removal of indwelling urinary catheters and ureter stents, of systemic application of antifungals, which penetrate well into the urinary tract [12]. In selected cases antifungal bladder irrigation may be appropriate.

For systemic treatment of urinary tract infections caused by fluconazole-susceptible organism in this population, fluconazole (3–6 mg/kg, daily for 24 days) is recommended. Fluconazole-resistant organism should be treated with amphotericin B (AmB) deoxycholate (0.3 0.6 mg/kg, daily for 1–7 days), with oral flucytosine (25 mg/kg, four times daily for 14 days), or with a combination of AmB deoxycholate and oral flucytosine [12]. One major drawback of AmB deoxycholate in this setting is its nephrotoxicity, which can limit the use of AmB especially in patients receiving CNI for immunosuppression. In severely immunocompromised patients and in suspected systemic dissemination of the infection, antifungal therapy should be expanded with an echinocandin without delay. AmB deoxycholate (50 mg/L sterile water) is recommended for daily bladder irrigation for a period of 5 days [12].

13.2.3 Pancreas Transplantation

The incidence of fungal infections in pancreas transplant recipients is between 3.4 and 38% [3, 8, 9, 13]. Almost all infections are caused by *Candida* spp. [3]. General risk factors are long-standing diabetes, concomitant renal insufficiency with RRT, enteric pancreas drainage, and induction therapy with antithymocyte globulins. Special risk factors for fungal infections are vascular graft thrombosis, posttransplant pancreatitis, posttransplant re-laparotomy, enteric anastomosis insufficiency, and re-transplantation [10]. It is recommended to use a universal prophylaxis for all pancreas recipients with fluconazole (4–6 mg/kg q24 h) [4, 10]. Due to the interaction of fluconazole and the CNI levels, the increase in fluconazole-resistant candida species, as well as the growing number of patients exhibiting special risk factors for IFI, the use of an echinocandin in the prophylactic setting appears as reasonable.

13.2.4 Liver Transplantation (LT)

The population of liver transplant recipients shows a large heterogeneity related to the risk profile for IFI. Transplant candidates with oncological indications (i.e., hepatocellular carcinoma), who present with a normal liver function and who did not undergo prior abdominal surgery, exhibit no increased risk for IFI. On the other hand, patients, who were referred to transplantation because of acute or acute on chronic liver failure and who are treated on intensive care units prior to transplantation, show a tremendous risk for suffering from fungal infection. IFI in LT recipients are despite maximal antifungal therapy accountable for mortality rates up to 72% [14, 15].

The overall incidence of fungal infection in liver transplant recipients is described as high as 5–42% [14, 16]. In recent published studies, the incidence of IFI in LT declines due to improved perioperative management and broader use of antifungal prophylaxis. An analysis of 386 LTs performed between 2006 and 2013 at one single center showed without using universal antifungal prophylaxis an overall incidence of IFI of 10.1% and an incidence of 4.1% in the group of low-risk recipients [17]. Most fungal infections in the setting of LT are caused by *Candida* spp. (80%), followed by *Aspergillus* spp. (15%), and other rare fungi. Within the *Candida* spp. infections, an increase of IFI due to non-*albicans Candida* species is reported. *Infections due to Candida* spp. occur earlier after LT then caused by *Aspergillus* spp., *Mucormycetes*, *Cryptococcus* spp., or other filamentous fungi. Despite the later onset of infections due to filamentous fungi, up to 75% of IFI due to *Aspergillus* spp. were diagnosed within the first 6 months after LT [6]. In a retrospective study, Raghuram et al. demonstrated that within 1, 3, and 6 months after LT, 67%, 81%, and 91%, respectively, of the IFI were observed [14].

Risk factors for IFI in patients undergoing LT were identified by many authors and are accepted as basis for decisions to initiate antifungal prophylaxis. The following factors predispose LT recipients for fungal infections: re-transplantation, prolonged operation time, need for re-laparotomy, transfusion requirements ≥40 blood products, impaired graft function, renal insufficiency, RRT, pretransplant ICU dependency, choledochojejunostomy, model of end-stage liver disease (MELD) score ≥25, prior fungal colonization or infection, pretransplant treatment with antibiotics, prior spontaneous bacterial peritoneal infections, and CMV infections, accumulating more than 6 g of prednisone within the first 12 weeks after LT [10, 14, 18, 19].

Considering these factors it is possible to grade the risk for fungal infections of the potential LT recipients into a low- and high-risk group. Universal antifungal prophylaxis should only be applied to patients belonging to the high-risk group. The recommended antifungal prophylaxis can be maintained with an echinocandin or a lipid formulation of amphotericin B. The prophylaxis should be applied for 2–4 weeks and should not be terminated if the risk factors did not resolve [10].

Early treatment of suspected fungal infections in LT recipients is crucial. Because of the high mortality rates due to IFI in these patients, also empiric treatment should be initiated with antifungals which exhibit broad activity against *Candida* spp. After identification of the fungus, a step-down therapy, if possible, is recommended. In cases where the transplantation was done more than 3 months before the onset of the suspected fungal infection, an agent with activity against *Aspergillus* spp. should be considered. Despite the possible hepatotoxicity of antifungal agents, the number of therapy discontinuations in LT recipients is low. The highest number of discontinuation of antifungal treatment has been described for AmB formulations and for itraconazole [20]. The rise of liver enzymes in conjunction with the use of echinocandins is reversible and in the clinical setting of LT is mostly irrelevant (Fig. 13.1).

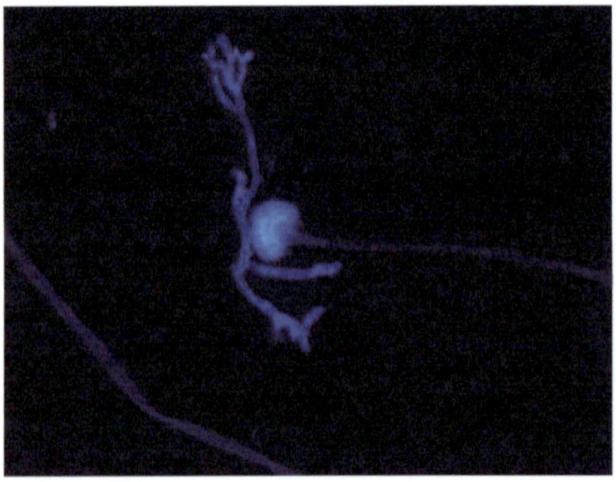

Fig. 13.1 Mixed fungal infection with *Aspergillus* spp. and *Mucormycetes* in a highly immunocompromised patient after liver re-transplantation. Courtesy of Dr. Maria Aigner, Division of Hygiene and Medical Microbiology, Medical University of Innsbruck, Innsbruck, Austria

13.2.5 Heart Transplantation

Besides kidney transplantation the recipients of heart transplants show the lowest incidence of fungal infections. In the literature the overall incidence of IFI in heart transplantation (HT) is described with 5% to 10.7% [9, 21, 22]. The majority of fungal infection is caused by molds. In up to 77% of heart recipients suffering from IFI, *Aspergillus* spp. can be diagnosed as responsible pathogen. The highest incidence of IFI in HT is seen within the first 3 months after transplantation [23]. Because of the comparatively low incidence of IFI, there is no recommendation for universal antifungal prophylaxis. In high-risk HT recipients, prophylaxis with an antifungal agent which exhibits activity against *Aspergillus* spp. (i.e., voriconazole, itraconazole, posaconazole, isavuconazole, or amphotericin B) is indicated [10]. Identified risk factors for fungal infection in HT are reoperation, delayed chest closure, pre- or perioperative mechanical circulatory support, RRT, concomitant CMV infection, colonization with *Aspergillus* spp., rejection episodes, and prolonged leukopenia after induction therapy [10, 23, 24].

Many patients were bridged to HT by implantation of a left ventricular assist device or by using other mechanical circulatory support. The number of patients treated with any circulatory support device exceeds 5000 per year in Europe and the USA, and the time patients stay on such a device extends constantly [25]. The prevalence of IFI in patients on mechanical circulatory support decreased over the last decades and is now 4.4% [25]. In contrast to HT recipients, most fungal infections in these patient groups are caused by *Candida* spp., a fact that should be considered for empirical therapy in this setting. Patients with implanted devices suffering from IFI should be treated as patients with fungal endocarditis. After successful treatment an antifungal suppressive therapy with an azole should be considered as long as the device is in place [12].

13.2.6 Lung Transplantation

The continuous open contact of the airways to the environment facilitates colonization and infection of lung transplant recipients with fungal spores. So, not surprisingly, the incidence of all IFI is as high as 15–35%, and the incidence of IA was described to reach a portion of up to 60–72% [9, 26]. Recent data show a decline in the incidence of all IFI (26%) as well as in the incidence of IA (44%) in lung transplantation [3]. At the same time, the number of non-*Aspergillus* mold infections is increasing. This trend might be caused by the broader application of a universal antifungal prophylaxis in the setting of lung transplantation. IFI and especially IA cause a tremendous mortality rate (IA up to 68%) in this population.

Besides the permanent exposure of the airway mucosa to inhaled pathogens and an impaired mucociliary clearance, other risk factors for the development of IFI in lung recipients were identified: pre- and posttransplant colonization with *Aspergillus* spp., re-transplantation, unilateral lung transplantation, prolonged bronchial anastomotic ischemia or insufficiency, induction therapy with antithymocyte globulins or monoclonal antibodies, rejection therapy, concomitant cytomegalovirus (CMV) infection, or tracheobronchial stent placement [5, 9, 10, 26].

The strong recommended prophylaxis for lung transplant recipients consists of inhaled nebulized AmB lipid complex or nebulized liposomal AmB. A weaker recommendation for universal prophylaxis with voriconazole also exists. The duration of the prophylactic therapy is indefinite but should, depending on the persistence of risk factors, last for a minimum of 4 months with voriconazole and 12 months with nebulized AmB formulations.

13.2.7 Small Bowel Transplantation

Of all SOT patients, the recipients of small bowel transplantation (SBT) show the highest incidence of both all-cause infections and fungal infections. This group of patients is characterized by long-standing diseases with the need of frequent hospitalizations, parental nutrition, and recurrent infections of central vein catheters. Immunosuppression in SBT consists of a highly effective induction therapy followed by immunosuppression at a higher level as in any other SOT. Due to these factors, the incidence of infectious complications in SBT is 100% [27]. Fungal infections were reported to occur in 40–62% of SBT recipients with a preponderance of yeast infections [3, 27, 28]. The share of candida infections exceeds 80% of all fungal infections with a high number of non-*albicans Candida* species [28].

Besides the underlying predisposition for IFI, several additional risk factors have been identified. A delayed or poor graft function, repeated abdominal surgery, insufficiency of the bowel anastomoses, rejection episodes, or RRT further increases the probability of manifestation of IFI [10].

Universal antifungal prophylaxis should be administered to all SBT recipients. Also fluconazole is still one recommended options, the use of echinocandins for prophylactic treatment seems reasonable due to the high number of non-*albicans Candida* spp. in SBT [10].

References

1. Ison MG, Nalesnik MA (2011) An update on donor-derived disease trans-mission in organ transplantation. Am J Transplant 11:1123–1130
2. Echenique IA, Ison MG (2013) Update on donor-derived infections in liver transplantation. Liver Transpl 19(6):575–585. https://doi.org/10.1002/j.idc.2013.02.001
3. Pappas PG, Alexander BD, Andes DR, Hadley S, Kauffmann CA, Freifeld A et al (2010) Invasive fungal infections among organ transplant recipients: results of the Transplant-Associated Infection Surveillance Network (TRANSNET). Clin Infect Dis 50(8):1101–1111. https://doi.org/10.1086/651262
4. Silveira FP, Kusne S, The AST Infectious Diseases Community of Practice (2013) Candida infections in solid organ transplantation. Am J Transplant 13:220–227. https://doi.org/10.1111/ajt.12114
5. Singh NM, Husain S, The AST Infectious Diseases Community of Practice (2013) Aspergillosis in solid organ transplantation. Am J Transplant 13(Suppl 4):228–241. https://doi.org/10.1111/ajt.12115.
6. Neofytos D, Fishman JA, Horn D, Anaissie E, Chang CH, Olyaei A et al (2010) Epidemiology and outcome of invasive fungal infections in solid organ transplant recipients. Transpl Infect Dis 12(3):220–229. https://doi.org/10.1111/j.1399-3062.2010.00492.x
7. Bush WW (1999) Overview of transplantation immunology and the pharmacotherapy of adult solid organ transplant recipients: focus on immunosuppression. AACN Clin Issues 10(2):253–269
8. Shoham S, Marr KA (2012) Invasive fungal infections in solid organ transplant recipients. Future Microbiol 7(5):639–655. https://doi.org/10.2217/fmb.12.28
9. Singh N (2000) Antifungal prophylaxis for solid organ transplant recipients: seeking clarity. Clin Infect Dis 31(2):545–553
10. Gavaldà J, Meije Y, Fortún J, Roilides E, Saliba F, Lortholary O et al (2014) Invasive fungal infections in solid organ transplant recipients. Clin Microbiol Infect 20(Suppl 7):27–48. https://doi.org/10.1111/1469-0691.12660
11. Delgado J, Calvo N, Gomis A, Pérez-Flores I, Rodríguez A, Ridao N et al (2010) Candiduria in renal transplant recipients: incidence, clinical repercussion, and treatment indication. Transplant Proc 42(8):2944–2946. https://doi.org/10.1016/j.transproceed.2010.08.019
12. Pappas PG, Kauffman CA, Andes DR, Clancy CJ, Marr KA, Ostrosky-Zeichner L et al (2016) Clinical practice guideline for the management of candidiasis: 2016 update by the Infectious Diseases Society of America. Clin Infect Dis 62(4):e1–e50. https://doi.org/10.1093/cid/civ933
13. Benedetti E, Gruessner AC, Troppmann C, Papalois BE, Sutherland DE, Dunn DL et al (1996) Intra-abdominal infections after pancreatic transplantation: incidence, treatment, and outcome. J Am Coll Surg 183(4):307–316
14. Raghuram A, Restrepo A, Safadjou S, Cooley J, Orloff M, Hardy D et al (2012) Invasive fungal infections following liver transplantation: incidence, risk factors, survival, and impact of fluconazole-resistant Candida parapsilosis (2003-2007). Liver Transpl 18(9):1100–1109. https://doi.org/10.1002/lt.23467
15. Husain S, Tollemar J, Dominguez EA, Baumgarten K, Humar A, Paterson DL et al (2003) Changes in the spectrum and risk factors for invasive candidiasis in liver transplant recipients: prospective, multicenter, case-controlled study. Transplantation 75(12):2023–2029
16. Liu X, Ling Z, Li L, Ruan B (2011) Invasive fungal infections in liver transplantation. Int J Infect Dis 15(5):e298–e304. https://doi.org/10.1016/j.ijid.2011.01.005
17. Unterpertinger R, Sieger J, Schneeberger S, Bosmuller C, Aigner M, Lass-Floerl C et al (2016) Inzidnez invasiver fungaler infektionen nach lebertransplantation. Transpl Int 29(Suppl S4):1–23
18. Fischer L, Sterneck M (2005) Invasive fungal infections in patients after liver transplantation. Mycoses 48(Suppl 1):27–35
19. Lichtenstern C, Hochreiter M, Zehnter VD, Brenner T, Hofer S, Mieth M et al (2013) Pretransplant model for end stage liver disease score predicts posttransplant incidence of fungal infections after liver transplantation. Mycoses 56(3):350–357. https://doi.org/10.1111/myc.12041
20. Wang JL, Chang CH, Young-Xu Y, Chan KA (2010) Systematic review and meta-analysis of the tolerability and hepatotoxicity of antifungals in empirical and definitive therapy for invasive fungal infection. Antimicrob Agents Chemother 54(6):2409–2419. https://doi.org/10.1128/AAC.01657-09
21. Echenique IA, Angarone MP, Gordon RA, Rich J, Anderson AS, McGee EC et al (2017) Invasive fungal infection after heart transplantation: a 7-year, single-center experience. Transpl Infect Dis 19(1). https://doi.org/10.1111/tid.12650
22. Hummel M, Thalmann U, Jautzke G, Staib F, Seibold M, Hetzer R (1992) Fungal infections following heart transplantation. Mycoses 35(1-2):23–34
23. Rabin AS, Givertz MM, Couper GS, Shea MM, Peixoto D, Yokoe DS et al (2015) Risk factors for

invasive fungal disease in heart transplant recipients. Transpl Infect Dis 17(2):259–266. https://doi.org/10.1111/tid.12362
24. Husain S, Sole A, Alexander BD, Aslam S, Avery R, Benden C et al (2016) The 2015 International Society for Heart and Lung Transplantation Guidelines for the management of fungal infections in mechanical circulatory support and cardiothoracic organ transplant recipients: executive summary. J Heart Lung Transplant 35(3):261–282. https://doi.org/10.1016/j.healun.2016.01.007
25. Gustafsson F, Rogers JG (2017) Left ventricular assist device therapy in advanced heart failure: patient selection and outcomes. Eur J Heart Fail 19(5):595–602. https://doi.org/10.1002/ejhf.779
26. Kubak BM (2002) Fungal infection in lung transplantation. Transpl Infect Dis 4(Suppl 3):24–31
27. Kusne S, Manez R, Bonet H, Abu-Elmagd K, Furukawa H, Irish W et al (1994) Infectious complications after small bowel transplantation in adults. Transplant Proc 26(3):1682–1683
28. Florescu DF, Islam KM, Grant W, Mercer DF, Langnas A, Botha J et al (2010) Incidence and outcome of fungal infections in pediatric small bowel transplant recipients. Transpl Infect Dis 12(6):497–504. https://doi.org/10.1111/j.1399-3062.2010.00542.x

14 Mycotoxins and Human Disease

Aleksandra Barac

Abbreviations

AFB1	Aflatoxins B1
IARC	International Agency for Research on Cancer
HBV	Hepatitis B
AFM1	Aflatoxin M1
DON	Deoxynivalenol
OTA	Ochratoxin A
BEN	Balkan endemic nephropathy
GI	Gastrointestinal
WDB	Water-damaged buildings
NAC	*N*-Acetylcysteine

14.1 History

Mycotoxins are secondary fungal metabolites that can be produced in crops and other food commodities. When ingested, mycotoxins may cause a mycotoxicosis, the term first used by Forgacs and Carll [1], which can result in an acute or chronic disease episode [2]. The oldest recognized mycotoxicosis of humans is ergotism caused by the plant parasitic fungus, *Claviceps purpurea*. After periodic outbreaks in central Europe, the disease became epidemic in the Middle Ages, where it was known as St. Anthony's fire [3, 4]. Gangrenous symptoms were described in medieval episodes of ergotism in humans, where early symptoms were hallucinations and swollen limbs with burning sensations, with subsequent necrosis leading to loss of appendages [4].

Today, the word *mycotoxin* simply means a toxin produced by a fungus. Modern mycotoxicology began with the discovery of the aflatoxins in the early 1960s [3]. Since that time, numerous other mycotoxins have been discovered [5].

14.2 Introduction

Mycotoxins are a relatively large, diverse group of naturally occurring, fungal toxins, many of which have been strongly implicated as chemical agents of toxic disease in humans and animals. The history and use of mycotoxins are very long and go back to antiquity, e.g., the philosopher Socrates was executed by drinking of a mixture containing poison hemlock. Today, there are potentially 20,000 to 300,000 known mycotoxins of micro- and macrofungi. Microfungi are the surrogate for the fungus itself that produces mycotoxins on the cellular level. Macrofungi refer to the fruiting bodies (mushrooms) that are appreciated deli food but may be poisonous and deadly. The diversity of toxic mechanisms will be equally as great. The number of mycotoxins actually known to be involved in disease is considerably less, but even this number is difficult to

A. Barac
Clinic for Infectious and Tropical Diseases, Clinical Centre of Serbia, Faculty of Medicine, University of Belgrade, Belgrade, Serbia

E. Presterl (ed.), *Clinically Relevant Mycoses*, https://doi.org/10.1007/978-3-319-92300-0_14

assess due to the diversity of effects of these unique compounds on humans [6–9].

The usual route of mycotoxin exposure is ingestion as food or feed contaminants. However, dermal and inhalation also may be important routes of exposure. Direct effects of mycotoxins range from acute disease where severe conditions of altered health may exist prior to death as a result of exposure to the toxin. These conditions are more likely following exposure to high levels of a mycotoxin. Other, more insidious or occult conditions (e.g., growth retardation, impaired immunity, decreased disease resistance) or more chronic disease manifestations (e.g., tumor formation) may result from prolonged exposure to small quantities of toxin [7, 10, 11]. Awareness is growing regarding the hazards of mycotoxins as contaminants of food and feed.

14.3 Microfungi

14.3.1 Classes of Mycotoxins

The mycotoxins that pose the greatest potential risk to human and animal health as food and feed contaminants are aflatoxins, trichothecenes, fumonisins, zearalenone, ochratoxin A (OTA), and ergot alkaloids. However, other mycotoxins should be included because of their frequency of occurrence in commodities, their products, or their co-occurrence with other important mycotoxins. This expanded list includes cyclopiazonic acid, sterigmatocystin, gliotoxin, citrinin, penitrems (perhaps other tremorogenic mycotoxins), patulin, and miscellaneous mycotoxins such as fusarin C, fusaric acid, penicillic acid, mycophenolic acid, roquefortine, Penicillium roqueforti (PR) toxin, and isofumigaclavines A and B [7, 9–11].

14.3.1.1 Major Classes of Mycotoxins

Aflatoxins are naturally occurring mycotoxins that are produced by various species of *Aspergillus*. The major aflatoxins commonly isolated from foods and feeds are aflatoxins B1 (AFB1), B2, G1, and G2 [12]. Aflatoxin is considered as hepatotoxic, carcinogenic, immunosuppressive, and antinutritional contaminant of many staple food commodities. Mutation of the P53 gene is considered as a key event in aflatoxin-induced carcinogenesis [10, 13, 14]. The endo-epoxide primarily binds to cellular proteins and is associated with direct cytotoxicity and the impairment of liver function. AFB1 is classified as a group 1 carcinogen by the International Agency for Research on Cancer (IARC) (Table 14.1) [15]. Epidemiological evidence suggest a synergistic effect of AFB1 and chronic hepatitis B (HBV) infections in the prevalence of liver cancer in humans [11, 13, 16]. Animal studies show that AFB1 also interferes with vitamins A, D, B12, iron, selenium, and zinc nutrition [10, 13, 17].

Table 14.1 Classification of food mycotoxins as potential human carcinogens

Group	Classification of food mycotoxins
1	Aflatoxin B1, B2, G1, G2
2A	–
2B	Aflatoxin M1, ochratoxin A, sterigmatocystin
3	Citrinin, patulin, luteoskyrin, cyclochlorotine, deoxynivalenol
4	–

Group 1, carcinogenic to humans; Group 2A, probably carcinogenic to humans; Group 2B, possibly carcinogenic to humans; Group 3, not classifiable as to its carcinogenicity to humans; Group 4, probably not carcinogenic to humans (classified by the International Agency for Research on Cancer)

Another important hepatic metabolite is aflatoxin M1 (AFM1), which is excreted into milk both in animals and in humans. This results in an undesirable exposure of infants. AFM1 is less biologically active than AFB1 but can also be converted into epoxide forms that lead to hepatotoxicity and hepatocarcinogenicity [9, 12, 13]. IARC has classified AFM1 as a group 2B carcinogen (possibly carcinogenic to humans) (Table 14.1) [15].

Trichothecenes are a family of nearly 150 structurally related compounds produced by several fungal genera: *Fusarium*, *Cephalosporium*, *Myrothecium*, *Stachybotrys*, *Trichoderma*, and others [18]. The most common trichothecene mycotoxin is deoxynivalenol (DON, sometimes referred to as vomitoxin), which is common contaminant of corn and wheat in Europe [18, 19].

Fumonisins are mycotoxins produced by *Fusarium verticillioides* [19–21]. There is evidence linking *F. verticillioides* infected corn to the high incidence of human esophageal cancer in South Africa and China [19, 21–23]. *F. verticillioides* is an almost universal inhabitant of corn [19, 21, 22, 24].

Ochratoxins are a group of structurally similar metabolites commonly produced by *Aspergillus ochraceus* and *Penicillium verrucosum*. The major mycotoxin in this group is OTA. OTA has been suggested as the etiological factor of the Balkan endemic nephropathy (BEN) [18].

Ergot alkaloids are produced by several species of *Claviceps* that infect grains or grain products. These mycotoxins are involved in either nervous or gangrenous syndromes in humans. Ergotism is one of the oldest mycotoxicoses known, although occurrence of the disease has declined over time [2–4].

14.3.1.2 Minor Classes of Mycotoxins

Cyclopiazonic acid is mycotoxin isolated from molds commonly found on agricultural commodities or used in fermented food production (*Aspergillus flavus*, *Aspergillus versicolor*, *Aspergillus tamarii*, and several *Penicillium* species used in the production of fermented sausages in Europe). This includes *Penicillium camemberti*, used in the production of Camembert cheese, and *Aspergillus oryzae*, used in the production of soy sauce in the Far East. This mycotoxin has been shown to occur naturally in corn, cheese, peanuts, and sunflower seeds [2, 7].

Sterigmatocystin is produced by several species of *Aspergillus* and *Bipolaris* and by *Penicillium luteum*. Sterigmatocystin has been detected at low concentrations in green coffee, moldy wheat, and in the rind of hard cheese [2, 7].

Citrinin is a yellow mycotoxin produced by several *Penicillium* and *Aspergillus* species, including *Penicillium verrucosum* strains that produce OTA. Like OTA, citrinin causes kidney damage in laboratory animals [2, 7].

Patulin is produced primarily by species of *Penicillium* and *Aspergillus*, and its limited toxic properties are of major concern because it occurs in apples and, subsequently, applesauce and juice [2, 7].

Citreoviridin originally was isolated from molds obtained from rice associated with a disease called "cardiac beriberi" that has occurred for three centuries in Japan (2). This mycotoxin also occurs in corn and other foods and feeds infected by some species of *Penicillium* and *Aspergillus* [2, 7].

Fusaproliferin has been detected in corn samples infected by *Fusarium proliferatum*, and *Fusarium subglutinans* that have been tested are capable of fusaproliferin production in culture [19, 21]. Although the significance of this compound in animal and human health remains to be determined, its acute toxicity to brine shrimp exceeds that of more familiar compounds such as the fumonisins.

14.3.2 Mycotoxin-Producing Fungi

Mycotoxins are produced by a wide array of diverse fungal species that generally are not aggressive pathogens. Most of the mycotoxins that are considered to be important are produced primarily by three genera of fungi: *Aspergillus*, *Penicillium*, and *Fusarium*. *Claviceps* and *Stachybotrys* also are important producers of mycotoxins [7, 10, 12, 22, 24].

Within the genus *Aspergillus*, the major class of mycotoxins is the aflatoxins. The crops most usually affected are corn, cotton, peanuts, and certain tree nuts. Although not conclusive in all crops, high temperatures seem to play a role in aflatoxin contamination [10, 14].

Within the genus *Fusarium*, there are a number of important mycotoxin-producing species. The major causative agents are *Fusarium graminearum*, *F. verticillioides*, *F. proliferatum*, and *F. subglutinans*. These latter agents may produce fumonisins during the pathogenic state in corn. *Fusarium graminearum* is a significant pathogen on wheat, barley, corn, and oats and is a major producer of DON in these grains [19, 21, 24].

Penicillium spp. are more typically associated with storage of crops and the production of

Table 14.2 Human diseases in which analytic and/or epidemiologic data suggest or implicate mycotoxin involvement

Disease	Substrate	Etiologic agent (spp.)	Ref.
Akakabio-byo	Wheat, barley, oats, rice	*Fusarium*	[8]
Alimentary toxic aleukia (septic angina)	Cereal grains (toxic bread)	*Fusarium*	[19]
Balkan endemic nephropathy	Cereal grains	*Penicillium*	[41]
Cardiac beriberi	Rice	*Aspergillus, Penicillium*	
Dendrodochiotoxicosis	Fodder (skin, inhalation)	*Dendrodochium toxicum*	
Ergotism	Rye, cereal grains	*Claviceps purpurea*	[4]
Esophageal tumors	Corn	*Fusarium moniliforme*	[20]
Hepatocarcinoma (acute aflatoxicosis)	Cereal grains, peanuts	*Aspergillus flavus, A. parasiticus*	[37–39]
Kashin-Beck disease, "Urov disease"	Cereal grains	*Fusarium* spp.	[8]
Kwashiorkor	Cereal grains	*Aspergillus flavus, A. parasiticus*	[32]
Onyalai	Millet	*Phoma sorghina*	[7]
Reye's syndrome	Cereal grains	*Aspergillus* spp.	[60]
Stachybotryotoxicosis	Hay, cereal grains, fodder (skin contact, inhalation)	*Stachybotrys atra*	[25]

mycotoxins such as OTA. OTA usually is formed in storage or during drying of certain commodities for processing [22, 23].

A number of fungi are capable of producing toxic alkaloids, and *Claviceps* spp. are the most notable in this regard. Toxic alkaloids also are produced by the genera *Epichloe* and *Neotyphodium*, both of which can be endophytic in certain plant species such as fescue and ryegrass [2].

Stachybotrys is a cellulolytic saprophyte that can be found in a variety of commodities, and the trichothecene metabolites of this organism can produce disease similar to some of those produced by *Fusarium* spp. Recently, this organism seemed to be involved in human disease where building materials were contaminated with the organism and possibly its toxic metabolites [25].

14.3.3 Impact of Mycotoxins on Human Diseases

Mycotoxicosis, the disease resulting from exposure to a mycotoxin, may be manifested as acute to chronic and ranges from rapid death to tumor formation [6, 9]. More occult disease may occur when the mycotoxin interferes with immune processes, rendering the patient more susceptible to infectious diseases. Humans likely are exposed to mycotoxins through several routes such as ingestion by contaminated food (the most prominent means of exposure), contact, and inhalation [2, 6, 9]. There are many diseases that have been described in humans for which either analytic or epidemiologic evidence implicates a mycotoxin etiology (Table 14.2) [9–11, 14]. The aflatoxins are known causes of acute aflatoxicosis in humans, as well as potential cofactor of hepatic carcinoma, together with HBV [11, 16]. OTA has been conjecturally associated with the Balkan endemic nephropathy (BEN). The rural populations in the Balkans have a high incidence of chronic kidney problems and tumors of the excretory organ system [18, 42–44]. The most likely toxic products of the *Fusarium* spp., the trichothecenes, are conjecturally associated with the most prominent disease described alimentary toxic aleukia. The trichothecene, DON, is capable of producing a disease in mice that is similar in histological descriptions to human glomerulonephropathy [18, 22, 23]. Stachybotryotoxicosis is a disease that occurs in humans and is suspected to be caused by toxins of the organism *Stachybotrys chartarum* [25]. The fumonisins have been associated with esophageal cancer in certain human populations [22]. Of interest to many investigators is that a number of mycotoxins are immunosuppressive and likely could be involved in human disease. Today, there is an apparent growing concern within the medical community regarding mycotoxin involvement in human diseases [6, 9]. The following section discusses mycotoxicoses for which there is considerable evidence for involvement of a specific mycotoxin(s). These and other human diseases where mycotoxin involvement is likely are presented in Table 14.2.

14.3.3.1 Acute Illness and Death

The symptoms of severe mycotoxicosis include hemorrhagic necrosis of the liver, bile duct proliferation, edema, and lethargy. Adult humans usually have a high tolerance of aflatoxin, and, in the reported acute poisonings, the children are those who die [26]. Acute poisonings, about 25% of which result in death, occur as a result of high levels of exposure [26, 27]. Reports of death and serious illness usually originate from developing countries within the zone of risk [28, 29].

14.3.3.2 Chronic Effects of Mycotoxins in Human Populations

In many regions of the world, dietary staples, especially cereal grains, contain low levels of mycotoxins. The impact of regular low-level intake of mycotoxins on human health is likely to be significant with a number of possible consequences including impaired growth and development, immune dysfunction, and the disease consequences of alterations in DNA metabolism [19].

14.3.3.3 Growth and Development

Numerous animal studies have shown that one of the first effects of mycotoxin ingestion is reduced feed intake and growth [22, 30]. There are facts revealing a very strong association between exposure to aflatoxin in the children and both stunting and being underweight. Both conditions reflect significant malnutrition and exposure of the children to aflatoxin in utero and subsequently after birth [30]. In West Africa, the aflatoxin exposure of children between 9 months and 5 years of age examined their growth, development, and height [30]. The children were also co-exposed to a number of infectious diseases, and it is likely that the exposure to disease and aflatoxin would significantly compromise growth and development through reduced food intake and also the repartitioning of nutrients to maintain an upregulated immune system and away from growth and development [31, 32].

14.3.3.4 Immunosuppression

Immunosuppression is a likely major economic effect of mycotoxins. Mycotoxins known to have this effect are aflatoxins, certain trichothecenes, OTA, and gliotoxin. These mycotoxins can be immunotoxic and exert effects on cellular responses, humoral factors, and cytokine mediators of the immune system and can cause a variety of immune-related changes, including thymic aplasia and inhibition of phagocytosis by macrophages, delayed cutaneous hypersensitivity, lymphocyte proliferation, and leukocyte migration [23, 33, 34]. The effects on immunity and resistance are often difficult to recognize in the field because signs of disease are associated with the infection rather than the toxin that predisposed the individual to infection through decreased resistance and/or reduced vaccine or drug efficacy. There are evidences who reveal strong association between aflatoxin exposure and reduced immunocompetence in children [35] and adults [36], suggesting that aflatoxin ingestion decreases resistance to infection in human populations. DON can both stimulate and suppress the immune system, with dysregulation of IgA and the development of kidney disease in animal models that closely resembles human glomerulonephritis IgA nephropathy [33, 34].

14.3.3.5 Carcinogenicity, Mutagenicity, and Teratogenicity

Several food-contaminating mycotoxins have been defined as harmful carcinogens by the IARC (Table 14.1), that is, DON/nivalenol, zearalenone, ochratoxin, fumonisins, and aflatoxins [2, 15]. There is significant body of evidence demonstrating human exposure in utero to a number of mycotoxins, but the relevance of this exposure to birth defects or impaired embryonic development has received relatively little attention [19]. Recent epidemiological investigations of human populations in Texas, China, Guatemala, and Southern Africa that rely on foods prepared from maize, which is often contaminated with fumonisins, found a significantly higher incidence of neural tube defects in babies [19].

14.3.3.6 Hepatocellular Cancer and Mycotoxins

Two major factors, aflatoxin and HBV, which commonly occur in the same populations, influence the risk of liver cancer. Independently, each factor significantly increases the relative risk of cancer, and most studies report them, together, to be synergistic [37, 38]. The suggested mechanism for this synergy is that aflatoxin suppresses DNA repair mechanisms that help limit the development of hepatocellular cancer from HBV, and HBV prevents detoxification, but it is also possible that the immunotoxicity of aflatoxin interferes with the suppression of cancer. AFB1 is the most well-known bioaccumulative toxin with strong mutagenic effect, involved in the development of hepatocellular cancer [37–39]. When individuals are exposed to AFB1 for a long time, monooxygenases produce reactive epoxide in the liver, leading to formation of toxic derivatives with nucleic acids and proteins [39, 40].

14.3.3.7 Mycotoxins and Balkan Endemic Nephropathy

There are convincing evidence that chronic poisoning with OTA is possible causative agents of BEN [41–44]. OTA, produced primarily by *Aspergillus ochraceous* or *Penicillium verrucosum*, occurs on several commodities prevalent in human diets, including barley and green coffee beans [42, 44]. OTA-mediated nephropathy is endemic, and outbreaks have been associated with weather conditions [43, 44]. This mycotoxin is considered a possibly carcinogenic to humans particular in the role of developing BEN-associated cancer (Table 14.1). However, the mechanism of OTA-derived tumor formation is unknown, and conflicting results regarding the potential of OTA to react with DNA to form covalent DNA adducts have been reported [45, 46].

14.3.3.8 Mycotoxins and Gastrointestinal Infections

The gastrointestinal (GI) tract, as the primary targeting organ, is exposed directly to mycotoxins with a higher concentration than other tissues and organs, which can affect the regeneration, proliferation, differentiation, and repair of intestinal epithelial cells. Some mycotoxins, such as AFB1, OTA, and DON, could reduce the expression of zonula occludens protein and increase intestinal mucosal permeability, thus damaging the barrier functions of intestinal epithelial cells and inducing bacterial translocation [21, 47]. Moreover, mycotoxins can influence the immune system of the GI tract [21, 48]. Mycotoxins could trigger mucosal immunoregulatory mechanisms such as the secretion of mucus, antimicrobial peptides, and immunoglobulins and directly induce inflammation by inducing intestinal epithelial cells to secrete chemotactic factors and pro-inflammatory cytokines [49]. Mycotoxins may be associated with chronic inflammation of the intestine in genetically susceptible patients with inflammatory bowel disease or coeliac disease [5, 47]. The long-term exposure of trichothecene toxins can increase intestinal colonization by aerobes [48]. The definite disturbance of human GI fungal and bacterial microbiota induced by mycotoxins still remains largely unknown.

14.3.3.9 Mycotoxins and Airway Diseases

Inhalation of mycotoxins is especially hazardous to those living inside damp, wet, and moldy buildings [50]. These toxins, mostly produced by fungi *Stachybotrys*, elicit recruitment of alveolar macrophages and neutrophils, pulmonary hemorrhage, and cytokine production and could trigger chronic obstructive pulmonary disease, while inhalation of a toxic dose of mycotoxin leads to systemic effects exclusive of lung injury [51, 52]. The most frequently recovered mycotoxins in nasal washings of individuals with respiratory diseases living in water-damaged buildings (WDB) are macrocyclic trichothecenes, found in 44% of the nasal washing specimens, whereas aflatoxin is present in 17% of these cases. On the other hand, mycotoxins were not found in nasal washings of a healthy control population. Other positive findings for the presence of mycotoxins in various tissues include trichothecenes in sera, breast milk, placenta, umbilical cord, and tissues (sinus) of individuals exposed in WDB [53, 54]. Clinical symptoms expressed by individuals living in WDB contaminated by *Stachybotrys*, mostly *S. atra* and *S. chartarum*, are pulmonary irritation and headaches, fatigue, malaise, diarrhea, inflammation of the nose, chest pain, or leukopenia [54, 55]. Strategy for prevention of this mycotoxicosis is using of polycarbonate membrane filters that could retain airborne particles of trichothecenes contaminated materials [50].

14.3.3.10 Mycotoxins and Deficiency of Vitamin B12

There are several pieces of evidence to show that mycotoxins affect cellular activities of the brain for which vitamin B12 plays a major role. Vitamin B12 possibly interacts with mycotoxins to effect some of the biochemical and neurological changes [56, 57]. It is believed that the biochemical consequences of fumonisin disruption of sphingolipid metabolism are increased free sphingoid bases and their 1-phosphates, alterations in complex sphingolipids, and decreased ceramide biosynthesis [24]. It is not yet clear whether vitamin B12 deficiency precludes fungal infection or vice versa. However, the factors commonly believed to predispose to recurrent chronic fungal infections included deficiency in whole blood folate, iron, and vitamin B complex [57]. These diseases occur as result of metabolic disorders and are due to inactivity of enzymes that are characteristic of vitamin B complex deficiencies (Table 14.3) [58].

Table 14.3 Signs, symptoms, and clinical neurologic indications of vitamin B12 deficiency

Signs and symptoms	Clinical neurological indications
Headache, fatigue, loss of appetite	Nerve damage and demyelination
Pinky-red sore or smooth tongue	Degeneration of perip heral nervous system leading to paralysis
Growth failure in children	Progressive peripheral neuropathy
Psychosis, confusion	Spinal degeneration and macrocytic cells
Depression, memory loss	Alzheimer's disease, allergies, asthma
Anxiety, insomnia	Crohn's disease, multiple sclerosis, insomnia, sciatic neuritis, trigeminal neuralgia, osteoarthritis

14.4 Macrofungi

14.4.1 Overview

Macrofungi, well known as mushrooms, are diverse group of the visible fruit of fungi, with known toxic effect on human [59, 61–63]. Approximately 100 of the known species of mushrooms are poisonous to humans, with new toxic species continually being identified [65, 66]. The geographical distribution of toxic mushrooms as well as toxicity of different mushrooms within the same genus may vary greatly (Table 14.4). Some mushrooms initially classified as edible have recently been reclassified as toxic [59]. Mushroom poisoning, termed mycetism or mycetismus, most commonly ensues after mushrooms are foraged, misidentified, and then consumed [64–66]. Worldwide, hundreds of mushroom poisonings are fatal each year [59, 65–67]. Most fatalities are secondary to *Amanita phalloides* ingestions [63, 65–67].

Some toxic mushroom ingestions will produce self-limited toxicity. Others will prove fatal. Generally, most toxic mushrooms produce some GI distress, and commonly GI symptoms are the first symptoms reported [59, 65]. A latency of <6 h to development of GI symptoms was utilized to predict that a mushroom ingestion should produce limited toxicity. This practice has limitations, and these limitations have become more apparent as new toxic mushrooms are recognized and more cases are reported. A study from Turkey reported 317 cases of mycetism, without delineating which mushrooms produced toxicity, and found that common symptoms include nausea (86.6%), vomiting (79.8%), and diarrhea (21.1%). More than 20% of patients who eventually developed hepatic failure had a latent phase of <6 h [62–65]. Similarly, there are reports about severe mushroom-induced hepatitis, 33% with initial symptoms within <6 h of ingestion [59, 63]. Not all patients presenting with symptoms within 6 h of ingestion have a benign course [59, 62, 63, 65]. Interestingly, if *A. phalloides* ingestion is known, or strongly suspected, to have occurred and diarrhea develops in <8 h, the prognosis is poorer [63–65]. Conversely, GI symptoms occurring >6 h after ingestion remain concerning for a possible serious clinical course and possible fatality [59, 62, 64–67].

14.4.2 Neurotoxins

Neurotoxic mushrooms may produce cholinergic, epileptogenic, inebriating, encephalopathic, or hallucinogenic syndromes [59, 63]. Many of these syndromes have associated visual disturbances. Some contain toxins that affect vasculature and are classified under neurovascular toxins (Table 14.4).

14.4.2.1 Cholinergic Syndromes

Some mushrooms contain muscarine that stimulates peripheral muscarinic receptors. Muscarine acts like acetylcholine, but is not degraded by cholinesterase, and therefore has a longer duration of action [63]. The amount of muscarine in *Amanita muscaria* is very low, and muscarinic symptoms are rarely seen after its consumption [59, 65]. *Inocybe*, *Clitocybe*, *Boletus*, and *Rubinoboletus* species can contain sufficient muscarine to produce muscarinic toxicity. Onset of toxicity is 15 min to 5 h after ingestion. Flushing, vasodilation, diaphoresis, lacrimation,

Table 14.4 Geographical distribution of recently described toxic mushroom

Primary system affected by toxins (effects)	Geographical location of mushroom harvest[a]	Mushrooms
Neurological (encephalopathy)	Germany	*Hapalopilus rutilans* (purple dye polypore)
Neurological (convulsive encephalopathy)	Japan	*Pleurocybella porrigens* (angel's wing)
Neurovascular (red, swollen, painful extremities)	Japan, South Korea	*Clitocybe acromelalgia*
Neurovascular (red, swollen, painful extremities)	France, Italy, Morocco	*Clitocybe amoenolens* (poison dwarf bamboo or burn mushroom)
Cardiac (sudden death)	Yunnan Province, China	*Trogia venenata* (little white)
Cardiac (sudden death)	Jiangxi Province, China	*Amanita franchetii, Ramaria rufescens*
Renal	Canada (South-West), USA (Pacific Coast to North-West)	*Amanita smithiana* (toxic lepidella or North American lepidella)
Renal	France (South), Spain, Italy	*Amanita proxima* (Mediterranean Amidella)
Renal	Japan	*Amanita pseudoporphyria Hongo*
Muscular (rhabdomyolysis, myocarditis)	France, Poland	*Tricholoma equestre* (yellow trich or yellow knight or man on horseback)
Muscular (rhabdomyolysis, myocarditis)	Taiwan, Japan, Korea, China, Nepal	*Russula subnigricans* (blackening russula)
Immune/heme (hemolysis, hepatorenal failure)	Northern Hemisphere	*Paxillus involutus* (poison pax or brown roll rim)
Immune/heme (pancytopenia)	Northeastern Asia	*Ganoderma neojaponicum Imazeki*[b]
Immune/heme (pancytopenia)	Japan, China, Korea, Java	*Podostroma cornu-damae*

[a]Copyright: J. Med. Toxicol. (2014) 10;173-189; Reference: [59]
[b]Newly reported and association not as well established as other causes of mycetism

miosis, blurred vision, hypersalivation, bronchorrhea, bronchospasm, vomiting, diarrhea, abdominal pain, tremor, restlessness, and bladder contraction can follow ingestion. Hallucinations, bradycardia or tachycardia, hypotension or hypertension, syncope, shock, and confusion are common [66, 67]. Treatment is supportive: fluid and electrolyte replacement, vasopressors, and atropine in case of bronchorrhea and bradycardia. Toxicity generally resolves within 12 h of ingestion [59, 63].

14.4.2.2 Epileptogenic Syndromes

The classic epileptogenic mushroom is *Gyromitra esculenta* (false morel), which may be confused with *Morchella* sp. (true morel, which is deemed edible but which can produce neurological symptoms if poorly cooked) or *Verpa bohemica* (early morel) [68]. Symptoms begin 4–12 h after ingestion. Clinical progression is vomiting and diarrhea followed by neurological symptoms (vertigo, ataxia, nystagmus, tremor, convulsions, and coma), sometimes followed by hepatic necrosis, jaundice, methemoglobinemia, hemolysis, and rhabdomyolysis [66–69]. Approximately 10% of poisoned patients die [70]. Treatment is supportive, while pyridoxine is recommended for neurologic symptoms including seizures with dosing regimen of 70 mg/kg up to 5 g, intravenously [66–69, 71]. Seizures may be resistant to benzodiazepines and barbiturates prior to GABA repletion aided by pyridoxine treatment [69]. In Japan, 2004, convulsive encephalopathy occurred epidemically, with latency of 1–31 days, when patients with hemodialysis-dependent renal failure ingested *Pleurocybella porrigens* (also called *Nothopanus porrigens*, Sugihiratake, and angel's wing). Patients exhibited convulsions (78%), myoclonus (47%), dysarthria (31%), ataxia (25%), and paresis or paralysis (22%) [72]. Intractable status epilepticus has also been reported [73–76]. Magnetic resonance imaging may reveal intracranial lesions involving the subcortical white matter of the insular cortex, claustrum, external capsule, putamen, and globus pallidus [76]. The mortality rate is approximately 30% [72, 73].

14.4.2.3 Encephalopathic Syndromes

In Germany, encephalopathy and hepatorenal insufficiency associated with purple urine have been reported following ingestion of *Hapalopilus rutilans* (Purple Dye Polypore) [59, 63, 65, 74]. The syndrome begins with nausea, vomiting, and abdominal pain approximately 12 h after ingestion. Hepatorenal laboratory abnormalities and neurological symptoms, such as vertigo, ataxia, drowsiness, hypotonia, and visual complaints, follow [66, 74]. *P. porrigens*, *Grifola frondosa*, and *Pleurotus eryngii* poisonings may be also presented with encephalopathy. Any mushroom that produces fulminant hepatic failure (e.g., *A. phalloides*) or that is epileptogenic (e.g., *G. esculenta*) may be associated with encephalopathy [63, 69].

14.4.2.4 Hallucinogenic Syndromes

Hallucinogenic mushrooms generally contain psilocybin and include *Psilocybe* spp., *Panaeolus* spp., and *Stropharia aeruginosa* [64]. Psilocybin-containing species may turn bluish (bruise) upon handling especially the stalks; however, this is nonspecific, as some other species that do not contain psilocybin bruise similarly [64]. Symptoms reflected in altered time-space perceptions, auditory, and visual hallucinations begin 15–30 min after ingestion and generally last up to 6 h and rarely last 12 h [66]. Mydriasis, hypertension, tachycardia, dysrhythmias, and myocardial infarction have also been reported [59, 63, 75]. Seizures and hyperthermia have been reported in children [75]. Treatment is supportive. Benzodiazepine and barbiturates have been used to control agitation and seizures [69, 75].

14.4.2.5 Neurovascular Toxins

Clitocybe amoenolens (burn mushroom) and *Clitocybe acromelalga* are associated with erythromelalgia. Erythromelalgia involves erythema, swelling, and pain of the distal extremities. Ingestion of only a few mushrooms can produce toxicity. In humans, symptoms appear 24 h after ingestion, and patients present with paresthesia of the digits followed by paroxysmal burning pain [63, 74]. Paroxysmal dilation of the blood vessels of the skin occurs, what is associated with tactile and burning pain and red, swollen hands and feet. Heat and a position decline induced paroxysmal crisis, which generally occurs nocturnally. Cyanosis or erythema may worsen during pain paroxysms. More severe cases are associated with local diaphoresis and trophic changes of the digits. The pain can be incapacitating. Dipping the extremities in cold water often provides relief, while traditional analgesics may be ineffective. The syndrome can last for weeks to months [59, 63, 69, 74].

14.4.2.6 Cardiotoxins and Sudden Death

A seasonal illness, called "Yunnan" sudden unexplained death, has been epidemiologically traced to *Trogia venenata* (little white) consumption. The exact toxin responsible for the syndrome is not yet known [77, 78]. Patients report nausea, vomiting, diarrhea, abdominal pain, and fatigue, while recurrent syncope and sudden unexpected death may occur. Many patients report palpitations, chest discomfort, dizziness, syncope, seizures, ventricular tachycardia, fibrillation, and elevated plasma enzymes in the hours preceding death [77, 78]. Postmortem examination revealed focal lymphocytic myocarditis, with breakage of the muscle fibers, lymphocytic infiltration of the liver, pulmonary alveolar edema, acute kidney necrosis, hepatocyte necrosis, and congestion of the liver, lung, or spleen [78].

14.4.2.7 Hepatotoxins

Amatoxins and gyromitrin are protoplasmic poisons that produce hepatotoxicity [77]. Many *Amanita* spp. contain amatoxin, in the first place *A. phalloides* (death cap), as well as some *Galerina* and *Lepiota* (e.g., *L. brunneoincarnata* and *L. helveola*). As little as 0.1 mg amatoxin/kg body weight may be lethal in adults [67, 77, 79].

In general, supportive care is the mainstay for mycetism [59, 79]. If a patient is actively vomiting, activated charcoal may not contribute to decontamination. Antiemetics may limit natural decontamination. Determining what mushrooms are likely to have been ingested, and therefore what treatments are most appropriate, will likely be based on the geographic location of mushroom harvesting (see Table 14.5) [63]. If a hepatotoxic mushroom, such as *A. phalloides*, has been ingested or is suspected, prompt treatment with an antidote seems prudent (Table 14.5) [67, 79].

Table 14.5 Antidotes for amatoxin in poisoning (recommended doses based on previously published reports)

Antidote	Mechanism of action[a]	Dose
Silibinin[b]	Competes with amatoxins for transmembrane transport; inhibits penetration of amanitin into hepatocytes; scavenges free radicals; produces anti-inflammatory effects; increases ribosomal RNA synthesis, increases protein synthesis	5 mg/kg IV over 1 h; then 20 mg/kg/24 h continuous infusion (diluted in 5% glucose to a concentration of 2 mg silibinin/ml) for 3 days (alternatively, 20 mg/kg/24 h can be divided into 6 doses)
N-acetylcysteine (NAC)	Promotes glutathione regeneration; scavenges free radicals	Follow dosing for APAP treatment: 150 mg/kg IV over 1 h, followed by 12.5 mg/kg/h for 4 h, followed by 6.25 mg/kg/h until hepatic failure resolution

[a]Retrieved from: J. Med. Toxicol. (2014) 10;173-189; Reference: [59]

[b]Silibinin is not approved as a therapeutic treatment for hepatic disease by the Food and Drug Administration in the USA; it is approved and available in Europe and Australia

References

1. Forgacs J, Carll WT (1962) Mycotoxicoses. Adv Vet Sci 7:273–382
2. Council of Agricultural Science & Technology (CAST) (2003) Mycotoxins: risks in plant, animal and human systems. task force report No. 139. Council of Agricultural Science & Technology, Iowa, USA
3. Matossian MK (1989) Poisons of the past: molds, epidemics, and history. Yale University Press, New Haven, p 190
4. Van Rensburg SJ, Altenkirk B (1974) Claviceps purpurea: ergotism. In: IFH Purchase (ed) Mycotoxins. Elsevier, New York, pp 69–96
5. Alonso VA, Pereyra CM, Keller LA et al (2013) Fungi and mycotoxins in silage: an overview. J Appl Microbiol 115(3):637–643
6. Paterson RR, Lima N (2010) Toxicology of mycotoxins. EXS 100:31–63
7. Wambacq E, Vanhoutte I, Audenaert K, De Gelder L, Haesaert G (2016) Occurrence, prevention and remediation of toxigenic fungi and mycotoxins in silage: a review. J Sci Food Agric 96(7):2284–2302
8. Bryden WL (2007) Mycotoxins in the food chain: human health implications. Asia Pac J Clin Nutr 16(1):95–101
9. Marin S, Ramos AJ, Cano-Sancho G, Sanchis V (2013) Mycotoxins: occurrence, toxicology, and exposure assessment. Food Chem Toxicol 60:218–237
10. Ahmad M, Ahmad MM, Hamid R, Abdin MZ, Javed S (2013) Use of response surface methodology to study the effect of media composition on aflatoxin production by Aspergillus flavus. Mycotoxin Res 29(1):39–45
11. Wu HC, Santella R (2012) The role of aflatoxins in hepatocellular carcinoma. Hepat Mon 12(10):e7238
12. Leong YH, Latiff AA, Ahmad NI, Rosma A (2012) Exposure measurement of aflatoxins and aflatoxin metabolites in human body fluids. A short review. Mycotoxin Res 28(2):79–87
13. Bedard LL, Massey TE (2006) Aflatoxin B1-induced DNA damage and its repair. Cancer Lett 241(2):174–183
14. Wild CP, Turner PC (2002) The toxicology of aflatoxins as a basis for public health decisions. Mutagenesis 17(6):471–481
15. IARC Working Group on the Evaluation of Carcinogenic Risks to Humans (2002) Some traditional herbal medicines, some mycotoxins, naphthalene and styrene. IARC Monogr Eval Carcinog Risks Hum 82:1–556
16. Nordenstedt H, White DL, El-Serag HB (2010) The changing pattern of epidemiology in hepatocellular carcinoma. Dig Liver Dis 42(3):S206–S214
17. Anyanwu EC, Kanu I (2007) Biochemical impedance on intracellular functions of vitamin B12 in chronic toxigenic mold exposures. Sci World J 7:1649–1657
18. Staneva R, Rukova B, Hadjidekova S et al (2013) Whole genome methylation array analysis reveals new aspects in Balkan endemic nephropathy etiology. BMC Nephrol 14:225
19. Voss KA, Gelineau-vanWaes JB, Riley RT (2006) Fumonisins: current research trends in developmental toxicology. Mycotoxin Res 22:61–69
20. Yoshizawa T, Yamashita A, Luo Y (1994) Fumonisin occurrence in corn from high- and low-risk areas for human esophageal cancer in China. Appl Environ Microbiol 60(5):1626–1629
21. Bouhet S, Hourcade E, Loiseau N et al (2004) The mycotoxin fumonisin B1 alters the proliferation and the barrier function of porcine intestinal epithelial cells. Toxicol Sci 77:165–171
22. Dersjant-Li Y, Verstegen MWA, Gerrits WJJ (2003) The impact of low concentrations of aflatoxin, deoxynivalenol or fumonisins in diets on growing pigs and poultry. Nutr Res Rev 16:223–239
23. Pestka JJ, Zhou RR, Moon Y, Chung YJ (2004) Cellular and molecular mechanisms for immune modulation by deoxynivalenol and other tricothecenes; unraveling a paradox. Toxicol Lett 153:61–73
24. Riley RT, Enongene E, Voss KA et al (2001) Sphingolipid perturbations as mechanisms for fumonisin carcinogenesis. Environ Health Perspect 109(2):301–308
25. Kuhn DM, Ghannoum MA (2003) Indoor mold, toxigenic fungi, and Stachybotrys chartarum: infectious disease perspective. Clin Microbiol Rev 16(1):144–172
26. Cullen JM, Newberne PM (1993) Acute hepatotoxicity of aflatoxins. In: Eaton DL, Groopman JD (eds) The toxicology of aflatoxins: human health, veterinary, and agricultural significance. Academic, London, pp 1–26
27. Eaton D, Ramsdell HS, Neal G (1993) Biotransformation of aflatoxins. In: Eaton D, Groopman JD (eds) The toxicology of aflatoxins: human health, veterinary, and agricultural significance. Academic, London, pp 45–72
28. Vargas EA, Preis RA, Castro L, Silva CM (2001) Co-occurrence of aflatoxins B1, B2, G1, G2, zearalenone and fumonisin B1 in Brazilian corn. Food Addit Contam 18:981–986
29. Henry SH, Bosch FX, Bowers JC (2002) Aflatoxin, hepatitis and worldwide liver cancer risks. Adv Exp Med Biol 504:229–233
30. Gong Y, Cardwell K, Hounsa A et al (2002) Dietary aflatoxin exposure and impaired growth in children from Beninand Togo: Cross sectional study. Br Med J 325:20–21

31. Elsasser TJ, Klasing KC, Filipov N, Thompson F (2000) The metabolic consequences of stress: targets for stress and priorities of nutrient use. In: Moberg GP, Mench JA (eds) The biology of animal stress. CABI Publishing, New York, pp 77–110
32. Hendrickse RC (1991) Kwashiokor: the hypothesis that incriminates aflatoxin. Paediatrics 88:376–379
33. Oswald IP, Marin DE, Bouhet S, Pinton P, Taranu I, Accensi F (2005) Immunotoxicological risk of mycotoxins for domestic animals. Food Addit Contam 22:354–360
34. Bondy G, Pestka JJ (2000) Immunomodulation by fungal toxins. J Toxicol Environ Health 3:109–143
35. Turner PC, Moore SE, Hall AJ, Prentice AM, Wild CP (2003) Modification of immune function through exposure to dietary aflatoxin in Gambian children. Environ Health Perspect 111:217–220
36. Jiang YI, Jolly PE, Ellis WO, Wang JS, Phillips TD, Williams JH (2005) AflatoxinB1 albumin adduct levels and cellular immune status in Ghanaians. Int Immunol 17:807–814
37. Chuang SC, La Vecchia C, Boffetta P (2009) Liver cancer: descriptive epidemiology and risk factors other than HBV and HCV infection. Cancer Lett 286:9–14
38. Llovet JM, Burroughs A, Bruix J (2003) Hepatocellular carcinoma. Lancet 362:1907–1917
39. Gomaa AI, Khan SA, Toledano MB, Waked I, Taylor-Robinson SD (2008) Hepatocellular carcinoma: epidemiology, risk factors and pathogenesis. World J Gastroenterol 14:4300–4308
40. Matsuda Y, Ichida T, Fukumoto M (2011) Hepatocellular carcinoma and liver transplantation: clinical perspective on molecular targeted strategies. Med Mol Morphol 44:117–124
41. Stiborova M, Arlt VM, Schmeiser HN (2016) Balkan endemic nephropathy: an update on its aetiology. Arch Toxicol 90(11):2595–2615
42. Anandagoda N, Lord GM (2015) Preventing aristolochic acid nephropathy. Clin J Am Soc Nephrol 10:167–168
43. Schmeiser HH, Kucab JE, Arlt VM et al (2012) Evidence of exposure to aristolochic acid in patients with urothelial cancer from a Balkan endemic nephropathy region of Romania. Environ Mol Mutagen 53:636–641
44. Stefanovic V, Toncheva D, Polenakovic M (2015) Balkan nephropathy. Clin Nephrol 83(1):64–69
45. Pfohl-Leszkowicz A (2009) Ochratoxin A and aristolochic acid involvement in nephropathies and associated urothelial tract tumours. Arh Hig Rada Toksikol 60:465–483
46. Mantle PG, Faucet-Marquis V, Manderville RA, Squillaci B, Pfohl-Leszkowicz A (2010) Structures of covalent adducts between DNA and ochratoxin A: a new factor in debate about genotoxicity and human risk assessment. Chem Res Toxicol 23:89–98
47. Pinton P, Braicu C, Nougayrede JP, Laffitte J, Taranu I, Oswald IP (2010) Deoxynivalenol impairs porcine intestinal barrier function and decreases the protein expression of claudin-4 through a mitogen activated protein kinase-dependent mechanism. J Nutr 140:1956–1962
48. Grenier B, Applegate TJ (2013) Modulation of intestinal functions following mycotoxin ingestion: meta-analysis of published experiments in animals. Toxins 5:396–430
49. Maresca M, Fantini J (2010) Some food associated mycotoxins as potential risk factors in humans predisposed to chronic intestinal inflammatory diseases. Toxicon 56:282–294
50. Eduard W (2009) Fungal spores: a critical review of the toxicological and epidemiological evidence as a basis for occupational exposure limit setting. Crit Rev Toxicol 39(10):799–864
51. Lichtenstein JH, Molina RM, Donaghey TC et al (2010) Pulmonary responses to Stachybotrys chartarum and its toxins: mouse strain affects clearance and macrophage cytotoxicity. Toxicol Sci 116(1):113–121
52. Liu C, Shen H, Yi L et al (2015) Oral administration of aflatoxin G(1) induces chronic alveolar inflammation associated with lung tumorigenesis. Toxicol Lett 232(3):547–556
53. Thrasher JD, Gray MR, Kilburn KH, Dennis D, Yu A (2012) A water-damaged home and health of occupants: A case study. J Environ Public Health 2012:312836
54. Brasel TL, Campbell AW, Demers RE et al (2004) Detection of trichothecene mycotoxins in sera from individuals exposed to Stachybotrys chartarum in indoor environments. Arch Environ Health 59:317–323
55. Layton RC, Purdy CW, Jumper CA, Straus DC (2009) Detection of macrocyclic trichothecene mycotoxins in a caprine (goat) tracheal instillation model. Toxicol Ind Health 25:693–701
56. Enongene EN, Sharma RP, Bhandari N, Voss KA, Riley RT (2000) Disruption of sphingolipid metabolism in small intestines, liver and kidney of mice dosed subcutaneously with fumonisin B (1). Food Chem Toxicol 38(9):793–799
57. Samaranayake LP (1986) Nutritional factors and oral candidosis. J Oral Pathol 15(2):61–65
58. Hitzig WH (1983) Protean appearances of immunodeficiencies: syndromes and inborn errors involving other systems, which express associated primary immunodeficiency. Birth Defects 19(3):307–312
59. Graeme KA (2014) Mycetism: a review of the recent literature. J Med Toxicol 10:173–189
60. Rogan WJ, Yang GC, Kimbrough RD (1985) Aflatoxin and Reye's syndrome: a study of livers from deceased cases. Arch Environ Health 40(2):91–95
61. Kirchmair M, Carrilho P, Pfab R et al (2012) Amanita poisoning resulting in acute, reversible renal failure: new cases, new toxic Amanita mushrooms. Nephrol Dial Transplant 27:1380–1386
62. Mendez-Navarro J, Ortiz-Olivera NX, Villegas-Rios M et al (2011) Hepatotoxicity from ingestion of wild mushrooms of the genus Amanita section Phalloideae collected Mexico City: two case reports. Ann Hepatol 10(4):568–574

63. French LK, Hendrickson RG, Horowitz BZ (2011) Amanita phalloides poisoning. Clin Toxicol 49:128–129
64. Hawksworth DL, Wiltshire PEJ (2011) Forensic mycology: the use of fungi in criminal investigations. Forensic Sci Int 206:1–11
65. Eren SH, Demirel Y, Ugurlu S, Korkmaz I, Aktas C, Guven FM (2010) Mushroom poisoning: retrospective analysis of 294 cases. Clinics 65(5):491–496
66. Lima ADL, Costa Fortes R, Carvalho Garbi Novaes MR, Percario S (2012) Poisonous mushrooms: a review of the most common intoxications. Nutr Hosp 27(2):402–408
67. Lukasik-Glebocka M, Druzdz A, Naskret M (2011) Clinical symptoms and circumstances of acute poisoning with fly agaric (Amanita muscaria) and panther cap (Amanita pantherina). Przegl Lek 68(8):449–452
68. Pauli JL, Foot CL (2005) Fatal muscarinic syndrome after eating wild mushrooms. Med J Aust 182:294–295
69. Karlson-Stiber C, Persson H (2003) Cytotoxic fungi-an overview. Toxicon 2(4):339–349
70. Michelot D, Toth B (1991) Poisoning by Gyromitra esculenta-a review. J Appl Toxicol 11(4):235–243
71. Lheureux P, Penaloza A, Gris M (2005) Pyridoxine in clinical toxicology: a review. Eur J Emerg Med 12:78–85
72. Gejyo F, Homma N, Higuchi N et al (2005) A novel type of encephalopathy associated with mushroom Sugihiratake ingestion in patients with chronic kidney diseases. Kidney Int 68(1):188–192
73. Kuwabara T, Arai A, Honma N, Nishizawa M (2005) Acute encephalopathy among patients with renal dysfunction after ingestion of "sugihiratake", angel's wing mushroom—study on the incipient cases in the northern area of Niigata Prefecture. Rinsho Shinkeigaku 45(3):239–245
74. Saviuc P, Danel V (2006) New syndromes in mushroom poisoning. Toxicol Rev 25(3):199–209
75. Satora L, Goszcz H, Ciszowski K (2005) Poisonings resulting from the ingestion of magic mushrooms in Krakow. Przegl Lek 62(6):394–396
76. Kurokawa K, Sato H, Nakajima K, Kawanami T, Kato T (2005) Clinical, neuroimaging and electroencephalographic findings of encephalopathy occurring after the ingestion of "sugihiratake" (Pleurocybella porrigens), an autumn mushroom: a report of two cases. Rinsho Shinkeigaku 45(2):111–116
77. Zhang Y, Li Y, Wu G et al (2012) Evidence against barium in the mushroom Trogia venenata as a cause of sudden unexpected death in Yunnan, China. Appl Environ Microbiol 78(24):8834
78. Shi GQ, Huang WL, Zhang J et al (2012) Clusters of sudden unexplained death associated with the mushroom, Trogia venenata, in rural Yunnan. PLoS ONE 7(5):e35894
79. Santi L, Maggioli C, Mastroroberto M, Tufoni M, Napoli L, Caraceni P (2012) Acute liver failure caused by Amanita phalloides poisoning. Int J Hepatol 2012:48748

MIX
Papier aus verantwortungsvollen Quellen
Paper from responsible sources
FSC® C105338

If you have any concerns about our products,
you can contact us on
ProductSafety@springernature.com

In case Publisher is established outside the EU,
the EU authorized representative is:
Springer Nature Customer Service Center GmbH
Europaplatz 3, 69115 Heidelberg, Germany

Printed by Libri Plureos GmbH
in Hamburg, Germany